Current Progress in Drug Discovery and Development

Current Progress in Drug Discovery and Development

Edited by Ned Burnett

hayle medical

New York

Hayle Medical,
750 Third Avenue, 9th Floor,
New York, NY 10017, USA

Visit us on the World Wide Web at:
www.haylemedical.com

ISBN: 978-1-63241-542-4

Cataloging-in-Publication Data

Current progress in drug discovery and development / edited by Ned Burnett.
    p. cm.
Includes bibliographical references and index.
ISBN 978-1-63241-542-4
1. Drugs. 2. Drug development. 3. Pharmacy. I. Burnett, Ned.
RS91 .C87 2019
615.1--dc23

Table of Contents

Preface

Over the recent decade, advancements and applications have progressed exponentially. This has led to the increased interest in this field and projects are being conducted to enhance knowledge. The main objective of this book is to present some of the critical challenges and provide insights into possible solutions. This book will answer the varied questions that arise in the field and also provide an increased scope for furthering studies.

Drug discovery is a significant part of medicine, pharmacology and biotechnology, which is concerned with the discovery of new and improved drugs. The process involves high-throughput screening (HTS), which refers to the testing of chemicals for their ability to modify the target. Other methods of drug discovery include de novo drug design, fragment-based lead discovery and protein-directed dynamic combinatorial chemistry. Drug development is the process of launching new drugs into the market after the lead compounds are identified during the drug discovery process. This stage involves two processes namely, pre-clinical development and clinical phase. Drug development ensures that all parameters of safety, pharmacokinetics, metabolism and toxicity of the new drug are analyzed prior to clinical trials. This book presents researches and studies performed by experts across the globe in the fields of drug discovery and drug development. The topics included herein are of utmost significance and bound to provide incredible insights to readers. A number of latest researches have been included to keep the readers up-to-date with the global concepts in these areas of study.

I hope that this book, with its visionary approach, will be a valuable addition and will promote interest among readers. Each of the authors has provided their extraordinary competence in their specific fields by providing different perspectives as they come from diverse nations and regions. I thank them for their contributions.

Editor

Edible and Medicinal Mushrooms as Promising Agents in Cancer

Ken Yasukawa

Additional information is available at the end of the chapter

1. Introduction

Conquering cancer is one of the major challenges facing mankind in the 21st century. The advancement of diagnostic techniques has made discovering miniscule tumors feasible, and early treatment of many types of cancers has consequently become a reality. However, while the development of anticancer drugs progresses, the number of people diagnosed with cancer continues to rise. The drug, tamoxifen, has been approved in the US to prevent breast cancer relapse. In addition, cancer prevention has become an important part of conquering cancer, with both primary and secondary prevention strategies. The former entails the prevention of cancer itself, while the latter involves the prevention of death once an individual has already developed cancer.

Edible mushrooms such as *Lentinula edodes* (shiitake) and *Grifola frondosa* (maitake) have been known from ancient folklore to possess properties that enhance biological defense responses (immune functions), and have been used in people with decreased immune function such as those with cancer, allergies and other disorders, and in elderly people. Many of these mushrooms contain compounds called β-glucans, which are high molecular weight polysaccharides of glucose linked together by glycosidic bonds. β-glucans are contained in mushrooms, yeast, fungi, and higher plants. In Japan, several mushroom-derived pharmaceutical products have been developed, and include schizophyllan from *Schizophyllum commune*, krestin from *Trametes versicolor*, and lentinan from *L. edodes* an anticancer polysaccharide from shiitake. In South Korea, meshima, a mycelia culture of *Phellinus linteus*, was developed as an anticancer drug. Antitumor activities of polysaccharides and peptide polysaccharides in these mushrooms have been reported. In addition to polysaccharides, unique substances such as sterols and triterpenes are reportedly present in mushrooms. Some of these compounds are promising anticancer agents. Please refer to a review published elsewhere for a description on herbal medicine extracts that have been anticipated for their cancer prevention effects [1]. In this chapter, we will introduce the anticancer activities of polysaccharides as well as the cancer prevention activities of sterols and triterpenes.

2. Mushroom-derived anticancer polysaccharides

Research on mushroom-derived β-glucans began when Chihara, Hamuro, and others at the National Cancer Center Research Institute in Japan isolated and purified lentinan, a β-1,3-glucan with branched chains formed by β-1,6-glycosidic bonds, from L. edodes in 1968 [2, 3]. Subsequently, many efficacy studies on lentinan, primarily concerning its antitumor activities, have been reported [4-6]. Ikekawa et al. intraperitoneally administered aqueous extracts of six types of edible mushrooms, and demonstrated their antitumor effects on cancer cell line sarcoma S-180 [7].

Upon such discoveries, polysaccharides lentinan and schizophyllan, glycoprotein krestin, and P. linteus mycelia extract meshima have been utilized as anticancer drugs.

Lentinan (Figure 1) demonstrated an effect to prolong the survival of patients with inoperable and relapsed stomach cancer in combination with a chemotherapeutic agent in a human double-blind controlled clinical trial. It has been revealed that its oral consumption, however, does not exhibit efficacy. In 1985, this compound was approved as an anti-malignant tumor agent (injectable solution), and has been prescribed to cancer patients as a pharmaceutical product. Subsequently, the antitumor effects of various mushroom extracts that contain β-glucan were reported in animal experiments [8]. However, most of these studies administered mushroom extracts that contain β-glucan to animals via injection, and there are very few reports that showed its effect via oral consumption. There is, however, one such rare report; an epidemiological study that suggests mushroom intake via oral consumption may be effective [9]. Intraperitoneal administration of lentinan suppressed 3-methylcolanthrene-induced tumor expression [5]. In Lentinula edodes, α-(1,4)-glucan binds with TLR-4, thereby inducing monocyte differentiation and exhibiting cytotoxic effects in A549 human lung carcinoma cells [10].

Schizophyllan derived from Schizophyllum commune (Figure 2) is typically structured with β1 → 3 linkage and on rare occasions with β1 → 6 linkage between D-glucose monomers [11]. Due to such structure, a rigid triple-helical structure is formed. In addition, this compound is used in anticancer drugs since it possesses antitumor activities [12]. However, it is administered via intramuscular injection, and its effects via oral route in the manner of food consumption have not been elucidated. Although the mechanism of the antitumor activities of β-glucans including schizophyllan is not completely understood, it is thought that they activate macrophages and natural killer (NK) cells through respective β-glucan receptors, induce a helper T1 cell-dominant immune response state, and consequently exhibit antitumor activities [13, 14].

Krestin, an anti-malignant tumor agent, is a protein-bound polysaccharide derived from the mycelia of Trametes versicolor CM-101 strain. Since this drug does not cause serious side effects

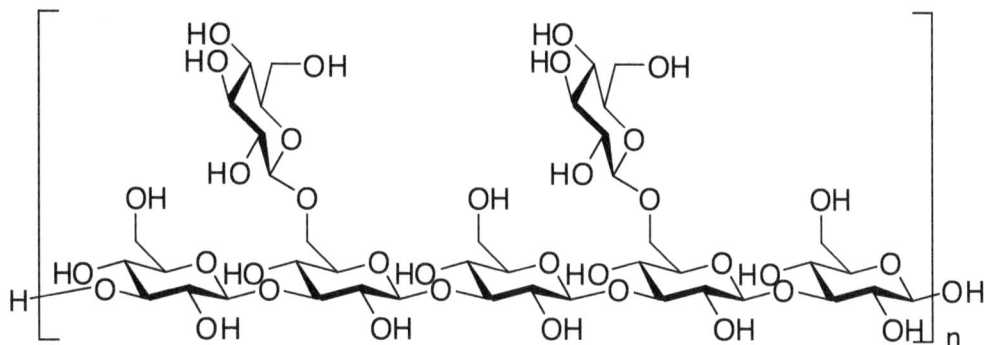

Figure 1. Structure of lentinan

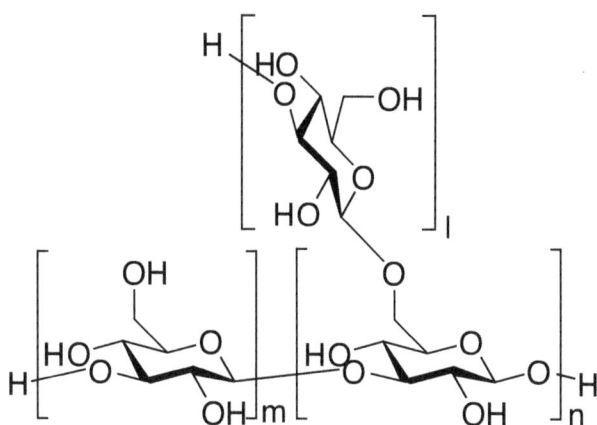

Figure 2. Structure of schizophyllan

with oral administration, there was a period of time in which it was used alone after its release in 1977. However, it is now evident that it has no effect by itself, and is now used in conjunction with other drugs. Krestin is thought to exhibit its antitumor actions by acting on the immune response mechanism that has decreased due to a cancer-bearing state. Krestin has a mean molecular weight of 9.4×10^4, and its sugar chain moiety consists of glucose (74.6%), galactose (2.7%), mannose (15.5%), xylose (4.8%), and fucose (2.4%), but mostly glucose in the form of β-glucans. The glucans have main chain β1 → 4 bond, and side chain β1 → 3 and 1 → 6 bond structures, and it has been suggested that branching occurs per number of sugar residues. Proteins and sugar chain moeities in Krestin are linked with each other by either O- or N-glycosidic bond [15]. In addition, coriolan, another antitumor polysaccharide derived from *Trametes versicolor*, was reported in 1971 [16].

P. linteus belongs to *Hymenochaetaceae* family, and is called *souou* in traditional Japanese medicine, and has been highly valued since ancient times. It has been referred to as the "mythical" mushroom since it grows extremely slowly in nature and artificial cultivation is also difficult. Research in South Korea succeeded in the mass cultivation of *P. linteus* Yoo (HKSY-PL2) strain, which has been shown to be more effective than most other strains. *P.*

linteus has properties to enhance the natural healing capability of the body, and was developed as a pharmaceutical product called meshima. Mycelia culture of *P. linteus* activated dendritic cells and macrophages through increased secretions of interleukin 12 (IL-12), interferon gamma (IFN-γ), tumor necrosis factor alpha (TNF-α) by T-cells, and enhanced the antitumor effects of NK cells [17]. A proteoglycan generated by *P. linteus* acted as an immunostimulant and disrupted the Reg IV/EGFR/Akt signaling pathway, thereby exhibiting tumor-inhibitory effects [18]. In addition, polysaccharides from *P. linteus* activated the P27kip1-cyclinD1/E-CDK2 pathway and induced S-phase cell cycle arrest in HT-29 cells, resulting in cellular damage [19].

Through their immunostimulatory properties, mushroom-derived polysaccharides and glycoproteins augment anticancer drugs, alleviate side effects, and contribute greatly to quality of life (QOL) improvement.

3. Chemical carcinogenesis and two-stage carcinogenesis theory

It has been acknowledged that many types of cancers are caused by environmental carcino-genic agents. In 1915, Yamagiwa and Ichikawa succeeded in inducing cancer by rubbing coal tar on rabbit ears [20]. The significance from this study was the skin cancer had metastasized to the rabbit lung. In 1941, Berenblum *et al.* applied carcinogenic agent benz[*a*]pyrene (B[*a*]A) and croton oil (seed oil of *Croton tiglium*) on mouse skin, and proposed a two-stage carcino-genesis theory that tumorigenesis occurs similarly to when B[*a*]A is applied continually [21, 22]. Specifically, changes due to a carcinogenic agent were termed initiation, and changes due to croton oil were termed promotion. Later, Hecker reported the cancer-promoting ingredient of croton oil as 12-*O*-tetradecanoylphorbol-13-acetate (TPA). Many of these experiments are conducted using initiators 7,12-dimethylbenz[*a*]anthracene (DMBA) and TPA [23,24]. Fujiki *et al.* later reported on many mouse skin tumor promoters such as teleocidin [25]. Cancer begins when cells transform into latent cancer cells after undergoing initiation by receiving initiators or radiation. Subsequently, these cells become cancer cells after a long period of promotion process by promoters. Finally, after modifications through a process termed progression, the cells acquire the ability to divide infinitely, thereby clinically morphing to cancer. These steps occur in a continuous manner, and cannot be strictly distinguished from each other. When considering primary prevention, it is realistic to suppress the promotion process, which requires a long period of time and is known to be reversible to some degree. In addition, it has also become evident that cancer develops via similar mechanisms in many organs. Further-more, TPA is known to activate Epstein-Barr virus (EBV). Although the prevalence of EBV is extremely high in Africa, the incidence of Burkitt's lymphoma greatly differs depending on the village [26]. It has been revealed that villages with greater incidence regularly utilized *Euphorbia tirucalli* and phorbol-esters, which are constituents of *Euphorbia tirucalli* and closely related to TPA. It is suggested these phorbol-esters are involved in the onset of Burkitt's lymphoma [27, 28].

4. Screening for cancer preventative substances

We are conducting a screening for an antitumor substance using a method in which the suppressive effect against tumor promoter-induced inflammation is examined as a positive outcome index [29]. This method was utilized by Hecker *et al.* when they isolated and identified TPA and this method has been confirmed to be advantageous with high correlation as it employs a carcinogenesis experiment and skin from inbred (syngeneic) mice. Specifically, when TPA is applied on the auricle of female ICR mice, maximum swelling was observed 6-10 hours later. The mushroom extracts suppressed the TPA effects, as seen by swelling inhibition, and were confirmed by two-stage carcinogenesis experiments on mouse skin. We induced inflammation with TPA in mice and investigated methanol extracts of 27 edible mushrooms, 8 mushroom supplements, and 3 medicinal mushrooms, discovering the presence of promising mushrooms as shown in Table 1. Specifically, inhibitory effects were observed in: *Russula delica, Lactarius deliciosus, Hypsizigus marmoreus* (*H. marmoreus*), *Mycoleptodonoides aitchisonii* (*M. aitchisonii*), *Naematoloma sublateritium* for edible mushroom; *Inonotus obliquus* (chaga), meshima, *Ganoderma lucidum* (reishi), deer horn shape *Ganoderma amboinense* (rokkaku reishi), *Pleurotus cornucopiae* (golden oyster mushroom) for mushroom supplements; and *Poria cocos* (poria) and polyporus as medicinal mushrooms [30]. Of these mushrooms, the application of methanol extracts of *H. marmoreus* [31], *M. aitchisonii* [30], poria [32], chaga [33], and meshima [34] suppressed the promotion process. These results indicated that edible and medicinal mushrooms are effective cancer preventing foods. In addition, there is a method in which the suppressive effect against the EBV activation that is involved in the onset of Burkitt's lymphoma is examined as a positive outcome index [35]. Substances that were confirmed to have inhibitory effects through this method are thought to contribute to cancer prevention in those infected with EBV.

Scientific name	IR (%)
Polyporus confluens	35**
Russula delica	65**
R. cyanoxantha	38**
R. pseudodelica	41**
R. sanguinea	41**
Lactarius deliciosus	61**
L. volemus	17
Armillariella mellea	12
Flammulina velutipes	30**
Hypsizigus marmoreus	58**
Lyophyllum decastes	54**
L. connatum	53**
L. shimeji	40**
Pleurocybella porrigens	50**

Scientific name	IR (%)
Tricholoma japonicum	49**
T. matsutake	39**
T. portentosum	41**
Lycoperdon perlatum	20*
Agaricus bisporus	36**
Macrolepiota procera	11
Phaeolepiota aurea	15
Sarcodon aspratus	22*
Mycoleptodonoides aitchisonii	62**
Rhodophyllus crassipes	23*
Naematoloma sublateritium	55**
Pholiota squarrosa	33**
Hygrophorus russula	36*
Ganoderma lucidum	82**
Ganoderma amboinense	79**
Polyporus mylittae	33**
Phellinus linteus	73**
Inonotus obliquus	84**
Pleurotus cornucopiae var. *citrinopileatus*	52**
Hericium erinaceum	19
Sparassis crispa	49**

IR: Inhibitory ratio at 1 mg/ear. * $p < 0.05$, $p < 0.01$ vs control group by Student's t test.

Table 1. Inhibitory effect of edible and medicinal mushrooms on TPA-induced inflammation in mice.

5. Cancer preventative effects of edible mushroom

Figure 3 illustrates the inhibitory effects of *M. aitchisonii* in mouse skin, two-stage carcinogenesis experiments. Specifically, Figure 3-A indicates the tumor incidence, where the vehicle control group showed the first tumor appearance in week 5 and tumor development in 93% of the mice in week 20. In contrast, mice that were given *M. aitchisonii* (*M. aitchisonii* group) showed the first tumor appearance in week 5 and tumor development in 53% of the mice in week 20. Figure 3-B shows the mean number of tumors at 20 weeks, where *M. aitchisonii* group presented 1.6 tumors in contrast to the vehicle control group that exhibited 11.2 tumors, confirming a 63% inhibitory effect [30]. Methanol extracts of *H. marmoreus* similarly suppressed the tumor promotion process [31].

A screening for suppressive ingredients was, therefore, conducted; using inhibitory effects against TPA-induced inflammation as an index, active ingredients were isolated and their

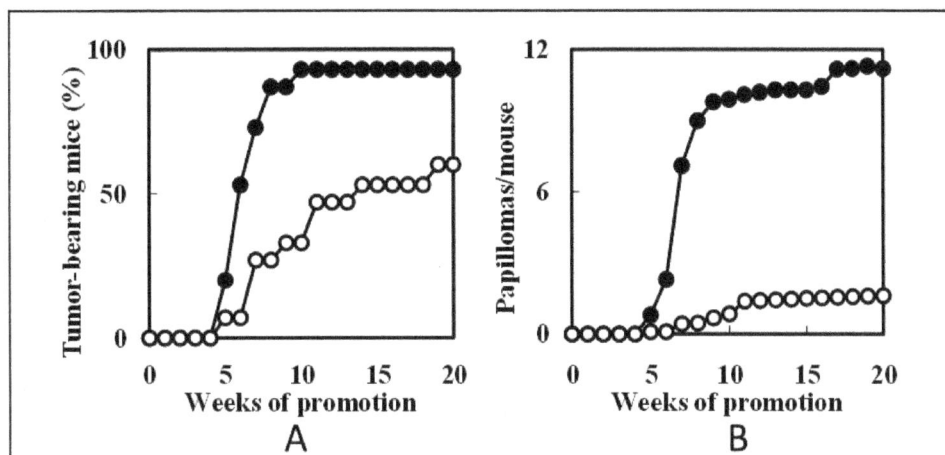

Data are expressed as percentage of mice bearing papillomas per mouse (A), and as average number of papillomas per mouse (B). ●, TPA + with vehicle alone;°, TPA with methanol extract of *M. aitchisonii*.

Figure 3. Inhibitory effect of the methanol extract from *Mycoleptodonoides aitchisonii* on the promotion of skin papillomas by TPA in DMBA-initiated mice [30].

chemical structures were elucidated. The active ingredients were ergosterol (**1**) and ergosterol peroxide (**2**) (Figure 4), which are normal ingredients of mushrooms, and these were stronger than non-steroidal anti-inflammatory drug indomethacin as shown by their 50% inhibitory effects (ID_{50}: 756 and 467 nM/ear, respectively vs. 908 nM/ear). These two sterols have been demonstrated to suppress the promotion process in mouse skin two-stage carcinogenesis experiments [31, 36]. Other sterols (**6-10**) have been reported to inhibit the TPA-induced EBV activation (Table 2.) [37].

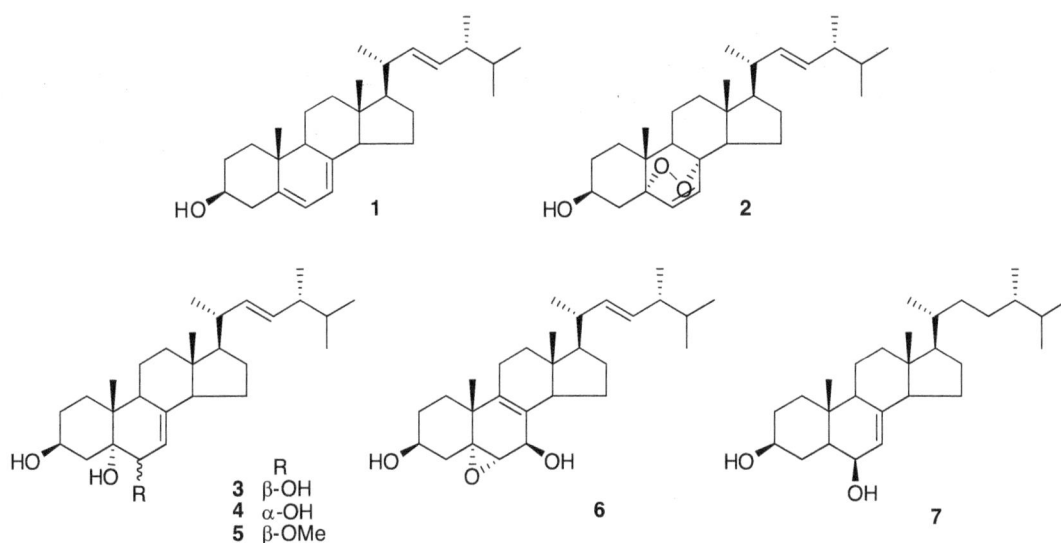

Figure 4. Structures of sterols from *Hypsizigus marmoreus*.

Compound	IC_{50}
Ergosterol (1)	520
Ergosterol peroxide (2)	525
Cerevisterol (3)	518
6-Epicerevisterol (4)	512
22,23-Dihydrocerevisterol (5)	515
6-O-Methylcerevisterol (6)	298
(22E,23R)-5α,6α-Epoxyergosta-8,22-diene-3β,7β-diol (7)	192
β-Carotene	397

IC_{50}: Mol ratio/32 pmol TPA.

Table 2. Inhibitory effects of sterols from *Hypsizigus marmoreus* on induction of the Epstein-Barr virus early antigen.

6. Cancer preventative effects of mushroom supplements

Mushroom supplements, such as meshima, chaga, and almond mushroom, are all believed to be beneficial for cancer, and utilized based on the wishes of cancer patients and their families. As shown in Table 1, supplements including reishi, rokkaku reishi, meshima, and chaga strongly suppressed TPA-induced inflammation [30]. Methanol extracts of Meshima and chaga strongly suppressed the promotion process in experiments involving DMBA and TPA carcinogens [33, 34]. Furthermore, chaga and meshima suppressed the promotion process through oral administration [38, 39].

Lanostane-type triterpenes depicted in Figure 5 were isolated and identified from chaga, and these triterpenes are known to show inhibitory effects in TPA-induced EBV activation (Table 3) [40, 41]. Eight types of lanostane-type triterpenes were isolated as active ingredients, and using the inhibitory effects against TPA-induced inflammation as an index, their 50% inhibitory effects (ID_{50}: 125-458 nM/ear) indicated that they are stronger than non-steroidal anti-inflammatory drug indomethacin (908 nM/ear) (Tasble 4) [33]. Of these triterpenes, inotodiol (13) and 3β-Hydroxylanosta-8,24-dien-24-al (15) suppressed the tumor promotion process [40, 41].

Compound	IC_{50}
Uvariol (10)	392
3β-Hydroxylanosta-8,24-dien-21-al (12)	232
Lanosta-8,23E-diene-3β,22R,25-triol (14)	231
Lanosta-7:9(11),23E-triene-3β,22R,25-triol (15)	228
Oleanolic acid	389

IC_{50}: Mol ratio/32 pmol/TPA.

Table 3. Inhibitory effects of lanostane-type triterpenes from *Inonotus obliquus* on induction of the Epstein-Barr virus early antigen.

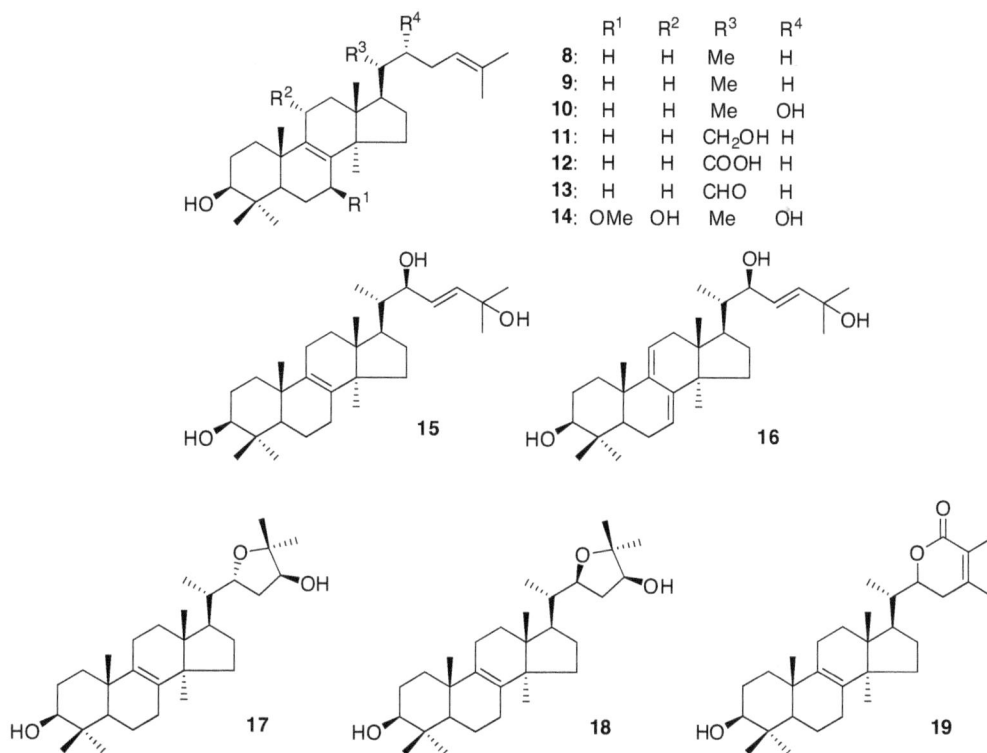

Figure 5. Structures of lanostane-type triterpenes from *Inonotus obliquus*.

Compound	ID_{50} (nM/ear)
Lanosterol (8)	458
Inotodiol (9)	125
Uvariol (10)	134
3β-Hydroxylanosta-8,24-dien-21-al (12)	389
Methoxyinonotsutriol (14)	272
3β,22-Dihydroxylanosta-7,9(11),24-triene (16)	335
Inotolacton B (19)	265
Indomethacin	908

ID_{50}: 50% Inhibitory dose.

Table 4. Inhibitory effects of lanostane-type triterpenes from *Inonotus obliquus* on TPA-induced inflammation in mice.

Reishi belongs to the *Ganodermataceae* family, and is cut into appropriate sizes to be brewed in hot water and consumed as an extract since the fruiting body is woody and not suitable for direct consumption, or is consumed as medicinal alcohol. It has been described in *Shennong Ben Cao Jing* (or *The Classic of Herbal Medicine*) compiled in the Eastern Han Dynasty (25-220), as a life-prolonging miracle drug that nourishes life, and since then, it has been used for various medicinal purposes in China. Akihisa *et al.* isolated multiple lanostane-type triterpene acids from its fruiting body, and reported that they suppress EBV activation as shown in Table 5 [42-44]. Of these compounds 20-Hydroxylucidenic acid N (**21**) suppressed the promotion process in mouse skin two-stage carcinogenesis [42]. With regards to triterpenes from reishi, ganoderic acid T (**49**) exhibited anticancer activities by inducing apoptosis in metastatic lung cancer cells mediated through mitochondria dysfunction and p53 expression [45]. In addition, ganoderic acid T (**49**) suppressed the nuclear translocation of NF-κB and expression of MMP-9 and iNOS, thereby inhibiting invasion by cancer cells [46]. Ganoderic acid DM (**46**) displayed anticancer activities by inducing G1-phase cell cycle arrest and apoptosis in MCF-7 cancer cells [47]. Ganoderic acid A (**44**) and ganoderic acid H (**42**) suppressed breast cancer cell invasion by inhibiting AP-1 and NF-κB and consequently down-regulating Cdk4 expression [48]. Ganoderic acid Me (**48**) inhibited tumor invasion by suppressing MMP2/9 expressions [49]. Lucidenic acid B (**26**) exhibited anti-invasive activity through suppressing TPA-induced NF-κB and AP-1 DNA-binding activities thereby downregulating MMP-9 expression in HepG(2) cells [50]. Lucidenic acid B (**26**) induced apoptosis through mitochondrial cytochrome release and the activations of caspase-9 and caspase-3 [51].

Compound	IC_{50}
Lucidenic acid F (**20**)	352
Methyl lucidenate F (**21**)	285
Lucidenic acid D_2 (**22**)	287
Methyl l ucidenic acid D_2 (**23**)	290
Lucidenic acid A (**24**)	280
Methyl l ucidenate A (**25**)	287
Lucidenic acid B (**26**)	354
Methyl lucidenate Q (**27**)	283
Methyl lucidenate L (**28**)	275
Lucidenic acid E_2 (**29**)	280
Methyl l ucidenate E_2 (**30**)	288
Lucidenic acid N (**31**)	332
Methyl l ucidenate C (**32**)	331
Lucidenic acid P (**33**)	286
Methyl l ucidenate P (**34**)	293
20-Hydroxy lucidenic acid F (**35**)	339
20-Hydroxy lucidenic acid D_2 (**36**)	350
20-Hydroxy lucidenic acid E_2 (**37**)	290
20-Hydroxy lucidenic acid N (**38**)	288
20-Hydroxy lucidenic acid P (**39**)	288
20(21)-Dehydrolucidenic acid A (**40**)	350
Methyl 20(21)-dehydrolucidenate A (**41**)	357
Ganoderic acid F (**42**)	293
Ganoderic acid C_1 (**43**)	336

Compound	IC$_{50}$
Ganoderic acid A (**44**)	291
Ganoderic acid C$_2$ (**45**)	290
Ganoderic acid DM (**46**)	352
Ganoderic acid T-Q (**47**)	281
Ganodermanondiol (**50**)	348
Ganolactone (**51**)	415
Ganoderic acid E (**52**)	281
Methyl ganoderate F (**53**)	289

IC$_{50}$: Mol ratio/32 pmol TPA.

Table 5. Inhibitory effects of lanostane-type triterpene acids from *Ganoderma lucidum* on induction of the Epstein-Barr virus early antigen.

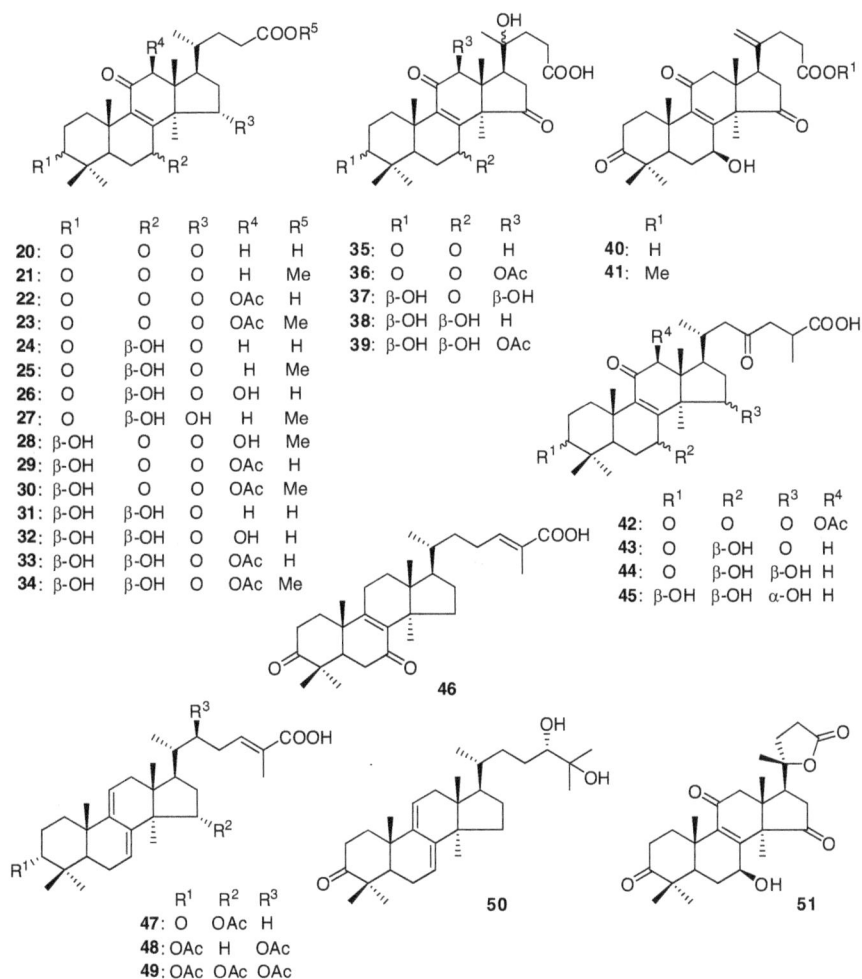

Figure 6. Structures of lanostane-type triterpene acids from *Ganoderma lucidum*.

Piptoporus betulinus is a fungus in the *Polyporaceae* family and the surface of its fruiting body had been used as a strop for razor blades. It is known that the Iceman, as evidenced by a mummy from 5,000 years ago found in the Tyrol region glacier, carried around this mushroom to prevent wound suppuration [52, 53]. Lanostane-type triterpenes (Figure 7) isolated from this mushroom suppressed TPA-induced inflammation [54].

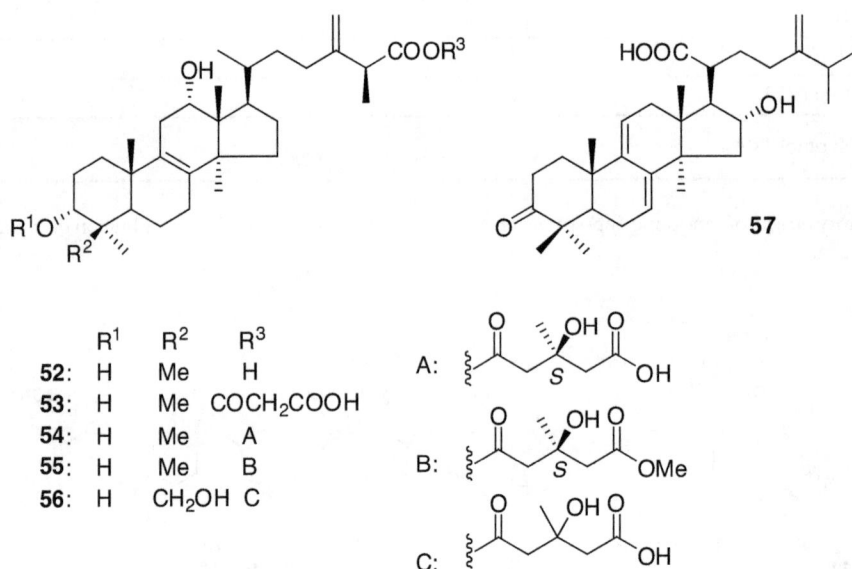

	R^1	R^2	R^3
52:	H	Me	H
53:	H	Me	COCH$_2$COOH
54:	H	Me	A
55:	H	Me	B
56:	H	CH$_2$OH	C

Figure 7. Structures of lanostane-type triterpenes from *Piptoporus betulinus*.

7. Cancer preventative effects and active ingredients of medicinal mushrooms

Of the medicinal mushrooms, polyporus (*Polyporus umbellatus; Polyporaceae* family) is an herbal medicine that possesses diuretic effects, but is also known to suppress TPA-induced inflammation. Screening for the active ingredients of this mushroom resulted in the isolation of insect metamorphosis hormone sterols, and the structures of eight compounds including new compounds polyporoid A (**58**), polyporoid B (**59**), and polyporoid C (**60**) were elucidated (Figure 8.) As shown in Table 6, the effects of these compounds in inhibiting TPA-induced inflammation (ID_{50}) were 117-682 nM/ear, which were greater than that of indomethacin [55].

The sclerotia of *Poria cocos* (*Polyporaceae* family) are referred to as poria, and due to their diuretic properties, and they are formulated in traditional Japanese medicine prescriptions. Additionally, they are also commonly formulated in traditional Japanese medicine prescriptions that are used as adjuvants. The oral administration of Juzentaiho-to and Rikkunshi-to, Japanese Kampo medicines, suppressed cancer promotion in mouse skin two-stage carcinogenesis experiments [56, 57]. It has been shown that, for an effect to appear, the immune response that

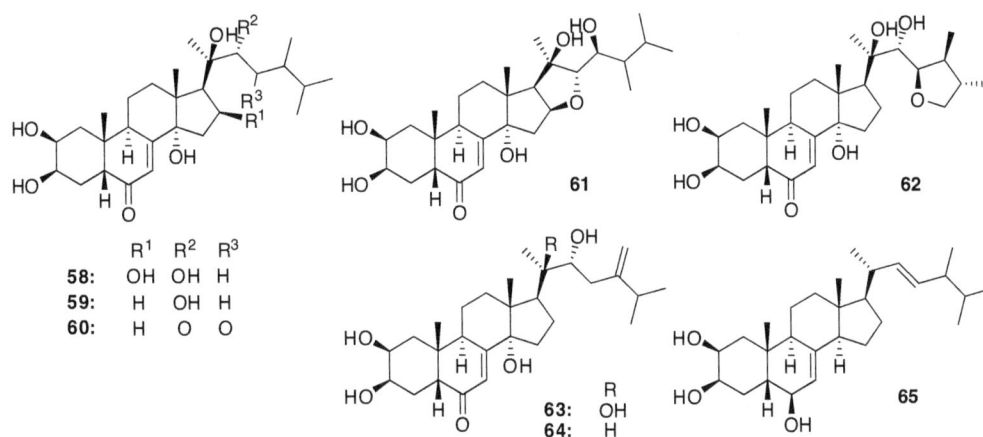

	R¹	R²	R³
58:	OH	OH	H
59:	H	OH	H
60:	H	O	O

Figure 8. Structures of ecdysteroids from *Polyporus umbellatus*.

Compound	ID_{50} (nM/ear)
Polyporoid A (**58**)	531
Polyporoid B (**59**)	682
Polyporoid C (**60**)	184
Polyporusterone A (**61**)	141
Polyporusterone C (**62**)	289
Polyporusterone B (**63**)	117
Polyporusterone G (**64**)	207
Ergosta-7,22-diene-3β,5α,6β-triol (**65**)	666
Indomethacin	838

ID_{50}: 50% Inhibitory dose.

Table 6. Inhibitory effect of ecdysterolids from *Polyporus umbellatus* on TPA-induced inflammation in mice.

is decreased during carcinogenic process be activated [57]. Of the formulated ingredients in these prescriptions, hoelen showed the strongest effect in suppressing TPA-induced inflammation [58]. A screening for the active ingredients of hoelen was therefore conducted, and multiple lanostane-type triterpene acids were isolated and identified (Figure 9) [32]. Of the poria-derived triterpenes, pachymic acid (**71**), 3-*O*-acetyl-16α-hydroxytrametenolic acid (**70**), dehydropachymic acid (**79**), 3β-hydroxylanosta-7,9(11),24-trien-21-oic acid (**75**), dehydroebuliconic acid (**81**), and poricoic acids A (**97**) and B (**94**) had inhibitory effects against TPA-induced inflammation (ID_{50}: 31-83 nM/ear), that were greater than that of indomethacin but similar to that of hydrocortisone (ID_{50}: 69 nM/ear). With regards to pachymic acid (**71**), 3-*O*-acetyl-16αhydroxytrametenolic acid (**70**), and poricoic acid B (**94**), all of which showed strong inhibitory effects, a mouse skin two-stage carcinogenesis experiment using DMBA and TPA demonstrated that they exhibited suppressive effects that were similar to that of the aforementioned ergosterol (**1**), ergosterol peroxide (**2**) and other triterpenes, even when 10% of the dosage of the latter compounds were administered [59]. These compounds have a carboxyl group (COOH) at the carbon 21 position (on side chain), and their suppressive effects decreased 90% when the COOH-group was methylated. It was discovered that COOH at the carbon 21 position plays an important role for activation [32]. Akihisa *et al.* isolated many new lanostane-type triterpene acids from poria, and reported their suppressive effects in TPA-induced EBV activation (Table 8) [60-62]. Moreover, they confirmed that 16-deoxyporicoic acid B (**93**), poricoic acid C (**95**), and 25-methoxyporicoic acid A (**102**) suppress the promotion process [60, 61]. Of these compounds, poricotriol A was revealed to induce apoptosis and possess antitumor effects [63]. Pachymic acid and dehydrotumulosic acid strongly suppress PL-A$_2$, which is related to inflammation [64].

Compound	ID$_{50}$ (nM/ear)
24-Dihydrolanosterol (**66**)	501
Lanosterol (**67**)	469
Tumulosic acid (**69**)	440
3-*O*-Acetyl-16α-hydroxytrametenoic acid (**70**)	31.1
Pachymic acid (**71**)	83.2
3β-Hydroxylanosta-7,9(11),24-trien-21-oic acid (**75**)	59.4
Dehydropachymic acid (**79**)	38.0
Dehydroeburiconic acid (**81**)	57.9
Polyporenic acid C (**82**)	201
3-Epidehydrotumulosic acid (**84**)	188
Poricoic acid B (**94**)	35.1
Poricoic acid A (**97**)	56.1
Poricoic acid AM (**98**)	148
Poricoic acid D (**100**)	243
Indomethacin	908
Hydrocortisone	68.9

ID$_{50}$: 50% Inhibitory dose.

Table 7. Inhibitory effect of lanostane-type triterpene acids from *Poria cocos* on TPA-induced inflammation in mice.

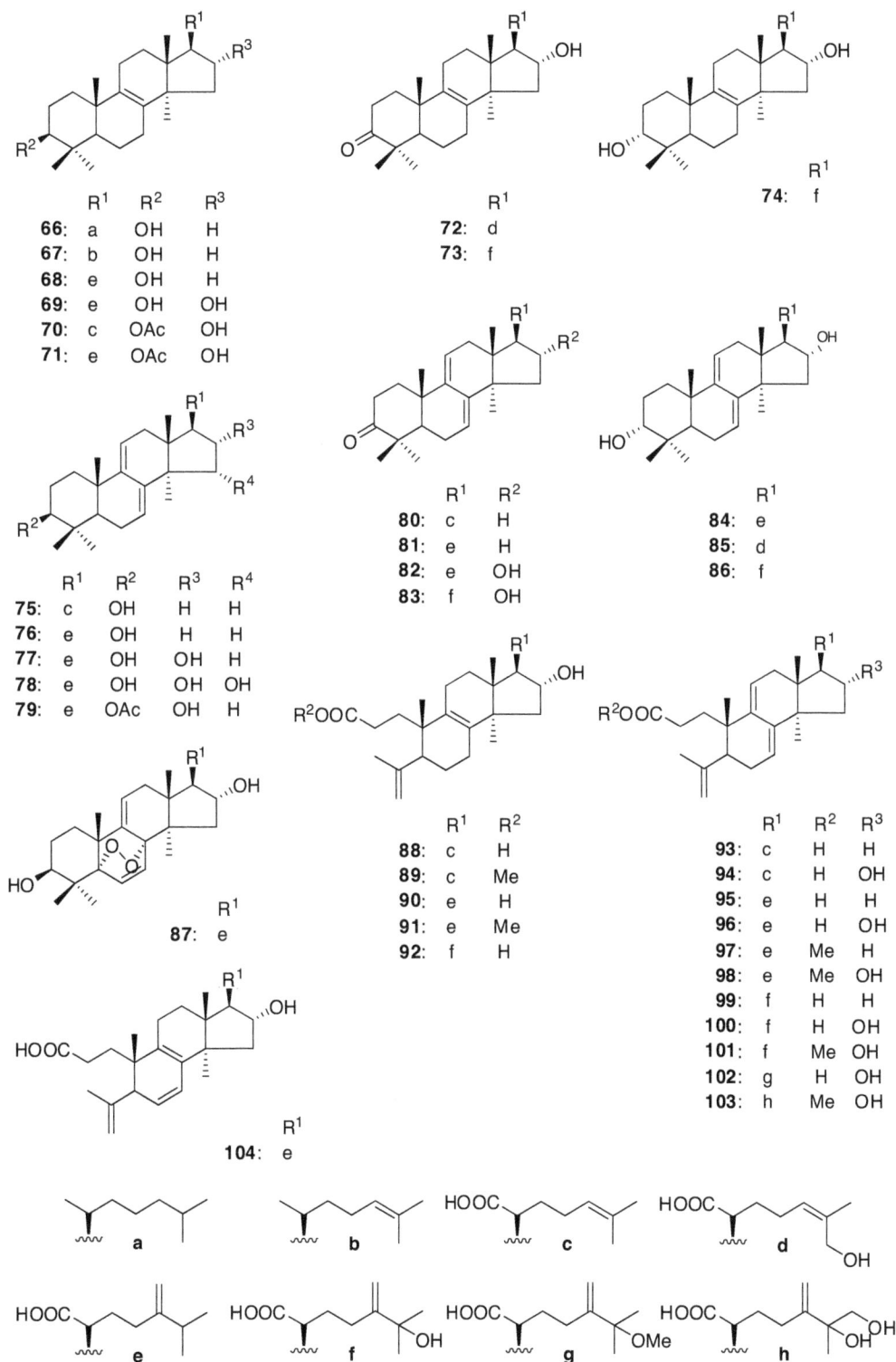

	R¹	R²	R³
66:	a	OH	H
67:	b	OH	H
68:	e	OH	H
69:	e	OH	OH
70:	c	OAc	OH
71:	e	OAc	OH

	R¹
72:	d
73:	f

	R¹
74:	f

	R¹	R²	R³	R⁴
75:	c	OH	H	H
76:	e	OH	H	H
77:	e	OH	OH	H
78:	e	OH	OH	OH
79:	e	OAc	OH	H

	R¹	R²
80:	c	H
81:	e	H
82:	e	OH
83:	f	OH

	R¹
84:	e
85:	d
86:	f

	R¹
87:	e

	R¹	R²
88:	c	H
89:	c	Me
90:	e	H
91:	e	Me
92:	f	H

	R¹	R²	R³
93:	c	H	H
94:	c	H	OH
95:	e	H	H
96:	e	H	OH
97:	e	Me	H
98:	e	Me	OH
99:	f	H	H
100:	f	H	OH
101:	f	Me	OH
102:	g	H	OH
103:	h	Me	OH

	R¹
104:	e

Figure 9. Structures of lanostane-type triterpene acids from *Poria cocos*.

Compound	IC_{50}
Eburicoic acid (**68**)	465
Pachymic acid (**71**)	286
16α-Hydroxyeburiconic acid (**72**)	348
16α,25-Dihydroxyeburiconic acid (**73**)	299
25-Hydroxy-3-epitumulosic acid (**74**)	238
3-Epidehydrotrametnolic acid (**75**)	464
Dehydroebricoic acid (**76**)	460
15α-Hydroxydehydrotumulosic acid (**78**)	268
Dehydropachymic acid (**79**)	284
Dehydrotrametenonic acid (**80**)	310
Dehydroebriconic acid (**81**)	405
16α,25-Dihydroxydehydroeburiconic acid (**83**)	340
16α,27-Dihydroxydehydrotrametenoic acid (**85**)	269
5α,8α-Peroxydehydrotumulosic acid (**87**)	202
Poricoic acid HM (**91**)	219
25-Hydroxyporicoic acid H (**92**)	202
16-Deoxyporicoic acid B (**93**)	262
Poricoic acid C (**95**)	273
Poricoic acid CM (**96**)	332
Poricoic acid AM (**98**)	195
25-Hydroxyporicoic acid C (**99**)	201
Poricoic acid D (**100**)	198
Poricoic acid DM (**101**)	207
25-Methoxyporicoic acid A (**102**)	268
26-Hydroxyporicoic acid DM (**103**)	187
6,7-Dehydroporicoic acid H (**104**)	193
β-Carotene	397

IC_{50}: Mol ratio/32 pmol TPA.

Table 8. Inhibitory effects of lanostane-type triterpene acids from *Poria cocos* on induction of the Epstein-Barr virus early antigen.

8. Conclusion

Mushroom polysaccharides and glycoproteins have antitumor mechanisms such as activating various immunocompetent cells and reinforcing the tumor aggressiveness of the host. Many mushroom-derived polysaccharides have very weak effects when administered orally.

However, with the advancement in food technology, the development of these polysaccharides as food products is progressing and their development as oral pharmaceutical products is also anticipated.

Poria and reishi are listed in the first treatise of Shennong Ben Cao Jing, and viewed as herbal medicines that help maintain health. Although some mushroom triterpenoids show strong suppressive effects similar to that of hydrocortisone, most result in a moderate antitumour promotor effect. It is expected that these triterpenoids, such as pachymic acid, may inhibit phospholipase A_2. Nonetheless, since these mushrooms are edible and are used as supplements and herbal medicines, they are considered to have extremely low or no toxicity. Therefore, these triterpenoids from poria and reishi are a promising group of compounds. In particular, pachymic acid, ganoderic acid T, and lucidenic acid B, are leads in the search for cancer prevention drugs; the development of cancer prevention drugs with properties akin to tamoxifen is desired. When developing a preventative drug, the safety of the substance must first and foremost be considered.

There are many other challenges, such as further elucidating the mechanism, ascertaining the appropriate intake level, and supplying large amounts of the compound. The cooperation and collaboration of researchers from various fields will be necessary to address these issues.

Acknowledgements

Dr. Michio Takido, my mentor and professor emeritus at School of Pharmacy, Nihon University, passed away on August 25, 2014. My research and attitude towards this research were greatly influenced by his guidance. This article is dedicated to Dr Takido with profound gratitude.

Author details

Ken Yasukawa

Address all correspondence to: yasukawa.ken@nihon-u.ac.jp, yasukawa.ken@nihon-.ne.jp

School of Pharmacy, Nihon University, Funabashi, Chiba, Japan

References

[1] Yasukawa K. Medicinal and edible plants as cancer preventive agents. In: Vallisuta O, Olimat SM (eds) Drug Discovery Research in Pharmacognosy. Rijeka: InTech; 2012. p181–208.

[2] Chihara G, Maeda Y, Hamuro J, Sasaki T, Fukuoka F. Inhibition of mouse sarcoma 180 by polysaccharides from Lentinus edodes (Berk.) sing. Nature 1969;222(5194) 687–688.

[3] Chihara G, Hamuro J, Maeda Y, Arai Y, Fukuoka F. Fractionation and purification of the polysaccharides with marked antitumor activity, especially lentinan, from *Lentinus edodes* (Berk.) Sing. (an edible mushroom). Cancer Research 1970;30(11) 2776–2781.

[4] Zákány J, Chihara G, Fachet J. Effect of lentinan on tumor growth in murine allogeneic and syngeneic hosts. International Journal of Cancer 1980;25(3) 371–376.

[5] Suga T, Shiio T, Maeda YY, Chihara G. Antitumor activity of lentinan in murine syngeneic and autochthonous hosts and its suppressive effect on 3-methylcholanthrene-induced carcinogenesis. Cancer Research 1984;44(11) 5132–5137.

[6] Hamuro J, Chihara G. Immunopotentiation by the antitumor polysaccharide lentinan, its immunopharmacology and physiology. In: The reticuloendoyhelial system. Vol. 8 (Hadden JW, Szentivanyl A, eds) Plenum Publ., New York, 1985, pp. 285–307.

[7] Ikekawa T, Uehara N, Maeda Y, Nakanishi M, Fukuoka F. Antitumor activity of aqueous extracts of edible mushrooms. Cancer Research 1969;29(3) 734–735.

[8] Ikekawa T. Beneficial effects of edible and medicinal mushrooms on health care. International Journal of Medicinal Mushroom 2001;3(4); 291–298.

[9] Hamuro J, Chihara G. Effect of antitumor polysaccharides on the higher structure of serum protein. Nature 1973;245(5419) 40–41.

[10] Lo TC-T, Hsu F-M, Chang CA, Cheng JC-H. Branched α-(1,4) glucans from *Lentinula edodes* (L10) in combination with radiation enhance cytotoxic effect on human lung adenocarcinoma through the Toll-like receptor 4 mediated induction of THP-1 differentiation/activation. Journal of Agricultural and Food Chemistry 2011;59(22) 11997–12005.

[11] Komatsu N, Okubo S, Kikumoto S, Kimura K, Saito G, Sakai S. Host-mediated antitumor action of Schizophyllan, a glucan produced by *Schizophyllum commune*. Japanese Journal of Cancer Research (Gann) 1969;60(2) 137–144.

[12] Okamura K, Suzuki M, Chihara T, Fujiwara A, Fukuda T, Goto S, Ichinohe K, Jimi S, Kasamatsu T, Kawai N, Mizuguchi K, Mori S, Nakano H, Noda K, Sekiba K, Suzuki K, Suzuki T, Takahashi K, Takeuchi K, Takeuchi S, Yajima A, Ogawa N. Clinical evaluation of Schizophyllan combined with irradiation in patients with cervical cancer. Cancer 1986;58(4), 865–872.

[13] Ross GD, Vetvicka V. CR3 (CD11b, CD18): a phagocyte and NK cell membrane receptor with multiple ligand specificities and functions. Clinical and Experimental Immunology 1993;92(2) 181–184.

[14] Di Renzo L, Yefenof E, Klein E. The function of human NK cells is enhanced by β-glucan, a ligand of CR 3 (CD11b/CD18). European Journal of Immunology 1991;21(7) 1755–1758.

[15] Kobayashi H, Matsunaga K, Oguchi Y. Antimetastatic effects of PSK (Krestin), a protein-bound polysaccharide obtained from basidiomycetes: an overview. Cancer Epidemiol, Biomarkers & Prevention 1995;4(3) 275–281.

[16] Ito H, Hidaka H, Suigura M. Effects of coriolane, an antitumor polysaccharide, produced by *Coriolus versicolor* Iwade. Japanese Journal of Pharmacology 1979;29(6) 953–957.

[17] Huang H-Y, Chieh S-Y, Tso TK, Chien T-Y, Lin H-T, Tsai Y-C. Orally administered mycelia culture of *Phellinus linteus* exhibits antitumor effects in hepatoma cell-bearing mice. Journal of Ethnopharmacology 2011;133(2) 460–466.

[18] Li Y-G, Ji D-F, Zhong S, Zhu J-X, Chen S, Hu G-Y. Anti-tumor effects of proteoglycan from *Phellinus linteus* by immunomodulating and inhibiting Reg IV/EGFR/Akt signaling pathway in colorectal carcinoma. International Journal of Biological Macromolecules 2011;48(8) 511–517.

[19] Zhong S, Ji D-F, Li Y-G, Lin T-B, Lv Z-Q, Chen H-P. Activation of P27kip1-cyclin D1/E-CDK2 pathway by polysaccharide from *Phellinus linteus* leads to S-phase arrest in HT-29 cells. Chemico-Biological Interactions 2013;206(2) 222–229.

[20] Yamagiwa K, Ichikawa K. Experimental study of the pathogenesis of carcinoma. The Journal of Cancer Research 1918;3 (1) 1–29.

[21] Berenblum I. The cocarcinogenic action of croton resin. Cancer Research 1941;1(1) 44–48.

[22] Berenblum I. The mechanism of carcinogenesis. A study of the significance of cocarcinogenic action and related phenomena. Cancer Research 1941;1(10) 807–814.

[23] Hecker E. Phorbol esters from crotn oil, chemical nature and biological activities. Naturwissenschaften 1967;54(11) 282–284.

[24] van Duuren BL. Tumor-promoting agents in two-stage carcinogenesis. Progress in Expremental Tumor Research 1969;11(1) 31–68.

[25] Fujiki H, Suganuma M. Naturally-derived tumor promoters and inhibitors of carcinogenesis. Toxin Reviews 1996;15(2) 129–156.

[26] van den Bosch CA. Is endemic Burkitt's lymphoma an alliance between three infections and a tumour promoter? Lancet Oncology 2004;5(12) 738–746.

[27] Aya T, Kinoshita T, Imai S, Koizumi S, Mizuno F, Osato T, Satoh C, Oikawa T, Kuzumaki N, Ohigashi H, Koshimizu K. Chromosome translocation and *c-myc* activation by Epstein-Barr virus and *Euphorbia tirucalli* in B lymphocytes. Lancet 1991;337(8751) 1190.

[28] Imai S, Sugiura M, Mizuno F, Ohigashi H, Koshimizu K, Chiba S, Osato T. African Burkitt's lymphoma: A plant, *Euphorbia tirucalli*, reduces Epstein-Barr virus-specific cellular immunity. Anticancer Research 1994, 14(3A) 933–936.

[29] Yasukawa K, Takido M, Takeuchi M, Nakagawa S. Effect of chemical constituents from plants on 12-*O*-tetradecanoylphorbol-13-acetate-induced inflammation in mice. Chemical & Pharmaceutical Bulletin 1989;37(4) 1071–1073.

[30] Yasukawa K, Kanno H, Kaminaga T, Takido M, Kasahara Y, Kumaki K. Inhibitory effect of methanol extracts from edible mushroom on TPA-induced ear oedema and tumour promotion in mouse skin. Phytotherapy Research 1996;10(4) 367–369

[31] Yasukawa K, Aoki T, Takido M, Ikekawa T, Saito H, Matsuzawa T. Inhibitory effects of ergosterol isolated from the edible mushroom *Hypsizigus marmoreus* on TPA-induced inflammatory ear oedema and tumour promotion in mice. Phytotherapy Research 1994;8(1) 10–13.

[32] Kaminaga T, Yasukawa K, Takido M, Tai T, Nunoura Y. Inhibitory effect of *Poria cocos* on 12-*O*-tetradecanoylphorbol-13-acetate-induced ear oedema and tumour promotion in mouse skin. Phytotherapy Research 1996;10(7) 581–584.

[33] Akita A, Sun Y, Yasukawa K. Inhibitory effects of chaga (*Inonotus obliquus*) on tumor promotion in two-stage mouse skin carcinogenesis. Journal of Pharmacy and Nutrition Science 2015;5(1), 71-76.

[34] Yasukawa K, Kitanaka S, Takahashi H, Hirayama H, Shigemoto K. Inhibitory effect of natural fruit body of *Phellinus linteus* on tumor promotion in mice skin. The Japanese Journal of Pharmacognosy 2007;61(1), 14–17.

[35] Ohigashi H, Takamura H, Koshimizu K, Tokuda H, Ito Y. Search for possible antitumor promoters by inhibition of 12-*O*-tetradecanoylphorbol-13-acetate-induced Epstein-Barr virus activation; ursolic acid and oleanolic acid from anti-inflammatory Chinese medicinal plant, *Glechoma hederaceae* L. Cancer Letters 1986;30(2) 143–151.

[36] Yasukawa K, Akihisa T, Kanno H, Kaminaga T, Izumida M, Sakoh T, Tamura T, Takido M. Inhibitory effects of sterols isolated from *Chlorella vulgaris* on 12-*O*-tetradecanoyl- phorbol-13-acetate-induced inflammation and tumor promotion in mouse skin. Biological & Pharmaceutical Bulletin (Tokyo) 1996;19(4), 573–576.

[37] Akihisa T, Franzblau SG, Tokuda H, Tagata M, Ukiya M, Matsuzawa T, Metori K, Kimura Y, Suzuki T, Yasukawa K. Antitubercular activity and inhibitory effect on Epstein-Barr virus activation of sterols and polyisoprenepolyols from an edible mushroom, *Hypsizigus marmoreus*. Biological & Pharmaceutical Bulletin 2005;28(6) 1117–1119.

[38] Akita A, Yasukawa K. Inhibitory effect of chaga (*Inonotus obliquus*) on tumor promotion in two-stage mouse skin carcinogenesis, Japanese Journal of Complementary and Alternative Medicine 2011;8(1) 29–32.

[39] Yasukawa K, Takahashi H, Kitanaka S, Hirayama H, Shigemoto K. Inhibitory effect of an aqueous extract of *Phellinus linteus* on tumor promotion in mouse skin. Mushroom Science and Biotechnology 2007;15(2) 97–101.

[40] Nakata T, Yamada T, Taji S, Ohishi H, Wada S, Tokuda H, Sakuma K, Tanaka R. Structure determination of inonotsuoxides A and B in vivo anti-tumor promoting activity of inotodiol from the sclerotia of *Inonotus obliquus*. Bioorganic & Medicinal Chemistry 2007;15(1) 257–264.

[41] Taji S, Yamada T, Wada S, Tokuda H, Sakuma K, Tanaka R. Lanostane-type triterpenoids from the sclerotia of *Inonotus obliquus* possessing anti-tumor promoting activity. European Journal of Medicinal Chemistry 2008;43(11) 2373–2379.

[42] Akihisa T, Nakamura Y, Tagata M, Tokuda H, Yasukawa K, Uchiyama E, Suzuki T, Kimura Y. Anti-inflammatory and anti-tumor-promoting effects of triterpene acids and sterols from the fungus *Ganoderma lucidum*. Chemistry & Biodiversity 2007;4(2) 224–231.

[43] Akihisa T, Tagata M, Ukiya M, Tokuda H, Suzuki T, Kimura Y. Oxygenated lanostane-type triterpenoids from the fungus *Ganoderma lucidum*. Journal of Natural Products. 2005;68(4) 559–563.

[44] Iwatsuki K, Akihisa T, Tokuda H, Ukiya M, Oshikubo M, Kimura Y, Asano T, Nomura A, Nishino H. Lucidenic acids P and Q, methyl lucidenate P, and other triterpenoids from the fungus *Ganoderma lucidum* and their inhibitory effects on Epstein-Barr virus activation. Journal of Natural Products 2003;66(12) 1582–1585.

[45] Tang W, Liu J-W, Zhao W-M, Wei D-Z, Zhong J-J. Ganoderic acid T from *Ganoderma lucidum* mycelia induces mitochondria mediated apoptosis in lung cancer cells. Life Sciences 2006;80(3) 205–211.

[46] Chen N-H, Liu J-W, Zhong J-J. Ganoderic acid T inhibits tumor invasion in vitro and in vivo through inhibition of MMP expression. Pharmacological Reports 2010;62(1) 150–163.

[47] Wu GS, Lu JJ, Guo JJ, Li YB, Tan W, Dang YY, Zhong ZF, Xu ZT, Chen XP, Wang YT. Ganoderic acid DM, a natural triterpenoid, induces DNA damage, G1 cell cycle arrest and apoptosis in human breast cancer cells. Fitoterapia 2012;83(2) 408–414.

[48] Jiang J, Grieb B, Thyagarajan A, Sliva D. Ganoderic acids suppress growth and invasive behavior of breast cancer cells by modulating AP-1 and NF-κB signaling. International Journal of Molecular Medicine 2008;21(5) 577–584.

[49] Chen N-H, Liu J-W, Zhong J-J. Ganoderic acid Me inhibits tumor invasion through down-regulating matrix metalloproteinases 2/9 gene expression. Journal of Pharmacological Sciences 2008;108(2) 212–216.

[50] Wang C-J, Chau C-F, Hsich Y-S, Yang S-F, Yen G-C. Lucidenic acid inhibits PMA-induced invasion of human hepatoma cells through inactivating MAPK/ERK signal

transduction pathway and reducing binding activities of NF-κB and AP-1. Carcinogenesis 2008;29(1) 147–156.

[51] Hsu C-L, Yu Y-S, Yen G-C. Lucidenic acid B induces apoptosis in human leukemia cells via a mitochondria-mediated pathway. Journal of Agricultural Chemistry 2008;56(11) 3973–3980.

[52] Capasso L. 5300 years ago, the Ice Man used natural laxatives and antibiotics. The Lancet 1998;352(9143) 1864.

[53] Schlegel B, Luhmann U, Härtl A, Gräfe U. Piptamine, a new antibiotic produced by *Piptoporus betulinus* Lu 9-1. The Journal of Antibiotics 2000;53(9) 973–974.

[54] Kamo T, Asanoma M, Shibata H, Hirota M. Anti-inflammatory lanostane-type triterpene acids from *Piptoporus betulinus*. Journal of Natural Products 2003;66(8) 1104–1106.

[55] Sun Y, Yasukawa K. New anti-inflammatory ergostane-type ecdysteroids from the sclerotium of *Polyporus umbellatus*. Bioorganic & Medicinal Chemistry Letters 2008;18(9) 3417–3420.

[56] Haranaka R, Kosoto H, Hirama N, Hanawa T, Hasegawa R, Hyun SJ, Nakagawa S, Haranaka K, Satomi N, Sakurai A, Yasukawa K, Takido M. Antitumor activities of Zyuzen-taiho-to and Cinnamomi Cortex. Journal Medical and Pharmaceutical Society for Wakan-Yaku 1987;4(1) 49–58.

[57] Yasukawa K, Yu S-Y, Takido M. Inhibitory effect of oral administration of Rikkunshi-to on tumor promotion in two-stage carcinogenesis in mouse skin. Journal of Traditional Medicines 1996;13(2) 180–184.

[58] Yasukawa K, Yu S-Y, Kakinuma S, Takido M. Inhibitory effect of of Rikkunshi-to, a traditional Chinese herbal prescription, on tumor promotion in two-stage carcinogenesis in mouse skin. Biological & Pharmaceutical Bulletin 1995;18(5) 730–733.

[59] Kaminaga T, Yasukawa K, Kanno H, Tai T, Nunoura Y, Takido M. Inhibitory effect of lanostane-type triterpene acids, the components of *Poria cocos*, on tumor promotion by 12-O-tetradecanoylphorbol-13-acetate in two-stage carcinogenesis in mouse skin. Oncology 1996;53(5) 382–385.

[60] Akihisa T, Nakamura Y, Tokuda H, Uchiyama E, Suzuki T, Kimura Y, Uchikura K, Nishino H. Triterpene acids from *Poria cocos* and their anti-tumor-promoting effects. Journal of Natural Products 2007;70(6) 948–953.

[61] Akihisa T, Uchiyama E, Kikuchi T, Tokuda H, Suzuki T, Kimura Y. Anti-tumor-promoting effects of 25-methoxyporicoic acid A and other triterpene acids from *Poria cocos*. Journal of Natural Products 2009;72(10) 1786–1792.

[62] Ukiya M, Akihisa T, Tokuda H, Hirano M, Oshikubo M, Nobukuni Y, Kimura Y, Tai T, Kondo S, Nishino H..Inhibition of tumor-promoting effects by poricoic acids G

and H and other lanostane-type triterpenes and cytotoxic activity of poricoic acids A and G from *Poria cocos*. Journal of Natural Products 2002;65(4) 462–465.

[63] Kikuchi T, Uchiyama E, Ukiya M, Tabata K, Kimura Y, Suzuki T, Akihisa T. Cytotoxic and apoptosis-inducing activities of triterpene acids from *Poria cocos*. Journal of Natural Products 2011;74(2) 137–144.

[64] Cuéllar MJ, Giner RM, Recio MC, Just MJ, Máñez S, Ríos JL. Two fungal lanostane derivatives as phospholipase A_2 inhibitors. Journal of Natural Products 1996;59(10) 977–979.

2

Intranasal Drug Administration — An Attractive Delivery Route for Some Drugs

Degenhard Marx, Gerallt Williams and
Matthias Birkhoff

Additional information is available at the end of the chapter

1. Introduction

Intranasal drug administration has a long tradition and was and is still used for medical as well as recreational purposes. The most common use is for treatment of local symptoms e.g. nasal congestion in the course of a common rhinitis or inflammation linked to allergic rhinitis. The medications intended for local activity are well established and can be found across the globe in every pharmacy and drug store. Examples for topical treatment of rhinitis are decongestants (oxymetazoline, xylometazoline, naphazoline), anti-histamines (azelastine, levocabastine, olopatadine) and glucocorticoids (e.g. mometasone, budesonide, fluticasone). For this particular indication, drugs should act fast and only locally while systemic absorption should be as low as possible; this to avoid systemic side effects which are linked with typical oral formulations of comparable drug substances.

As described earlier [1] intranasal administration has much more potential. The nasal mucosa can be used for non-invasive systemic administration of drugs. The surface of the nasal mucosa in humans is around 150 cm^2, a tissue which is well supplied by blood vessels. This ensures a rapid absorption of most drugs, can generate high systemic blood levels and avoids the first pass metabolism which needs to be taken into account following oral administration. This bypassing of the gastrointestinal system even enables the delivery of peptide hormones [1]. Calcitonin and desmopressin are on the market for years now; insulin and glucagon were under clinical development for this administration route [2].

The rapid absorption of drugs via the nasal mucosa is also utilized for pain medications (e.g. fentanyl nasal sprays), rescue medications like naloxone for opioid overdosing or midazolam for seizures in children. An important aspect for such medications is that intranasal administration is considered a non-invasive administration route and easy to do for self-administration or for care-givers. It has a low potential for injuries or disease transmission (hepatitis B, HIV). This is of special importance if fast relief from severe symptoms is required and patient's ability to deal with injections is impaired. Intranasal triptanes for migraine treatment, fentanyl to stop cancer breakthrough pain and ondansetrone to relieve nausea are examples for this trend. For these indications, single dose systems or multi-dose pumps with counting or lock-out mechanisms are available to reduce the risk of unintended overdosing or misuse [1].

Vaccines may also benefit from the intranasal route. Existing vaccines commonly utilize the intramuscular and oral administration route. While the respiratory and gastrointestinal tract is very immune competent and fights with microbes permanently, the muscle is not the first choice. Intramuscular vaccination primarily induces systemic immune response, mainly via formation of vaccine-strain specific circulating antibodies. Injections of vaccines were done since the early days and they are indeed effective. So for most people today vaccination is equal to getting an intramuscular injection which is linked to pain. For the health care professional it is linked to fears of needle stick injuries, risk of disease transmission and dangerous medical waste.

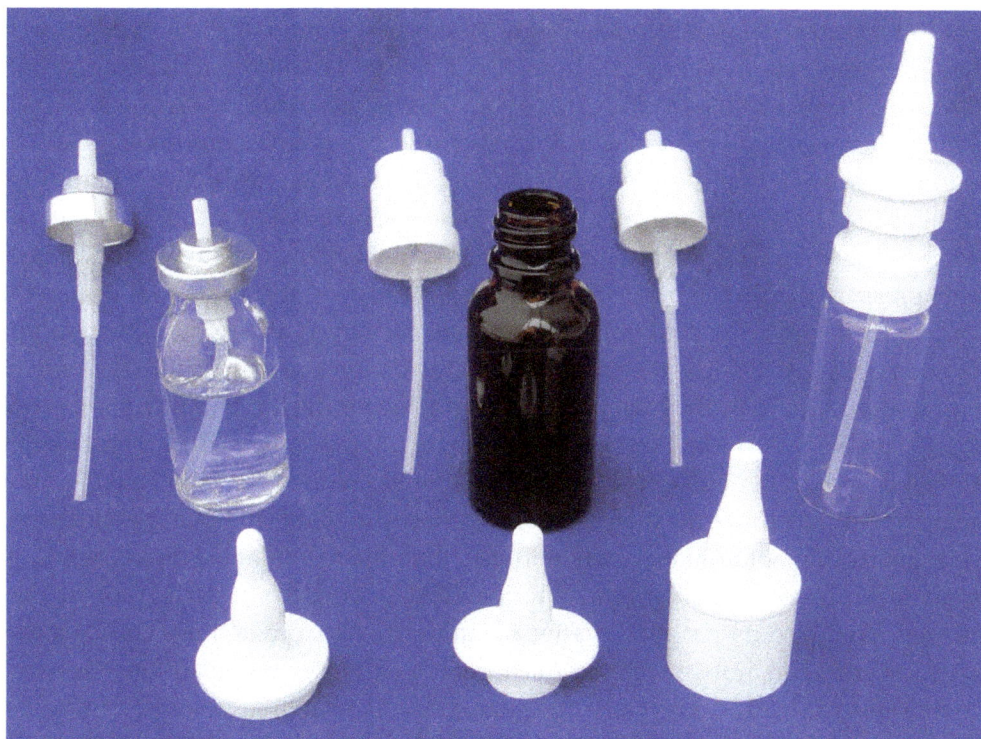

Figure 1. Multi-dose spray pumps can be fitted onto the bottles using a crimp ferrule, screwed-on or simply snapped on (from left to the right). In the forefront different types of nasal spray actuators.

Intranasal vaccination provides a promising non-invasive and gentle alternative. The nasal mucosa is continuously exposed to dust and microbes and therefore extremely immune competent. Due to the presence of the so called nasal-associated lymphoid tissue (NALT), intranasal vaccination elicits broader protection. It induces mucosal (protection at the site of infection) and systemic immunity, which includes antibody formation as well as activation of circulating immune cells. It has also been reported that the nasal route induces cross-protection against variant strains of e.g. influenza viruses, an observation which may contribute to the development of so-called "universal vaccines". There is also evidence that this administration route may enable the development of therapeutic vaccines for chronic, hard-to-treat diseases such as hepatitis B [3].

Intranasal administration is an attractive route for a wide range of drugs and indications. With this review we will try to provide some insight into this technology and some considerations for a successful development of such drugs.

2. Evolution of multi-dose spray pumps

Multi-dose spray pumps represent the highest share of delivery systems for intranasal administration. This type of pumps was developed some 50 years ago and ousted step by step droppers and pipettes. These multi-dose spray pumps now dominate the market because they are very cost effective and convenient. The technical solution is quite simple: drug formulation is filled into multi-dose bottles made of glass or different plastic materials, which are closed by attaching the nasal spray pump including a dip tube. Nasal spray pumps are displacement pumps and when actuating the pump by pressing the actuator towards the bottle, a piston moves downward in the metering chamber. A valve mechanism at the bottom of the metering chamber will prevent backflow into the dip tube. So the downward movement of the piston will create pressure within the metering chamber which forces the air (before priming) or the liquid outwards through the actuator and generates the spray. When the actuation pressure is removed, a spring will force the piston and actuator to return to its initial position. This creates an underpressure in the metering chamber which pulls the liquid from the container by lifting up the ball from the ball seat above the dip tube at the bottom of the metering chamber [1]. The metering chamber ensures the right dosing and an open swirling chamber in the tip of the actuator will aerosolize the metered dose. In these pumps systems no measures are taken to prevent microbial contamination when in use, thus the formulation must contain preservatives, in most cases benzalkonium chloride (BAC). To date, most of the medications administered nasally contain a preservative to support long storage times and proper in-use stability. For some years now, most manufacturers of delivery systems offer so called "preservative free systems" (PFS) which are designed in such a way that no preservatives have to be added. At least in Europe, authorities support the use of preservative-free nasalia and request it for children and adolescents [4]. A switch from preserved to unpreserved medications is also often used as a life-cycle management measure and the products are clearly labeled as "without preservatives" or "does not contain preservatives". Today, preservative free systems are most widely used to moisturize the nasal mucosa using saline solutions or for nasal decongestants.

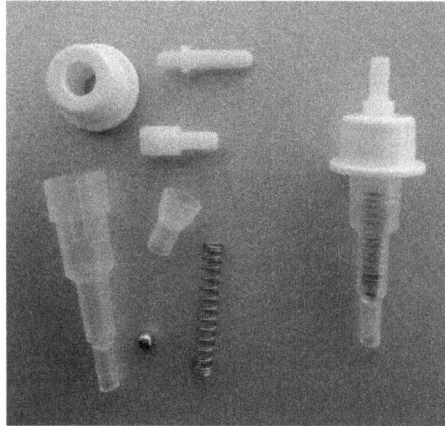

Figure 2. Components of a typical multi dose pump. For a fully functional system a dip tube, fixture and actuator need to be added.

In December 2012, the US Consumer Product Safety Commission (CPSC) issued a rule to require child resistant (CR) packaging for any over the counter or prescription product containing the equivalent of 0.08 milligrams or more of an imidazoline [5]. This class of drugs is widely used as decongestant for cough & cold medications. The reason for this request was the high number of accidental uptake of such medications by children and resulting serious health risks. The commission estimated that approximately 39 million units of nasal products containing imidazolines are sold annually in the US. A great proportion of the nasal products are presented with metering nasal spray pumps. In a comment [5] the CPSC stated that nasal spray pumps even when crimped onto the bottle are not considered CR and that either the pump action or the over cap must be child resistant. This forced the pharmaceutical industry to introduce child resistant features for nasal decongestants intended for the US market.

3. A short introduction on intranasal administration

Nasal sprays or drops are widely used and therefor easy-to-use and cost-effective solutions are already available for liquid or for dry powder formulated drug products. Also the basic requirements for the development of nasal sprays are well known. An important point when a development for nasal administration is considered: the product should have no unpleasant smell and should not be irritating or influence the sense of smell. There should be also no safety concern, if a dose is unintentionally shot into the eyes.

For most nasal spray pumps the dispensed volume per actuation is set between 50 and 140 µl, and an administered volume of 100 µl per nostril is optimum in adults. Higher volumes are prone to drip out immediately. So the anticipated dose should fit into a volume of roughly 100-200 µl when both nostrils are sprayed. Standard spray pumps will deposit most of the sprayed dose into the anterior region of the nasal cavity (see Fig. 3) [6]. Surface tension of the droplets and mucus layer will cause the immediate spread of the spray. Afterwards mucociliary clearance will distribute the liquid layer within the nasal cavity. Since the nasal mucus layer is continuously renewed and discarded into the throat, the nasal residence time of the administered drug depends on how fast it dissolves within the mucus layer and penetrates into the mucosa [7].

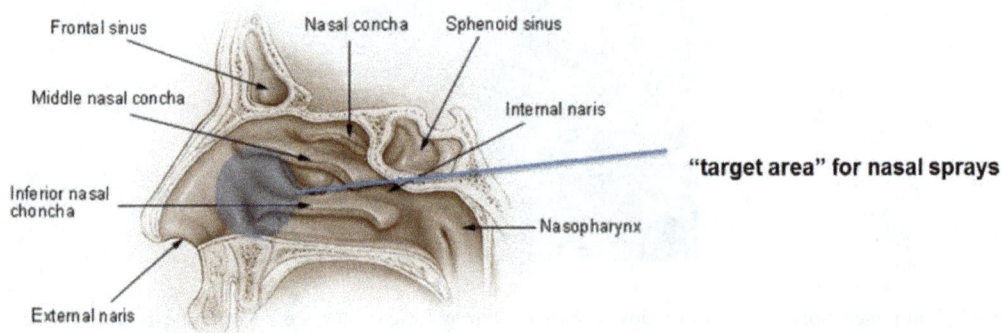

Some facts about the nasal cavity
➢ total surface area ~150 cm^2 (~10 % is olfactory epithelium)
➢ total cavity volume 15-20 ml
➢ mucus layer is completely renewed within 15-20 min and discarded into the pharynx

Figure 3. Anatomy of the nasal cavity.

If a nasal spray is considered, authorities will require a lot of data to describe the nasal spray pump and its performance as part of the container closure system [8, 9]. Most of these required parameters are used for quality control purposes. For nasal deposition efficiency, the spray plume angle and administration angle are critical factors, while many other spray parameters, including droplet particle size, have relatively minor influences on deposition within the nasal cavity [10].

The nose is a very effective filter and most particles and droplets will be caught within the nasal cavity. Only particles less than 10 µm median aerodynamic diameter, so called fine particles, can reach the lower airways during nasal breathing [11]. Most spray pumps will generate an aerosol with a mean particle size from 40-100 µm during the fully developed phase which is recognized as fine mist. Such an aerosol will deposit well in the nasal cavity.

To date, nearly all drugs for intranasal administration are liquids and just some recreational drugs are used as powders. Of course dry powder preparations can be used without the need for reconstitution to a liquid. The particle size should be in the same range as droplets from a nasal spray and fine particles should be minimized to avoid pulmonary deposition. The size and structure of the particles must be a compromise between safe administration (no fine particles, good deposition) and fast speed of dissolution of the particles within the mucus layer [3]. Powders for nasal administration will most likely need protection from moisture uptake though the moisture sensitivity may be formulation-dependent. Long term use of powder formulations may result in mucosal irritation and chronic use should be considered with caution, but single administration should be of much lower risk.

4. Which technology is on the market?

For intranasal administration of drugs a lot of delivery systems are available, simple and low cost as well as highly sophisticated. It ranges from droppers, to sprayers to be attached to a syringe, to so called unit- and bi-dose systems as well as multi-dose solutions for liquids. This wide range of available systems opens the door to tailored packaging.

There are some considerations to choose the right solution in a competitive environment. Convenient and safe use and cost of goods need to be balanced. Also the availability of high speed filling and packaging equipment for the selected presentation should be evaluated. There are of course some other considerations for the different types of systems which should be discussed here.

Droppers are the simplest and -just looking on packaging costs- the cheapest way to deliver medication into the nose. The blow-fill-seal (BFS) technology is widely used. The BFS droppers made of polyethylene or polypropylene are cheap but require special filling equipment. Also the material for the dropper (e.g. adhesion profile, evaporation rate) as well as processing temperatures during the BFS process may set some limitations. Splitting half doses from one single container may be a challenge and so for each nostril (if the medication requires this) one dropper needs to be considered. To deliver the right dose, some substantial overfilling is required which can be neglected for cheap formulations but may be important for expensive drugs.

Droppers for multi-dose presentations are still on the market but can be considered to be obsolete. A preserved formulation for multi-dose presentations is mandatory but preservatives will not solve all hygienic jaundices. Precise dosing is also close to impossible so that only drugs with a wide safety margin can be used with such systems. Intranasal administration using droppers is not very convenient. To get a good nasal deposition, the recipient should lie down or bend the head backwards to improve deposition.

For some rescue medications like naloxone or midazolam or some intranasal vaccines **spray tips** (see Fig. 4) attached to standard Luer-syringes are used to deliver the drug. The handling is somehow inconvenient, because in most cases the drug must be transferred from a vial into the syringe. Then the spray tip is attached and the system is ready for administration. The generated spray and the quality of the nasal deposition depend much on the characteristics of the spray tip and the smooth displacement movement of the plunger of the syringe. If no mechanical aid is employed (e.g. removable clips to split 2 half doses), it is difficult to separate doses for each nostril. Also, depending on the handling procedure, a dead volume of 70-130 µl for the spray tip + syringe combination must be considered. A concern for such kits may be a possible confusion of the administration route. The used syringes are easily fitted with a needle and there is some risk in real life, that the drug intended for intranasal administration is injected. Most of these disadvantages can be avoided if prefilled systems are used.

So called **unit/bidose systems** (see Fig. 5) for liquid formulations are state of the art for the intranasal administration of drugs requiring exact dosing. They have been on the market for more than 10 years for intranasal breakthrough pain and migraine management. The systems contain one or two separated half doses ready for administration. They are optimized for easy intuitive and safe handling. These systems will also ensure an optimal nasal deposition of the drug. These advantages are linked to a somehow higher price. The filling is similar to the procedure used for prefilled syringes and requires appropriate equipment.

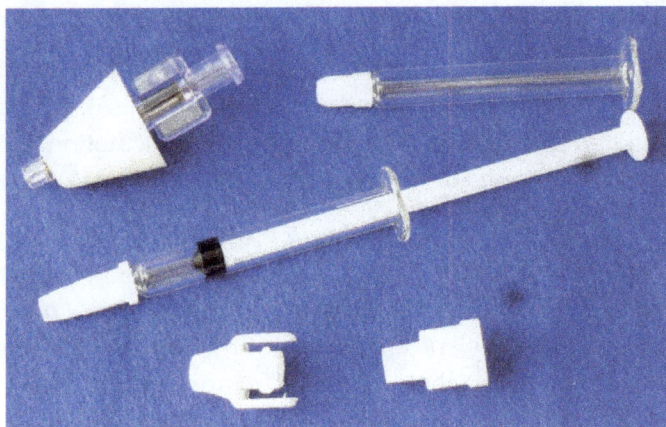

Figure 4. Spray tips for syringes which are used for the intranasal administration of naloxone, midazolam or some influenza vaccines.

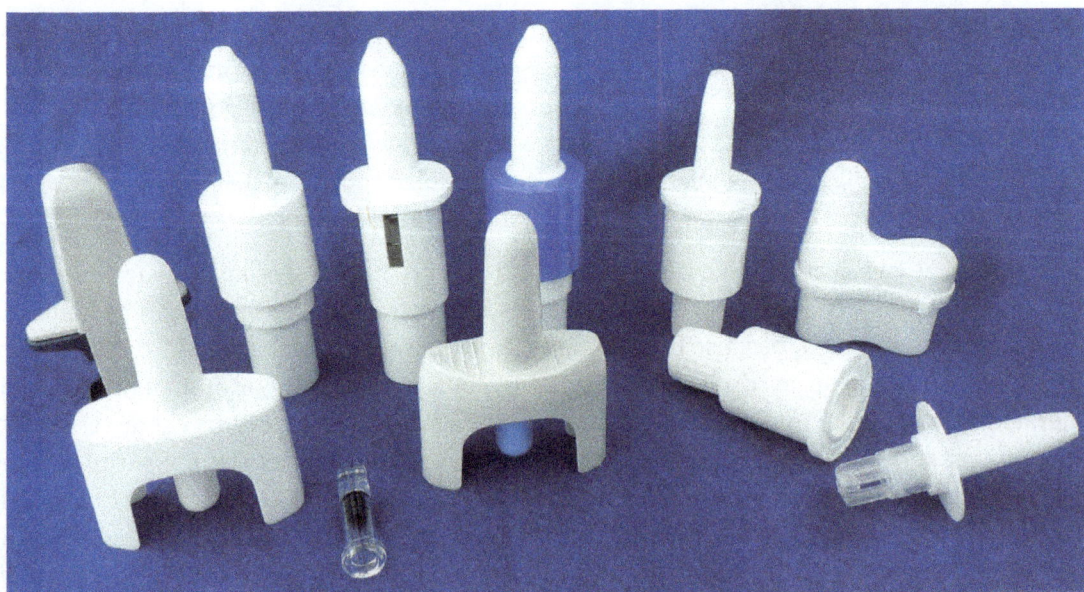

Figure 5. Examples of unit/bidose systems for liquids on the left with a glass vial which contains the one or two doses of the drug product and dry powder devices on the right.

Dry powder systems: In the near future, some drugs and vaccines will probably focus on dry powder formulations to take advantage of improved storage conditions. It may be a challenging task to generate a powder with the right particle size. As mentioned before, the particles must be designed for safe administration (no fine particle fraction), good deposition and fast dissolution within the mucus layer. For dry powders, electrostatic charge and moisture ingress must be considered. Systems which actively drive out the powder, using compressed air generated by a pump-like mechanism, seem to be better accepted than passive ones, where the powder is taken up by the nasal air flow. Dealing with dry powder needs of course different manufacturing and filling technologies, which are already available for other medications.

Multi-dose solutions are by far the most widely used package solution. In Asia, simple squeeze bottles are on the market which can be considered obsolete because exact dosing is not possible and during use mucus may be sucked back into the bottle. The current standard multi-dose solutions are metering nasal spray pumps attached to bottles containing 10-30 ml of a liquid formulation. For this reason we would like to provide a closer insight into the technology of spray pump systems. As mentioned earlier the manufacturer fills the drug formulation into multi-dose bottles made of glass or Pharma-grade plastic materials. These are then closed by attaching the spray pump including a dip tube. The pump may be fixed by a screw closure, crimped on or simply snapped onto the bottle [1]. Now the system should be tight and no leakage should be observed during subsequent handling. This filling process is done on high-speed lines which can easily fill and close 60-200 bottles per minute.

Before the system can be used, the pump must be primed. This is normally done by the patient just before first use. A number of priming strokes is required to purge the air off the system and dip tube and to deliver the product at the intended dose volume. Spray pumps are displacement pumps. When actuating the pump, a piston moves downward inside the metering chamber. A valve mechanism with a ball sealing the metering chamber against dip tube and container at the bottom of the metering chamber will prevent backflow into the dip tube. So the downward movement of the piston will create pressure within the metering chamber which forces the air (before priming) or the liquid outwards through the actuator and generates the spray. When the actuation pressure is removed, a spring will force the piston and the connected actuator to return to its initial position. This creates an underpressure in the metering chamber which pulls the liquid from the container by lifting up the ball from the ball seat above the dip tube at the bottom of the metering chamber [1]. For a proper repeated function the spray pump should be held in upright positions to ensure that the end of the dip tube is always submersed in the formulation.

4.1. Bottles

Bottles or containers are an integral part of multi-dose container closure systems and will also influence the general appearance of the final product. Special shapes may be used to differentiate a product from competitors. Glass bottles are less prone to cause interactions and will give good protection to the formulation even for long storage intervals. Sometimes the glass can influence the stability of the formulation (change in pH, release of trace metals). This depends of course on the quality of the glass which is described by its hydrolytic class (classes

I-III are normally used for pharmaceutical products). The disadvantages which glass bottles may have are the higher weight and the risk to breakage when dropped [1].

Bottles are also made of plastic material (e.g. polyethylene, polypropylene, polyethylene terephthalate). A pump supplier will most likely not manufacture these bottles because a complete different technology is used. Parts for spray pumps are quite exclusively made by injection moulding which gives high precision. Bottle manufacturers use a process referred to as blow-moulding. The general principle is to make a hollow raw part and then blowing up the material to the final dimensions. The most important disadvantage for all bottles made of plastic material is evaporation/weight loss during storage. Plastic materials are not a perfect barrier for gas or water evaporation. This problem can be tackled using laminated materials but these are more expensive. Another potential risk has to be considered: inks and adhesives from labels may migrate through the bottle wall and leach into the formulation [1].

Pure mechanics but critical for all types of bottles: the bottle opening must fit the pump exactly. It needs to be tested and dimensions need to be controlled because variations may cause leakages or damage the housing of the pump during final assembly. To avoid any issues, consultation of the pump system supplier is highly recommended as these companies are experienced in managing this interface. The pump supplier should be able to recommend a range of suited bottles from suppliers which provide reliable quality. Before switching to another bottle or bottle supplier, the compatibility with the pump system should be checked in advance [1].

5. First steps to identify the right delivery system

One of the first steps in approaching the development of an intranasal drug administration project is to select the appropriate system for delivering the drug formulation. The selection of the delivery system is strongly governed by the type of formulation envisaged for delivery. Most likely the formulation will be liquid (solution or suspension), but also powder or gel formulations are possible. Of course the dosing frequency as well as legal restrictions (e.g. for controlled substances) will influence the decision for a single or multi-dose presentation. Once the basic type of system has been selected, it is then prudent to do some basic compatibility investigation or studies in order to avoid any obvious incompatibilities between the components and the proposed active pharmaceutical ingredient (API) and any known excipients before moving on to the formulation development stage.

The materials used for the systems are selected by the manufacturer to warrant proper mechanical function and low likelihood of chemical interactions. In practice potential interactions between the formulation and parts of the spray pumps due to sorption or swelling should be excluded. Typical tests that could be considered at this stage include immersion tests of the functional parts of the pump in the formulation to detect swelling or discoloration. First tests with assembled pumps from this immersion test will provide data on potential effects on mechanical function (e.g. friction, metering).

Material	Typical functions
Polyethylene (PE)	Functional parts of the pump, actuator and fixtures, dip tube, bottles
Polypropylene (PP)	Functional parts of the pump, actuator and fixtures, dip tube, bottles
Polyoxy methylene (POM)	Functional parts (may release formaldehyde!)
Rubber or elastomers	Gaskets, seals, stopper
Stainless steel	Springs, balls for valve mechanism
Aluminum	Ferrules for crimped connections
Glass	Bottles, vials, balls for valve mechanisms

Table 1. Typical classes of materials used for nasal spray systems

A simple test for spray performance will assure that the formulation can be aerosolized by the considered pump and the delivered particle size is appropriate for effective nasal deposition. As mentioned earlier, the particle size should be in the range from at least 10 to a maximum of 150 μm. Particle sizes above 10μm assure that no product passes in to the lungs and impact in the nasal cavity. Droplets greater than 150 μl should be avoided as they are prone to run out of the nasal cavity immediately. It is not unwise to perform such preliminary compatibility tests with a certain range of different pumps to get an impression which may provide the best performance.

Type of materials
Chemical name / identity of the material
Chemical name of any monomer used
Supplier name
Compliance with relevant standards in relation to their intended use (e.g. pharmacopeias)
Complete qualitative composition when:
The material is not described in the European or national pharmacopeias
The monography authorizes the use of several additives (from which the manufacturer may choose)
Specifications
Identification
Reference to European Pharmacopeia or Member State monographs or in-house monograph (if not described in EP or Member State monographs)
Non-compendial methods (with validation) should be included where appropriate

Table 2. General information on the container closure system related to materials of construction which should be provided by the supplier of the system

At the end of the whole development process the requirements from authorities are straight forward: "For the final product (=formulation in combination with the whole container closure system) the suitability of the container closure system used for the storage, transportation (shipping) and use of the drug product should be discussed. This discussion should consider, e.g., choice of materials, protection from moisture and light, compatibility of the materials of construction with the dosage form (including sorption to container and leaching) safety of materials of construction, and performance (such as reproducibility of the dose delivery from the system when presented as part of the drug product)" [12].

6. Formulation development

Nasal drug formulations are broadly categorized into several types including solutions, suspensions, powders or gels. A key factor in selecting the type of nasal formulation to be developed is whether the therapy is intended for local or systemic application. Depending on the application, factors such drug absorption rate from the nasal mucosa into the systemic blood circulation and residence time in the nasal cavity become key elements in the formulation development process.

Taking as examples spray solutions and suspension type formulations, the following factors should be considered during nasal formulation development:

Drug, particles: consideration should be given to the desired therapeutic concentration for each dose, keeping in mind whether the total dose to the nasal cavity will be one (single nostril delivery) or two (one delivery into each nostril). For aqueous solutions and suspensions the typical dosing volume ranges are 50-140µl and for solution or suspension in pressurized metered dose inhalers (pMDIs) the typical delivery volumes are in the range of 25µl. The primary particle size of the API in suspension formulations also needs to be considered with regard to the droplet size delivered during dosing and any impact it may have on the dissolution of the particles once deposited in the nasal cavity.

pH/buffers: the pH inside the nasal cavity can influence the rate and extent of absorption of ionizable drugs. The average baseline human nasal pH is reported to be around 6.3 [13] and the pH of several commercially available nasal spray products are in the range of 3.5 to 7.0, and the optimal range for pH of these nasal formulations is suggested to be 4.5 to 6.5 [14]. The pH of the formulation can also affect the stability of the drug product during its shelf life so this also needs to be considered during development.

Osmolality: Studies have shown that hypotonic nasal spray formulations improve drug permeability through the nasal mucosa [15] and some marketed products report osmolality in the range 300-700mOsmol/K.

Viscosity/surface tension: the majority of commercially marketed products contain agents that modify the viscosity and surface tension of the formulations, they are included in order to manage factors such as thinning and thixotropic behavior and are key elements in the performance of the dispensed product such as drop particle size, spray angles and also influence the residence time of the product once delivered, in the nasal cavity.

Ingredients	IIG limit for nasal route, %w/w	Function
Alcohol, 200 proof	2	Co-solvent
Anhydrous dextrose	0.5	tonicity
Anhydrous trisodiumcitrate	0.0006	buffer
Benzyl alcohol	0.0366	preservative
Benzalkonium chloride	0.119	preservative
Butylated hydroxyanisole	0.0002	antioxidant
Cellulose microcrystalline	2	Suspending agent, stabilizer
Chlorobutanol	0.5	preservative
Carboxymethyl cellulose Na	0.15	Suspending agent
Edetate disodium	0.5	Chelator, antioxidant
Hydrochloric acid	Not reported	pH adjustment
Methylparaben	0.7	preservative
Oleic acid	0.132	Penetration enhancer
PEG400	20	Surfactant, co-solvent
PEG3500	1.5	surfactant
Phenylethyl alcohol	0.254	Preservative, masking agent
Polyoxyl 400 stearate	15	surfactant
Polysorbate 20	2.5	surfactant
Polysorbate 80	10	surfactant
Propylene glycol	20	Co-solvent
Propylparaben	0.3	Preservative
Sodium chloride	1.9	tonicity
Sodium hydroxide	0.004	pH adjustment
Sulfuric acid	0.4	pH adjustment

Table 3. Examples of key nasal formulation excipients and their inactive ingredient guidance (IIG) dosing levels

Other excipients: in addition to buffer salts several types of excipients may be required in order to develop a stable nasal spray formulation. These include solvents and co-solvents to keep the active pharmaceutical ingredient (API) in the dissolved or suspended state, as well as preservatives for non-sterile products. If the formulation is a suspension or emulsion, surfactants and/or emulsifying agents, stabilizers and suitable oil-phase components may be required. Although there are numerous surfactants, emulsifying agents, solvents, co-solvents, oils and preservatives available, only a limited number of excipients are listed in the US FDA inactive ingredient guide (IIG) for nasal products. Table 3 lists some key excipients and their IIG dosage levels, as reported in the FDA IIG database for nasal spray formulations [16].

Controlling residence time in the nasal cavity: increasing the residence time of the drug, once delivered on the nasal mucosa, can be beneficial especially for local applications and can aid drug absorption through the nasal mucosa. One approach is too increase the viscosity of the formulation but this should be balanced against any impact on droplet size distribution during delivery into the nasal cavity [17].

Penetration enhancers: these agents increase the penetration of drugs through the nasal mucosa. Typical penetration enhancing agents are solvents, co-solvents, ionic and some non-ionic surfactants, selected fatty acids, including oleic acid and certain lipids and cyclodextrin [18, 19].

Powder and gel nasal formulations: in formulating nasal powders the key elements to manage are controlling the primary particle size of the API as well as the excipients to get efficient nasal deposition, and selecting a system that provides acceptable protection of the powder during storage and efficient delivery to the nasal cavity during dosing. For nasal gel applications the formulations can be relatively simple and key elements will be stability and shelf-life and the selection of the dispensing system used to deliver the gel to the nasal cavity.

7. Performance parameters

Nasal drug product performance characterization is driven by regulatory requirements which allow for successful approval and marketing of these products. The most stringent regulatory standards for nasal drug products are issued in the USA [20] and in Europe [21]. During the development process information has to be documented on many factors in order to construct a regulatory dossier. Typical expectations for development characterizations in the US and Europe are detailed in Table 4.

Once approved and marketed these products have to be routinely controlled in order to assure ongoing performance and quality and the typical regulatory expectations for marketed nasal product specifications and testing are detailed in Table 5. The rationale behind these perform-ance characterization tests are related to factors such as dosing accuracy, shelf life, product robustness and user safety, the key ones being as follows:

Priming, re-priming: most nasal spray pumps need to be primed in order to fill the dosing chambers before use and to assure full dosing of the product. In addition, some pumps do not retain the dose in the metering chamber when stored for longer periods, i.e. 7 days, 1 month etc. and may need to be re-primed before use after a specified period of non-use which will be defined in the patient leaflet.

Characterization test	US	EU
Stability / shelf life	√	√
Temp. cycle testing	√	√
Priming re-priming	√	√
Micro/bioburden	√	√
Extractables	√	√
Leachables	√	N/A
USP tests, 601, 87, 88, 661, 381...	√	N/A
Drop testing, vibration, shipping, air transport tests	√	√
Effect of orientation	√	√
Plume geometry	√	N/A
Profiling near exhaustion	√	√
Performance in the hands of different users	√	√
Particulates	√	N/A

Table 4. Examples of product characterization test during development of nasal spray products.

Control test	US	EU
Priming, re-priming	√	√
Dose weight (through life)	√	√
Leakage	√	√
Dimensional, metrology	√	√
Droplet/particle size distribution	√	√
Spray pattern	√	N/A
Extractables	√	√
Microbial limits	√	√

Table 5. Examples of routine control testing for nasal spray products.

Dose weight through life: this test assures that the pump delivers the prescribed dose consistently throughout the use-life of the product, usually beginning middle and end of use. Regulatory requirements exist in most markets for limits on dosing accuracy and these can be found by referring to each country specific regulatory dosing limit specifications for nasal products.

Leakage: this assures that the product integrity is maintained throughout its proposed shelf life and that the contents are not lost during storage at various environmental conditions. The ICH stability test conditions [22] are the key reference with regard to stability testing.

Dimensional/metrology measurements: these assure that the spray pump meets specified critical quality dimensions in order to assure that the nasal product functions efficiently and meets the key performance tests assuring consistent quality.

Particle size distribution: this can refer to the primary particle size specification of the API itself in suspensions or to the droplet (liquid solution) or particle (powder) size distribution of the delivered spray. Specifications need to be put in place for this key parameter and the justified limits registered in the regulatory submissions as it is closely related to nasal deposition efficiency.

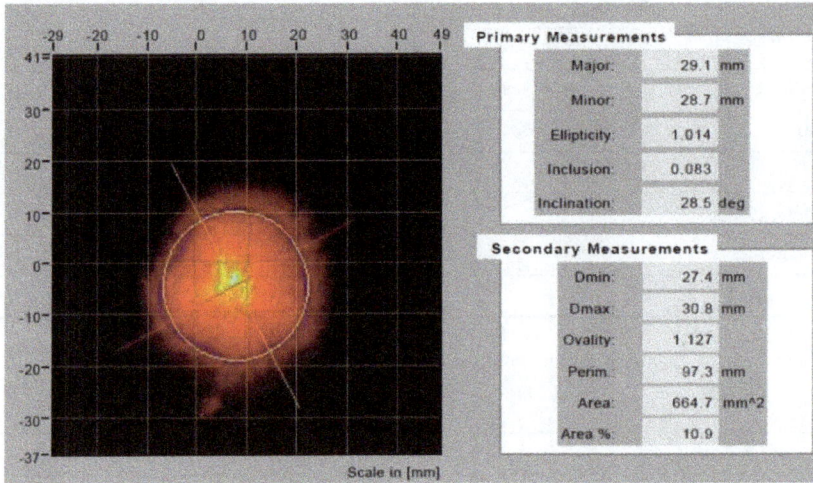

Figure 6. Typical display from a spray pattern test using laser imaging, which can give information about the ovality of the emitted spray.

Spray pattern: this is another test to assure consistent quality of the delivered nasal spray and characterizes parameters such as angle and plume shape, see Figures 6 and 7.

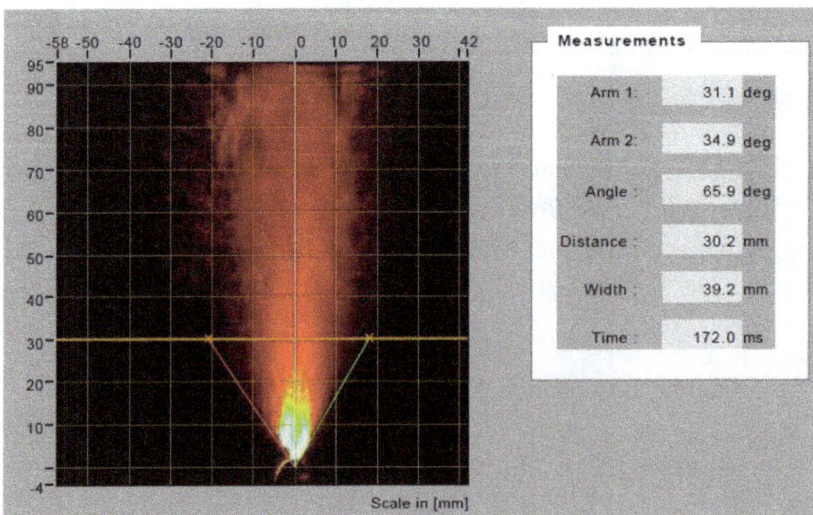

Figure 7. Typical display from a spray angle test using laser imaging, which can give information about the angle of the emitted spray.

Extractables/leachables: this test assures the safety of the product and specifically measures and controls the potential chemical contaminants which may come from the packaging or container closure system into the formulation and therefore be potentially toxic for the patients, if ingested. The PQRI [23] have issued detailed guidance documents on this subject in conjunction with the FDA which outline how to tackle this specific parameter.

Particulates: this test characterizes the contamination of the nasal formulation by any foreign particulates and is related to the overall safety of the product.

Microbial limits: specification and tests exist to measure and characterize this parameter, for preserved nasal formulations this will usually mean measuring the levels of preservatives, e.g. benzalkonium chloride in the product and during its proposed shelf life. The units of measurement are usually colony forming units (CFU's). For non-preserved nasal products the characterization tests are somewhat more complicated and include challenge testing with contaminated bacterial environments to assure the integrity of the system for protection against microbial contamination. Special drug delivery systems are needed in order to use non-preserved nasal formulations.

Robustness: here a number of different test are applied including dropping the whole packaging, exposure to vibration, simulation of shipping and transportation. These characterization tests are meant to assess the robustness of the product to normal transport and day to day use.

— Description of the assembled device and each individual component:
· Identification of the packaging component
— Product Name, Code / Item number
— Manufacturer
· Engineering drawings (with critical dimensions)
— Description of the manufacturing process
· Manufacturing process
· Operations performed after manufacture (washing, coating)
· Treatment procedures
— Description of the controls
· Incoming, in-process and release controls
· For materials of construction, the manufacturing process and the finished product (component or assembled device)

Table 6. General information on the container closure system which should be provided by the supplier [8,9].

User studies: these tests look at the ergonomic and human factor aspects of the systems and include investigation and data generation on potential issues such as orientation, patient handling (young, old, comprised dexterity etc.), actuation forces and many other factors.

Regulatory Guidance's have appeared in the last few years outlining how to tackle these 'human factor' issues [24].

As can be seen from the above list of tests, the development process for a nasal drug product can be quite long, intensive, and costly and depending on the complexity of the product can take upwards of 18 months keeping in mind that suitable real time stability data also need to be generated for regulatory submissions.

8. Trends for nasal drug administration

8.1. Use of preservatives in multi-dose products

For some years now, so called "preservative-free multi-dose" systems ("PFMD") are on the market and gain share. Such systems are certainly appreciated by the growing number of patients who experienced discomfort with preserved formulations. The issue of significance for the patient and consumer, however, is the high incidence of local side effects attributed to preservatives. The discussion is controversial, and published preclinical and clinical studies are not always consistent. It seems to be clear that short-term use of preparations containing preservatives at low concentrations is well tolerated, but preservatives can cause serious inflammatory effects with long-term use [25]. The responses may include chemical irritation, hyperreactivity and true allergies [26]. The German Authorities (BfArM) addressed the use of benzalkonium chloride for nasal sprays in 2003 [27] which encouraged the preservative free systems for this administration route. Today a range of technical solutions is available to overcome this issue. The highest risk of contamination obviously comes from the orifice of the nasal spray system, because it may come in contact with skin and mucosa as well as with infected mucus in the nose. Some marketed systems use the oligodynamic activity of a silver wire in the tip of the actuator, a silver coated spring and ball [28]. Such systems are able to keep microorganisms down between long dosing intervals, even when the tip is immersed into bacterial contaminated fluid [29].

The most recent preservative free systems follow a purely mechanical approach to minimize interactions between parts of the device and the formulation. One technical solution to prevent contamination via the orifice is referred to as "tip seal technology" [25]. A spring loaded valve is located directly below the opening of the tip orifice and does not allow any microbes to migrate from any surfaces or contacted liquids into the system, the orifice is "sealed" under resting conditions. The tip seal keeps the system closed until a defined pressure (for nasal sprays it is more than 3 bar) is reached by pressing down the actuator. Then the system will open and the formulation is forced through the orifice with a higher pressure than needed to open the valve. When the pressure drops at the end of the actuation the tip seal will immediately close the orifice with an outward movement. So no backflow of potentially contaminated medication or other liquid is possible. Depending on the pump system, the fluid path may even be "metal-free", which means the springs needed for the device operation do not come in contact with the formulation [25].

To avoid contamination of the formulation via venting air different technical solutions are used. The simplest way is sterile filtration of the venting air using separate filters or filter gaskets. For oxygen-sensitive formulations, so called collapsing bags or depressed systems are used. The formulation is filled in a special, microbial tight bag which is protected by a surrounding bottle. When dispensing the product, the bag collapses with the content not coming in contact with the ambient air. Some pumps are constructed in such a way, that the whole system is air-tight and during use some vacuum (up to -300 mbar) is generated within the bottle. Those systems allow even a purging with inert gases to reduce oxygen content in the container head space [25].

These described technical solutions to make the use of preservatives obsolete are well established and mature technologies.

8.2. Non-aqueous nasal formulations

The majority of prescription nasal spray products on the market are aqueous formulations. Just recently some so called "dry mist" nasal sprays (e.g. QNASL®, ZETONNA™) were introduced. For these products the technology of the pressurized metered dose inhalers (pMDI's) is utilized which are well established for the treatment of asthma bronchiale and chronic obstructive pulmonary disease. The active ingredient is dissolved or suspended into hydrofluoroalkane (HFA) propellant and typical delivery volumes are in the range of 25µl. Non-aqueous nasal spray formulations are suspected to have increased levels of safety risks due to the fact that they use excipient such as propylene glycol, isopropyl alcohol and PEG400, which are known to cause local irritation particularly for chronic use [30]. Nasal steroids such as beclomethasone and ciclesonide are formulated in such non-aqueous HFA propellants and in this case it is the same formulation approach as is used for inhalation suspension products using pressurized metered dose inhalers (pMDI's).

8.3. Side actuated spray pumps

An innovative development in nasal spray pumps are side actuated nasal spray devices designed to help improve patient compliance due to their reduced dependence on patient actuation force or speed. These devices are intended to be compact, ergonomic with intuitive design and have short and motionless nasal nozzles where the fingers are no longer in contact with the nostrils. They have softer actuation and are suitable for a wide range of applications including pediatrics and elderly patients who may have compromised dexterity.

8.4. Unit- and bi-dose sprayer

Unit dose devices can also be considered attractive options for certain types of therapy, especially for all kinds of rescue medications. The ready to use packaging will reduce stress (e.g. no fear for injuries, disease transmission) and handling errors which may happen in such situations. Such kind of packaging also limits the amount of drug which needs to be handled which is important for controlled substances.

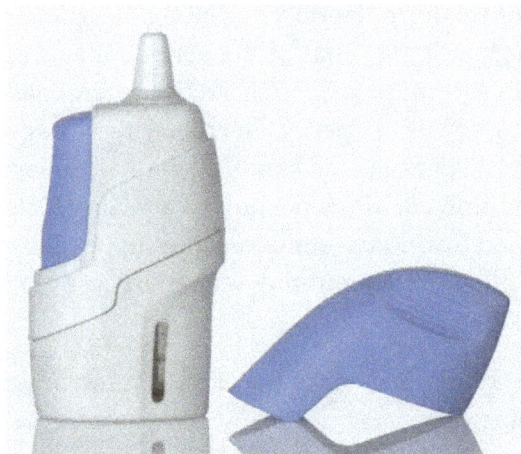

Figure 8. Example of a side actuated multi-dose spray pump

a. Pain management, e.g. migraine or cancer breakthrough pain episodes, here the molecules are often potent and the amount of dose should be limited in order to avoid any undesirable side-effects or risks of diversion or misuse.

b. Vaccines are often one-off treatments and they can be formulated in powder forms so as to avoid the cold chain logistics difficulties associated with liquid vaccines and can easily be used out the hospital environment, such as field vaccination stations.

By using such unit dose or single throw away devices, one can avoid many of the issues outlined above for pain or vaccination therapies.

9. Conclusion

Intranasal drug administration is a technology with an interesting past and a fascinating future. In only a few fields cooperation between developers of novel pharmaceutical remedies on one side and manufacturers of sophisticated delivery systems on the other side is equally essential. Precise metered dosing, maximum flexibility, product protection and, last not least, patient adherence are the key areas to work on. The increasing use of unpreserved formulations in both prescription and OTC (over the counter) products establishes additional challenges. Patients and consumers appreciate the convenient and intuitive handling of modern nasal delivery systems, properties which are important for further and sustainable success of nasal administration in general. However, with regulatory demands increasing, professional guidance is needed and should be provided by manufacturers of nasal drug delivery systems to support pharmaceutical companies in finding the optimum configuration. Even though such support can not exempt marketers form performing proper due diligence on the finished product, it is obvious that time to market can be reduced substantially if available resources are utilized in a proper cooperation mode.

Author details

Degenhard Marx[1*], Gerallt Williams[2] and Matthias Birkhoff[1]

*Address all correspondence to: degenhard.marx@aptar.com

1 Aptar Radolfzell GmbH, Radolfzell, Germany

2 Aptar France SAS, Le Vaudreuil, France

References

[1] Marx D and Birkhoff M (2011). Multi-Dose Container for Nasal and Ophthalmic Drugs: A Preservative Free Future?, Drug Development - A Case Study Based Insight into Modern Strategies, Dr. Chris Rundfeldt (Ed.), ISBN: 978-953-307-257-9, InTech, DOI: 10.5772/27767. Available from: http://www.intechopen.com/books/drug-development-a-case-study-based-insight-into-modern-strategies/multi-dose-container-for-nasal-and-ophthalmic-drugs-a-preservative-free-future

[2] Leary AC, Dowling M, Cussen K, O'Brien J, Stote RM. Pharmacokinetics and pharmacodynamics of intranasal insulin spray (Nasulin) administered to healthy male volunteers: infuence of the nasal cycle. J Diabetes Sci Technol. 2008, 2(6): 1054-60

[3] Marx D, Leitz M, Fagot C. Do We Need New Devices for Intranasal Vaccination? Drug Development & Delivery. 2011, 11 (3): 54-59

[4] Guideline on pharmaceutical development of medicines for paediatric use, 3 January 2013, EMA/CHMP/QWP/805880/2012 Rev. 2

[5] Consumer Product Safety Ccommission 16 CFR Part 1700, CPSC Docket No. 2012–0005, Requirements for child-resistant packaging: Products containing imidazolines equivalent to 0.08 milligrams or more. December 12, 2012

[6] Fagot Ch and Marx D. Intranasal vaccines -a platform technology for an innovative vaccine industry. December 2011, Express Pharma India, access at http://archive.expresspharmaonline.com/20111231/research02.shtml

[7] Suman JD, Laube BL, Lin TC, Brouet G, Dalby R. Validity of in vitro tests on aqueous spray pumps as surrogates for nasal deposition. Pharm Res. 2002;19(1): 1-6

[8] Guidance for Industry: Nasal Spray and Inhalation Solution, Suspension, and Spray Drug Products - Chemistry, Manufacturing, and Controls Documentation. US Department of Health and Human Services, Food and Drug Administration, Center for Drug Evaluation and Research (CDER). Rockville, MD; 2002

[9]   Committee for medicinal products for human use (CHMP). Guideline on the phar-
      maceutical quality of inhalation and nasal products. London: European Medicines
      Agency; 2006

[10] Foo MY, Cheng YS, Su WC, Donovan MD. The influence of spray properties on intra-
      nasal deposition. J Aerosol Med. 2007, 20(4): 495-508

[11] Stuart BO. Deposition and clearance of inhaled particles. Environ Health Perspect.
      1984; 55: 369-390

[12] ICH Harmonised Tripartite Guideline: Pharmaceutical Development Q8; Step 4 ver-
      sion, November 2005

[13] Washington N., et al, 'Determination of baseline human nasal pH and the effect of
      intranasally administered buffers', Int. J. Pharm. 198:139-146 (2000)

[14] Aurora R., et al, 'Development of nasal delivery systems: a review', Drug Del. Tech.
      2(7), 70-73 (2002)

[15] Farina D., 'Regulatory aspects of nasal and pulmonary spray drug products', pub-
      lished in handbook of non-invasive drug delivery systems, Ed. V.Kulkarni, Elsevier,
      Oxford, UK, 247-290 (2010)

[16] FDA IIG (Inactive Ingredient Guidance), http://accessdata.fda.gov/scripts/cder/iig/
      index.cfm

[17] Dayal P., et al, 'Evaluation of different parameters that effect droplet size distribution
      from nasal sprays using the Malvern Spraytech, J. Pharm. Sci., 93: 1725-1742 (2004)

[18] Law S.L., et al, 'Preparation of desmopressin-containing liposomes for intranasal de-
      livery', J. Control. Rel., 70: 375-382 (2001)

[19] Davis S., et al, 'Absorption enhancers for nasal drug delivery', Clin. Pharm., 42(13),
      1107-28 (2003)

[20] Nasal Spray and Inhalation Solution, Suspension, and Spray Drug Products Chemis-
      try, Manufacturing and Controls Documentation, U.S. Department of Health and
      Human Services, Food and Drug Administration, Center for Drug Evaluation and
      Research (CDER), May 1999

[21] EMEA-Heath Canada: Joint Guideline on the Pharmaceutical Quality of Inhalation
      and Nasal Products EMEA/CHMP/QWP/49313/2005

[22] Stability testing of new drug substances and products Q1A, ICH harmonized tripar-
      tite guideline, 6 February 2003

[23] Safety thresholds and best practices for extractables and leachables in orally inhaled
      and nasal drug products, PQRI Leachables and Extractables Working Group, 8 Sep
      2006

[24] Human factors engineering—Design of medical devices, ANSI/AAMI HE75, 2009/ (R)2013

[25] Marx D and Birkhoff M. Will the future be preservative-free? Manufacturing Chemist Pharma, published 17th May 2013, access at

[26] http://www.manufacturingchemist.com/technical/article_page/ Will_the_future_be_preservativefree/88155

[27] Hong J, Bielory L. Allergy to ophthalmic preservatives. Curr Opin Allergy Clin Immunol.

[28] 2009;9(5):447-453.

[29] Bescheid des Bundesinstitut für Arzneimittel und Medizinproduke für benzalkoniumchlorid-haltige Arzneimittel zur Anwendung in der Nase, A 37489/38186/03 Bonn, Dezember 2003

[30] Groß D. The COMOD-System – a preservative free drug therapy against glaucoma. 321-328, in Orgül/Flammer (Editors): Pharmacotherapie in glaucoma, Bern 2000

[31] Bagel S, Wiedemann B. Extension of in-use stability of preservative-free nasalia. Europ J Pharmaceutics and Biopharmaceutics. 2004, (57): 353–358

[32] Kibbe A.H., (Ed), Handbook of pharmaceutical excipients, 3rd Edition, Am. Pharm. Asso., 392-398, 442-444 (2000)

3

Nuclear Receptor Modulators — Current Approaches and Future Perspectives

Thales Kronenberger, Oliver Keminer,
Carsten Wrenger and Björn Windshügel

Additional information is available at the end of the chapter

1. Introduction

In multicellular organisms the regulation of growth, development and metabolic homeostasis involves extensive intercellular communication. This is achieved by diverse endocrine signal molecules that often address intracellular receptors which regulate gene expression in a ligand-dependent manner. Proteins involved in up- or down-regulation of gene expression are termed transcription factors. It is estimated that about 10 % of the human genome encodes proteins of this family [1]. An important class of transcription factors are nuclear receptors (NRs). So far, 48 different NRs have been identified in humans. However, due to alternative splicing the number of different functional NRs is substantially larger [2]. Similar to other protein families (*e.g.* G protein-coupled receptors) a unified nomenclature system has been established in order to overcome problems due to multiple names for the same gene [3].

NRs recognize and bind small molecules that comprise, for example, steroid and thyroid hormones, vitamins as well as fatty acids and their derivatives [4]. In fact, for only about half of human NRs an endogenous ligand has been identified so far. The involvement of several members of the NR superfamily in various diseases has made this class of transcription factors highly attractive for pharmaceutical industry. As described below, several members of the NR family are already addressed by drugs and more receptors are under investigation [5].

Understanding nuclear receptor function requires knowledge of the NR structure. The composition of nuclear receptors is modular and involves 5-6 domains with distinct functions (Figure 1). Evolutionary most conserved domains are the DNA-binding domain (DBD) and the ligand-binding domain (LBD). Other domains show a considerable variation in length and sequence such as the N-terminal domain, the hinge region - connecting DBD and LBD - as well as the C-terminal domain.

The N-terminal domain (NTD) possesses a ligand-independent activation function 1 (AF-1) and contains several post-translational modification sites [6, 7]. The NTD size may vary considerably, ranging from 23 to 602 residues. Although no X-ray crystal structures of this domain are available, circular dichroism studies have indicated the presence of some secondary structures upon posttranslational modifications [8]. The DBD domain consists of about 70 highly conserved amino acids and contains two zinc-finger motifs which are essential for DNA binding [9]. The DBD organisation allows binding to specific DNA sequences (responsive elements) [9]. The core region of the response elements is organised as hexameric motif with the consensus sequence 5'-AGGTCA-3' [8]. The number of motifs as well as their organisation and spacer length between the repetitive elements and the flanking regions affect the specificity of NR binding [10, 11]. A typical response element presents two repetitions of the core motif that can be organised in inverted, everted or direct repeats [12].

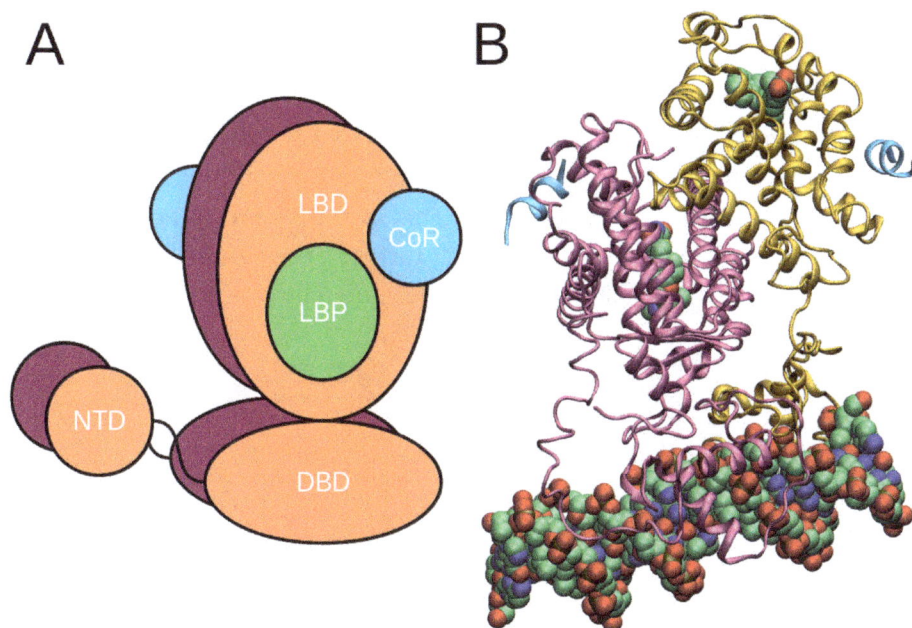

Figure 1. Assembly of nuclear receptor and their interaction partners. A: Nuclear receptors are composed of several domains. Main domains are i) the N-terminal domain (NTD) of variable length that carries the ligand-independent activation function 1 (AF-1), ii) the DNA-binding domain (DBD) that binds to the response elements in the promoter region of target genes and iii) the ligand-binding domain (LBD) that harbours the ligand-binding pocket (LBP), the ligand-dependent activation function (AF-2) as well as a binding site for coregulatory proteins (CoR) and other nuclear receptors.Most nuclear receptors bind as dimers to their response elements. B: X-ray crystal structure (PDB code 3DZY of the PPARγ (violet) and RXRα (orange) DBD and LBD (cartoon representation) bound to DNA (CPK representation). Structure was solved in complex with NR agonists (shown in CPK representation) rosiglitazone (PPARγ) and 9-cis retinoic acid (RXRα) as well as coactivator peptides (blue ribbons).

The second large domain is the ligand-binding domain (LBD) that is connected to the DBD via the hinge region. As the name already indicates, the LBD is capable to bind small molecules in its ligand-binding pocket (LBP) [12]. In addition, the LBD carries the ligand-dependent activation function 2 (AF-2), located on its C-terminal helix (helix 12, H12) [13]. In addition, the LBD contains a dimerisation motif that allows binding of other NRs and an interaction site for co-regulatory proteins that are important for activation and inhibition of target gene expression [14, 15]. The LBD comprises about 250 amino acids and is mainly composed of α-helices, arranged in a so-called three-layered helix sandwich. The ligand-binding pocket is found between both outer layers. Size and amino acid composition of the LBP differ substantially among different NRs resulting in LBP volumes ranging between 100 Å^3 (ERRα) and 1300 Å^3 (PPARγ) [13, 14]. In some cases, for example NURR1, no ligand-binding pocket is present, suggesting a ligand-independent mechanism of action [23].

Ligand-binding to the LBP modulates the conformation of helix 12 (AF-2). Agonists induce AF-2 to adopt a helical conformation that covers the ligand-binding pocket like a lid. By this process, a binding site for co-activator proteins is generated. These bind to the receptor via their nuclear receptor interacting domain (NRID) which contains a highly conserved LxxLL motif (L = leucine, x = any residue) [15]. Several co-activators (*e.g.* SRC-1) contain an intrinsic histone acetyltransferase function which results in decondensation of the chromatin at the promoter region, thereby improving accessibility of further transcription factors. In addition, co-activators recruit other proteins with histone modifying capabilities as well as proteins of the basal transcription machinery. Eventually, these processes initiate target gene expression. In contrast, NR antagonists displace H12 from the active conformation, which is often associated with partial unfolding of the helix. This event induces binding of co-repressor proteins to the receptor. Similar to co-activators, further proteins are recruited that lead to chromatin condensation (*e.g.* by histone deacetylases), thereby silencing gene expression.

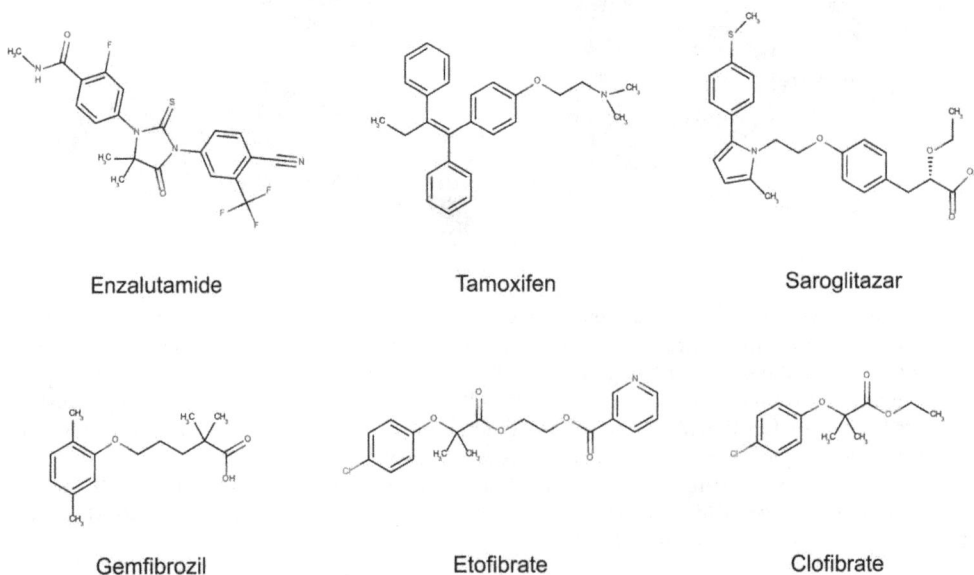

Enzalutamide	Tamoxifen	Saroglitazar

Gemfibrozil	Etofibrate	Clofibrate

Figure 2. Examples for approved drugs targeting nuclear receptors.

Besides other drug target classes such as G protein-coupled receptors, ion channels or receptor tyrosine kinases, nuclear receptors represent another major receptor target class. As of 2011, 76 approved drugs targeting 17 nuclear receptors were available (See Figure 2 for selected examples) of which several generate more than 1 billion dollar sales each year [5]. In this chapter we will highlight selected NRs which are targeted by approved drugs and provide insight into current efforts to address additional receptors using small molecules. A focus will be on novel mechanisms of receptor inhibition as shown by co-activator-binding inhibitors. In addition, currently used methods for studying nuclear receptor function in drug discovery are described.

2. Pharmaceutically relevant nuclear receptors and their drugs

Most nuclear receptors addressed by approved drugs belong to the subfamilies 1 (thyroid receptor like receptors) and 3 (estrogen receptor like receptors). Main indication areas are cancer, hormone replacement and metabolic diseases.

An NR that is targeted by both, agonists and antagonists, is the estrogen receptor (ER), belonging to the steroid hormone receptors. Two ER forms exist, called α and β (NR3A1, NR3A2). An endogenous ligand of both ERs is the steroid hormone 17β-estradiol. While estradiol preferentially binds to the α-form (Figure 3A & C), the third estrogen produced in humans (estriol) favors the β-form. Both ERα and ERβ bind as homodimers to their response elements. The natural ligand estrogen is also applied in hormone replacement therapy.

Of main pharmaceutical relevance is ERα. In the majority of breast cancers (~70 %), ERα is overexpressed in breast tissue (ERα-positive cancer). Since the natural ligand estradiol plays an important role in breast cancer development and progression, antagonists targeting ERα have been developed for treatment of ERα-positive breast cancer [16]. A frequently used drug that addresses ERα is tamoxifen (Figure 2), a potent antagonist of the receptor. Being a prodrug, tamoxifen requires conversion to the bioactive forms 4-hydroxytamoxifen and N-desmethyl-4-hydroxytamoxifen in the liver by cytochromes CYP2D6 and CYP3A4. Both metabolites possess up to 100-fold better affinity to the receptor than the prodrug [17]. Tamoxifen and its metabolites belong to the class of selective estrogen receptor modulators (SERMs), which are chemically different to the natural ligand estradiol. In breast tissue, tamoxifen metabolites act as competitive inhibitors of the natural ligand estradiol in the ER ligand-binding pocket, while in other tissues such as the endometrium, the compounds act as potent ER agonist [18]. This agonistic effect is problematic as it substantially increases the risk of uterine cancer and therefore the compound is not used for long-term treatment [27].

Another selective estrogen receptor modulator is the benzothiophene raloxifene which is applied for treatment and prevention of osteoporosis in postmenopausal women but also for reducing the breast cancer risk. The compound is not a prodrug like tamoxifen as it already contains two hydroxyl groups that form hydrogen bonds with the same LBP-residues as the tamoxifen metabolites. Also a difference is the mechanism of action as raloxifene does not show

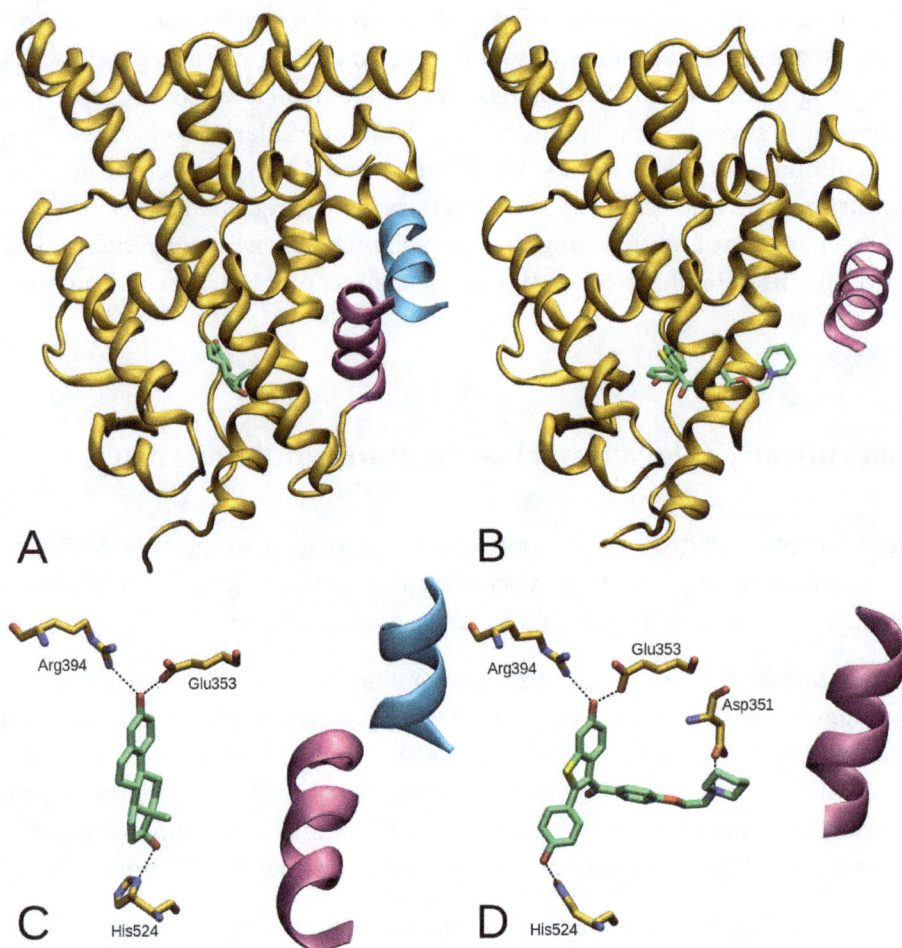

Figure 3. Protein-ligand interactions in estrogen receptor α (ERα). A: ERα (cartoon representation) in complex with the natural agonist estradiol (capped sticks representation, carbon atoms in green, oxygen atoms in red). Helix 12 (violet) is in the active conformation enabling coactivator binding (NRID in blue). B: Antagonist binding (raloxifene) displaces H12 from the active conformation thereby disrupting the coactivator binding site. C & D: Binding modes of estradiol (C) and raloxifene (D) within the ERα LBP. Both compounds have an identical hydrogen bond interaction pattern (black dotted lines). In addition, raloxifene forms a salt bridge with Asp351.

any antitumor activity. Instead, the compound is used for preventing osteoporosis and may also reduce the incidence of breast cancer in postmenopausal women.

Both SERMs are T-shaped molecules. X-ray crystal structures of estrogen receptor α co-crystallized with 4-hydroxytamoxifen and raloxifene have revealed the binding mode within the LBP (Figure 3B & D).The core structure of both compounds is planar and binds in a similar orientation into the ligand-binding pocket as the natural ligand estradiol (Figure 3A & C). Several hydrogen bonds shared with the receptor ensure tight binding. Hydrogen bond formation with the receptor is only possible for the metabolized forms of tamoxifen and explains why these molecules are much more potent compared to the prodrug. The side chain protruding from the core structure of tamoxifen metabolites and raloxifene sterically displaces H12 from the active conformation, resulting in an inactive NR [25, 26].

Another member of the nuclear receptor superfamily targeted by drugs is the androgen receptor (AR, NR3C4). Natural AR ligands are the androgens testosterone or dihydrotestosterone (Figure 4A), both activating the receptor. AR is expressed in several tissues of which the prostate and adrenal gland are representing the main expression sites [19]. Besides its role in sexual differentiation in utero and male pubertal genesis, AR is involved in maintenance of libido, spermatogenesis, muscle mass and strength, bone mineral density and erythropoiesis [20]. Several diseases such as prostate cancer or androgen insensitivity syndrome have been linked to AR [19]. For treatment of prostate cancer hormone deprivation using chemical (luteinizing-hormone-releasing hormone analogues, LHRHa) or surgical castration is a standard therapy that is initially effective in reducing the number of circulating tumor cells. But almost invariably resistance emerges after few years. This type of cancer is then referred to as castration-resistant prostate cancer (CRPC) with poor prognosis. By virtue of AR gene overexpression and amplification as well as mutations within the AR gene, androgen receptor activity is upregulated in CRPC. In order to treat CRPC, AR antagonists, also termed anti-androgens, have been developed.

Both steroidal and non-steroidal AR antagonists have been developed. Low efficacy and hepatotoxicity as well as cardiovascular side effects and problems with libido and potency have limited the use of steroidal antiandrogens. These side effects are largely due to the effect of the drugs on other nuclear receptors recognizing steroid hormones (e.g. progesterone receptor, or glucocorticoid receptor). Non-steroidal anti-androgens (NSAA), which have been introduced about 25 years ago, are mainly used in advanced and metastatic prostate cancer treatment [21]. First generations of NSAAs were flutamides and their derivatives bicalutamide or nilutamide, which are chemically related compounds. The mode of action of these drugs is to compete with the natural ligand for AR binding and thereby antagonizing the receptor and inhibiting tumor growth. While flutamide is usually used in combination with LHRH-a, bicalutamide is also applied as monotherapy. In contrast to steroidal anti-androgens, side effects due to binding to other steroid hormone receptors are less severe.

Enzalutamide (Figure 2), introduced in 2009, is a second generation NSAA used in treatment of CRPC. Besides competing with the natural ligands, the drug also reduces nuclear translocation and, as a consequence, DNA binding of the receptor [22]. Enzalutamide prolongs life of cancer patients, who did not receive chemotherapy before, with only a few registered side-effects [23]. However, in many CRPC-patients resistance occurs after several months of treatment which had been linked to a mutation within the LBD [24].

In order to overcome resistance problems and to establish therapeutics not targeting the ligand-binding pocket, an alternative approach is to address the protein-DNA interactions of the AR by molecules binding to the DBD. By now several studies have already reported successful identification of compounds targeting DBD of enzalutamide-resistant ARs [25, 26].

Another example for receptors targeted by already approved drugs is the group of peroxisome proliferator-activated receptors (PPARs). Three PPAR subtypes have been identified: PPARα, PPARδ (also termed PPARβ) and PPARγ. Unlike ER, all PPARs form heterodimers with the retinoid X receptor. Another difference to steroid hormone receptors is a considerably larger LBP. Natural ligands of PPARs include various fatty acids and eicosanoids. Some compounds

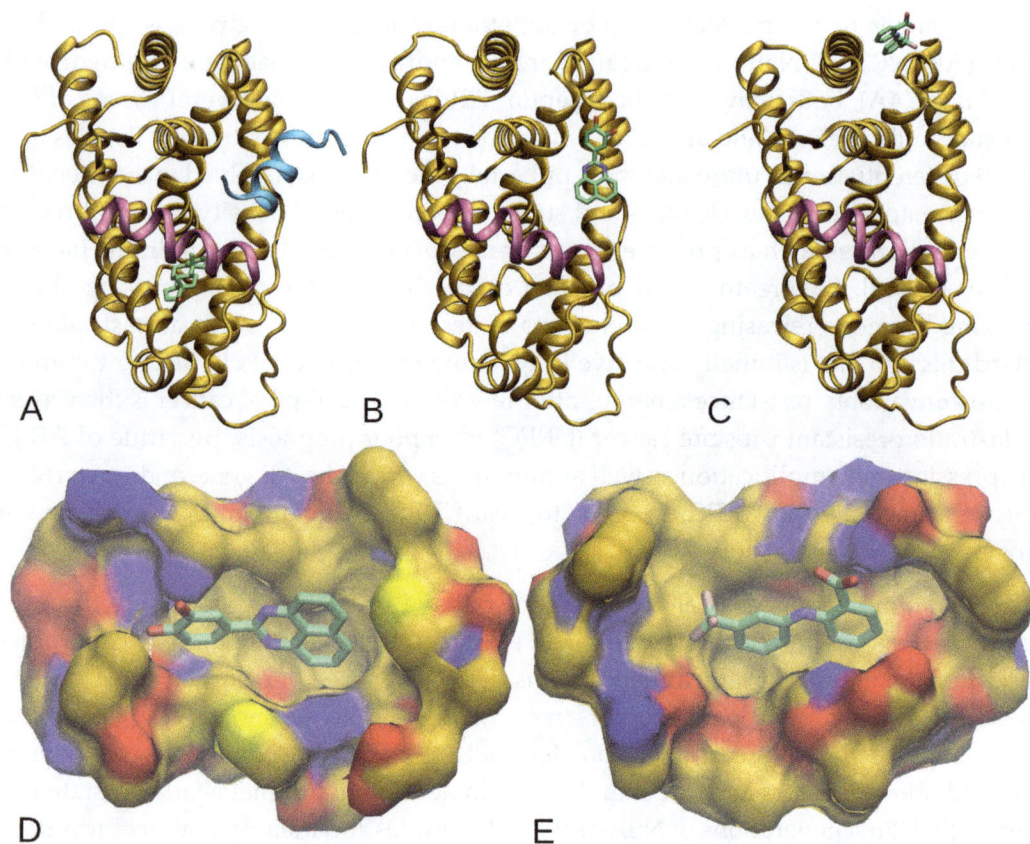

Figure 4. Protein-ligand interactions in androgen receptor (AR). A: AR in complex with testosterone (capped sticks representation) and coactivator peptide (blue). H12 is shown in violet. B: AR in complex with small molecule (AV6) bound to AF-2 site. C: AR in complex with flufenamic acid bound to BF-3 site. D & E: Binding modes of AV6 (D) and flufenamic acid (E) within AF-2 and BF-3 pockets (shown as surface). AV6 shares a hydrogen bond with the receptor as indicated by the white dotted line.

specifically address single PPAR subtypes. For example leukotriene B4 activates only PPARα while a variety of prostaglandins are ligands for PPARγ.

All currently approved PPAR drugs target α and γ subtypes and are used in treatment of metabolic diseases. PPARα is addressed by fibrates, *e.g.* clofibrate or gemfibrozil (Figure 2). Upon receptor activation, a large set of genes is upregulated, including many enzymes involved in lipid metabolism, *e.g.* lipid transport, oxidation, lipogenesis or cholesterol transport [27]. Compounds of the thiazolidinedione class have been developed for targeting the subtype PPARγ (*e.g.* rosiglitazone, pioglitazone, troglitazone). Rosiglitazone and pioglitazone are used in treatment of type II diabetes, both activating PPARγ and thereby increasing the sensitivity of adipocytes to insulin which lowers glucose blood levels. Due to liver toxicity, troglitazone has been completely withdrawn from the market.

Another class of PPAR-addressing molecules has been introduced recently. The so-called glitazars are dual PPAR agonists, activating PPARα and PPARγ. In 2013, the first glitazar (saroglitazar) was approved as drug in India while other glitazar research programs have been discontinued due to safety reasons. Saroglitazar (Figure 2) is used for treatment of diabetic dyslipidemia and hypertriglyceridemia.

Most nuclear receptors are addressed due to their direct involvement in a disease. However, some members of the NR superfamily are interesting because of their involvement in drug metabolism. This process comprises three phases that involve compound modification (e.g. oxidation by cytochrome P450 enzymes), coupling reactions with hydrophilic substances (e.g. glucuronic acid, glycine) and finally excretion of the metabolised molecules from the cell via transporter proteins. Both, pregnane X receptor (PXR) and the constitutive androstane receptor (CAR), are mainly expressed in liver and intestine and are responsible for ligand-dependent induction of gene expression of proteins involved in all phases of drug metabolism [50]. Due to their ability to bind structurally and chemically diverse molecules, including many prescription drugs and other synthetic compounds that enter the human body, CAR and PXR are also termed xenosensors [28].

Comparing both receptors, PXR is most promiscuous and recognizes a large set of prescription drugs, among them calcium channel blockers, statins, antidiabetic drugs, HIV protease inhibitors and also artemisinin and its derivatives [29, 30]. PXR X-ray crystal structures have unravelled the basis for the pronounced ligand promiscuity of the receptor. The receptor LBD deviates from the canonical NR fold (H6 unfolded, H7 broken, long H1-H3 loop which is part of LBP), resulting in a large LBP with considerable plasticity that adapts to structurally and chemically diverse molecules [31, 32]. The molecular weight of compounds binding to PXR varies from 200 to more than 800 Da. Rifampicin is the largest known PXR agonist.

Similar to PXR, CAR binds structurally diverse ligands, however the spectrum is less pronounced since the ligand-binding pocket is much smaller and less flexible [33]. Known ligands are 5-androstan-3-ol and 5-androst-16-en-3-ol as well as pregnanedione [34-36]. Also prescription drugs such as artemisinin and meclizine have been identified as CAR ligands, (meclizine acts as inverse agonist) [29, 37]. Besides direct activation upon ligand binding, CAR can be also indirectly induced in a yet unknown manner by compounds such as phenobarbital or phenytoin, respectively [38].

3. Current status of NR drug discovery research

3.1. Other nuclear receptors as potential drug targets

Current NR research not only continues to develop improved modulators for receptors already targeted by approved drugs as described before, but also intends to address other NRs that have been identified to be involved in various diseases with agonists or antagonists. Representative examples for these nuclear receptors are the liver X receptor (LXR), farnesoid X receptor (FXR) or PPARδ.

LXR exists in two isoforms: LXRα (NR1H3) and LXRβ (NR1H2). While LXRα is mainly expressed in the liver, LXRβ is ubiquitously expressed. Endogenous LXR ligands are oxysterols, oxigenated derivatives of cholesterol (e.g. 27-hydroxycholesterol, cholestenoic acid) and cholic acid [39]. Both isoforms are involved in transcriptional control of genes involved in uptake, transport, efflux and excretion of cholesterol in a tissue-dependent manner as well as inflammatory responses in the CNS [40, 41]. LXRα and LXRβ bind as heterodimers (RXRα) to the response elements of LXR target genes which comprise (among others) ABC transporters, apolipoprotein A and fatty acid synthase. Therefore, compounds modulating LXR are considered as potential therapeutics for metabolic and neurodegenerative diseases. Many small molecules targeting LXR have been identified in the last decades and several have reached clinical phases [42]. A problem of LXR agonists are adverse effects due to LXRα activation in the liver, resulting in increased hepatic lipogenesis, hypertriglyceridemia and liver steatosis. As both isoforms share 77 % sequence homology in DBD and LBD, the identification of selective agonists is not a trivial task. Nevertheless, some selective LXRβ agonists have been reported. The first identified selective agonists (N-acylthiadiazolines) activate the β-isoform several times more efficient than the α-isoform [43]. A phenylsulfone-substituted quinoxaline compound has been identified as partial agonist of LXRβ (potent activator in kidney cells, low induction in liver cells) and revealed poor affinity towards LXRα [44]. Very recently, LXRβ-selective compounds have been identified using pharmacophore modelling and shape-based virtual screening which activated LXRβ up to 1.8-fold over the α-isoform [45].

As described above, two members of the PPAR subfamily are already addressed by approved drugs. Current research also focuses on the third member, PPARδ. Expressed in most metabolically active tissues, the receptor regulates expression of a set of genes involved in glucose homeostasis and fatty acid synthesis/storage, mobilization and catabolism [46]. Due to its physiological functions, agonists of PPARδ are considered as potential therapeutics of the whole spectrum of metabolic syndromes including diabetes, atherosclerosis and obesity [46]. In addition, PPARδ agonists have been shown to stimulate oligodendrocyte differentiation and thus are considered as potential therapeutics in demyelinating disorders such as multiple sclerosis [47].

So far, a large bunch of receptor agonists have been identified that advanced research on this PPAR subtype and its physiological role [48]. Recently, a benzisoxazole has been identified as PPARδ-selective agonist with an EC_{50}-value of 4.5 nM as determined using a cell-based assay [49]. Another example is GW501516, a PPARδ ligand developed by GlaxoSmithKline that has been identified by combinatorial chemistry and structure-based design [50]. The compound revealed high affinity and potency against PPARδ while showing a more than 1000-fold selectivity over PPARα and PPARγ. Despite its favorable effect on the receptor and no toxicity in human trials, the compound was not developed further. Later studies in animal models revealed the compound to possess a substantial carcinogenic potential.

Besides the discovery of receptor-selective compounds, the development of dual agonists activating two PPAR subtypes or pan-agonists activating all members of the PPAR subfamily is also actively pursued. Although a compound of the glitazar class has recently been approved as drug, no further compounds have reached so far the market.

Another example of a promising nuclear receptor drug target is the farnesoid X receptor (FXR) which binds bile acids, the final product of the cholesterol metabolism [51]. Due to the toxic properties of bile acids their levels have to be tightly regulated. FXR can regulate the bile homeostasis by activating other nuclear receptors (such as CAR, PXR and VDR) [52], cell surface receptors (G protein-coupled bile acid receptor 1), receptor and calcium-gated potassium channels. FXR signaling is involved in the regulation of intestinal bacterial flora [53], liver regeneration [54] and - in case of misregulation - to hepatocarcinogenesis [55, 56]).

FXR is considered as a suitable drug target for the treatment of dyslipidemia, atherosclerosis and cholestatic disorders, and some effort has been spent on identification and development on agonists [57]. From the already approved drugs, the antiparasitic drug ivermectin has been identified as a FXR agonist [58]. In spite of some side effects related to trygliceride misbalance, FXR agonists are able to recover cholestasis and antidyslipidemic effects [59, 60].

3.2. Co-activator-binding inhibitors as a future therapeutic approach?

All currently approved drugs targeting NRs address the ligand-binding pocket. In recent years, novel approaches for inhibiting NRs have emerged in order to overcome limitations of LBP-targeting drugs. Problems may be side effects due to displacement of the natural ligand, thereby disturbing physiological homeostasis, but also limitations of the ligand diversity as imposed by the shape and composition of the LBP as well as resistance of the receptor due to mutations [61].

In order to overcome these limitations, non-LBP pockets have been investigated for their potential to harbour small molecules and thereby modulate receptor activity. In particular, sites involved in NR-co-activator interactions or receptor-DNA contacts have been investigated in detail. The modulation of NR-co-activator interactions has been studied extensively in recent years and several studies have reported the successful discovery of co-activator binding inhibitors (CBI) which confirms the applicability of this approach [62]. Nevertheless, the development of CBIs is challenging due to specificity issues (more than 300 coregulators have been identified in humans so far) as well as the general conformational flexibility of NRs.

Most studies have concentrated on the co-activator binding site (AF-2 site). Several alternate mechanisms have been proposed for explaining the deleterious effects of interference with AF-2. Besides inhibition of co-activator binding , this may involve corepressor recruitment, increase on the NR turnover levels, blockage of the dimer formation, or inhibition of interactions between the N- and C-terminal domain [8].

Because of the anti-androgen resistance phenomenon of prostate cancer [63], modulators addressing the AF-2 site have attracted attention. The effect of AR co-regulator binders is considered to function by inhibition of the N/C interaction that occurs between AF-1 and AF-2 which is considered as crucial for stabilization of the receptor-ligand complex in the active conformation [61]. Interestingly, AR not only binds co-activators carrying the LxxLL motif but also the more bulky FxxLF motif. X-ray crystal structures of the AR LBD revealed the presence of deep pockets at the AF-2 site, enabling accommodation of the large FxxLF side chains. Not only synthetic peptides, based on a pyrimidine core, were able to selectively displace AR co-activator molecules, as corroborated by FRET assays, and interfere with transcription activation [64], but also small molecules have been identified to disrupt co-activator binding using a virtual screening campaign with subsequent experimental validation (Figure 4B & D) [65].

Another receptor for which AF-2 binders have been identified is the thyroid hormone receptor (TR). TR subtypes are a target for treatment of hyperthyroidism or cardiac arrhythmias. The co-activator binding site of TRβ has been successfully targeted using macrolactam-constrained co-activator peptides [66]. Another approach to address TRβ is the use of suicide inhibitors. The proposed pro-drug, DHPPA (or 3-(dibutylamino)-1-(4-hexylphenyl)-propan-1-one)) is able to interact with the AF-2 surface in a similar way as he co-activator SRC-1 [67].

Also the xenosensor PXR has been investigated for inhibition by CBIs. As described before, the receptor has not been addressed for specific treatment. Instead, PXR AF-2 inhibitors are intended to prevent premature drug metabolism, leading to prolonged half-lifes that may result in lower dosages and less side effects. In addition, PXR antagonists may be applied to prevent drug-drug-interactions in patients treated with combination therapies or multimorbid patients exposed to a variety of drugs. Antibiotics such as fluconazole, enilconazole and ketoconazole inhibit PXR, resulting in reduced expression levels of CYP3A4 and MDR1 [68]. It has been shown that the compounds inhibit PXR-SRC-1 interactions by binding to the AF-2 site using site-directed mutagenesis [69]. Based on the proposed binding mode and the resulting receptor-ligand interactions, a pharmacophore has been generated [70]. In a follow-up study the pharmacophore has been utilized for the identification of several small molecule antagonists of PXR, including the FDA approved prodrug leflunomide [71].

In addition to the AF-2 site, other regions of the LBD also have been successfully targeted by small molecules that modulate the interaction of the receptor with co-activator proteins. Recently, a small hydrophobic pocket formed by amino acids located on helix 1, the H1-H3 loop as well as helix 9 has been identified on the AR surface (termed BF-3 site) to be addressable by small molecules [67]. By testing a set of approximately 55,000 compounds from various sources using fluorescence polarisation and X-ray crystallographic screenings, several small molecules such as 3,3′,5-triiodothyroacetic acid, T3 or flufenamic acid have been identified to bind to BF-3 (Figure 4C & E) [67]. The BF-3 site is conserved among steroid hormone receptors such as progesterone receptor, mineralocorticoid receptor and glucocorticoid receptor, suggesting that a similar approach could also lead to the identification of CBIs against these receptors [72]. Compounds binding to BF-3 seem to allosterically interfere with co-activator binding to the AF-2 site [73]. In the last years, several studies have reported the successful discovery of additional small molecules targeting the BF-3 pocket. Using virtual screening in combination with biochemical and cell-based tests, a set of structurally diverse AR inhibitors has been identified. Binding to BF-3 has been confirmed by solving the X-ray crystal structure of the receptor-ligand complex. In a follow-up study, one of these molecules was further developed to AR inhibitors with IC_{50} values at low micromolar range [74]. Subsequently the crystal structure of the AR in complex with 2-((2-phenoxyethyl)thio)-1H-benzimidazole confirmed molecule binding at the BF-3.

4. Methods to assess ligand binding and/or activation of nuclear receptors

In the last thirty years several molecular and cell biology standard methods have been applied to investigate nuclear receptor functions and regulations [75]. For example cDNA cloning has been used to identify the genes encoding orphan nuclear receptors. In order to discover hormone-response elements, electrophoretic mobility shift assays (EMSA) and chromatin-immunoprecipitation (ChIP) have been applied as well as different GST pull-down assays [76-78].

To investigate the biological effect of a compound, a variety of binding assays have been developed. A standard ligand-binding how a ligand competes with a known labeled ligand in binding to the receptor [79]. In recent years a variety of non-radioactive activity assays such as biochemical-based fluorescent polarization and time-resolved fluorescence assays have been developed [80]. Detailed analyses of the macromolecular interaction of ligand binding, including affinity- and binding kinetics, have been performed by the surface plasmon resonance (SPR) technology (see also below) [81].

Due to their relevance as therapeutic targets [83] the pharmaceutical industry prioritised the development of novel assay systems that allowed to accelerate the throughput and the screening of large compound collections. Therefore, a couple of academic laboratories as well as pharmaceutical and biotech companies have spent much effort in the development of high-throughput screening compatible screening assays in the last decade [84, 85]. These efforts led to modified methodologies with higher throughput and less variability. A couple of NR screening campaigns have used smal molecule libraries such as Sigma-Aldrich LOPAC, Biomol and Tocris/TimTec bioactive collection and U.S. Food and Drug Administration 1 and 2 collection [86]. Despite the fact that most of the assays have been designed for certain targets the principles could be expanded to any NR, making these assay formats accessible to drug discovery applications.

In the following, a selection of relevant biochemical and cell-based assays as well as *in silico* methods is presented that is frequently used in NR research, both in academia and pharmaceutical industry.

4.1. Transactivation assays

The most common test systems for nuclear receptor activation are cell-based transactivation assays. These assays rely on the potential of nuclear receptors to activate transcription upon ligand binding [87, 88]. In general, this is achieved by transfection of cells with an expression vector for the receptor and a reporter vector that contains the binding site for the receptor and also encodes for a protein that, when incubated with the appropriate substrate, result in a detectable signal.

Standard protocols involve transient transfection of the receptor and a response element-reporter gene construct [89]. The general advantage of these cell-based assays is that they allow screening of large compound libraries in a reproducible fashion [85]. Until now many cell lines have been described as possible recipients of these vectors, including CHO, HuH7, MCF-7, HEK293, HepG2 and Caco-2 cells [90]. Using transient transfection systems a couple of investigators identified activators for various nuclear receptors [62].

4.2. Corregulator-recruitment (mammalian two-hybrid, CARLA)

An alternative transactivation assay system is the mammalian two-hybrid system. This assay represents a powerful approach for detecting protein-protein interactions in cells, which has evolved from the original two-hybrid system into a method for identifying NR ligands. The system is based on the finding that co-activators and co-repressors are involved in the regulation of NR function. Following ligand binding, many NRs perform a conformational change and form a specific co-activator binding pocket, which permits co-activator binding. In the mammalian two-hybrid approach, chimerical receptors containing the LBD of interest are fused to the DBD of the yeast transcription factor GAL4, which binds to specific NR response elements. The interaction between the NR and its co-activator is detected using a reporter gene containing multiple copies of the GAL4 upstream activating system.

Examples are mammalian two-hybrid assays consisting of the LBD of human CAR and co-activator SRC-1 fused to GAL4 DBD. In this assay the ligand binding enhances the interaction between LBD and SRC-1, which is detected by the reporter gene activity [91]. Using a similar assay a set of agonists and inverse agonist were identified to bind to the human CAR even if some results were contradictory [92, 93]. It was speculated that the use of truncated chimerical receptors resulted in subtle conformational changes and unspecific protein-protein interactions [90], which led to the conclusion that utilization of full-length receptors is more sensitive and better reflects the *in vivo* situation [85].

An assay type that allows monitoring of co-activator recruitment is the Co-Activator-dependent Receptor Ligand Assay (CARLA) [100]. CARLA is based on the principle that ligand-binding stimulates interaction between the NR and a co-activator protein which is part of the normal pathway for transcriptional activation. Technically, CARLA is a GST pull-down assay using a GST-receptor fusion protein and a labelled co-activator. The GST fusion protein is immobilized on glutathione-sepharose beads and incubated with the co-activator in the presence or absence of potential ligands. In this setup an actual ligand of the receptor enhances the interaction of the receptor with the co-activator and thereby increases the amount of co-activator that is pulled down. In summary, CARLA is a functional binding assay that reports on the molecular consequence of ligand binding.

Originally, the assay has been developed for the PPARs [94-96]. However, with some modifications the assay format can be used for any nuclear hormone receptor and several co-activators including SRC-1, CBP/p300, Tif2, Rac3, GRIP-1, and RIP140 [97].

4.3. Surface plasmon resonance, biochemical assay formats, AlphaScreen® and LANCE®

Detailed analyses of the macromolecular interaction of ligand-binding including affinity and binding kinetics is performed by Surface Plasmon Resonance (SPR) [81]. This technology overcomes the common limitations of indirect non-equilibrium methods due to its high sensitivity [82]. In the standard SPR approach, only small amounts of receptor protein are immobilized onto solid phase while different concentrations of the ligand are passed in flow over the surface. In NR research, SPR has been applied to detect and quantify receptor-DNA, receptor-receptor, as well as receptor-ligand interactions [81]. In the past it has also been used to characterize binding of co-regulators of a variety of nuclear receptors including thyroid receptor, estrogen and androgen receptor [98-101]. With regard to high-throughput applications, a variety of non-cell based assay formats based on the AlphaScreen® or LANCE® technology have been described [102-104].

AlphaScreen® is a non-radioactive homogeneous proximity assay that relies on energy transfer between an acceptor and a donor bead brought into proximity via biological interaction. The donor beads are embedded with a photosensitizer, which converts oxygen to an excited state upon illumination. If a biomolecular interaction drags an acceptor bead into close proximity of a donor bead, the excited singlet oxygen will transfer its energy to the acceptor bead leading to emission of light depending on the fluorophore in the acceptor beads. Each donor bead is capable of generating up to 60,000 singlet oxygen molecules with a half-life of 0.3 seconds, allowing measurements in a time-resolved mode and with substantial signal amplification. The technology can used to rapidly develop high-throughput screening (HTS) assays for NRs [105-107].

A nuclear receptor AlphaScreen® assay is based on the ligand-activated biomolecular interaction between NR and its co-activator, followed by the detection of this interaction using AlphaScreen® compatible reader technology. For many NRs a consensus co-activator peptide sequence (LxxLL motif) is sufficient for the interaction of the agonist-bound receptor with LBD. The detection can be realised by various strategies depending on the nature of the involved binding partners. Rouleau & Bossé (2006) described such an AlphaScreen® Assays, for estrogen receptor α (ERα) and retinoic acid receptor γ (RARγ) [107]. Other configurations depending on the availability of respective detection reagents, tags and beads are also possible which have already been described for *e.g.* FXR receptor [105].

Another well validated assay type for studying NR-ligand interactions is based on the LANCE® Technology [102]. In the LANCE® assay, a signal is generated when a donor molecule labelled with chelate europium (Eu) gets into proximity of the acceptor molecule labelled with allophycocyanin (APC). When a biological interaction brings the donor and the acceptor into close proximity, excitation of the Eu-chelate at 340 nm allows Fluorescence Resonance Energy Transfer (FRET) to the acceptor APC molecule resulting in fluorescence emission at 665 nm. Long stakes shift and excited-state lifetimes of Europium complex (hundreds of microseconds) warrant Time-Resolved FRET (TR-FRET) analysis.

In LANCE® nuclear receptor assays the same biomolecular interactions between the ligand binding domain and the NR box are addressed. In principle different binding partners can be used depending on their stability and availability: Examples for combinations are: i) Interaction between agonist-bound receptor or receptor LBD and LxxLL motif-containing peptide and/or ii) interaction between an apo- or holo-receptor and the co-repressor interaction domain.

There are a few examples in literature where LANCE assays based on the interaction between receptor and co-activator-derived peptide have been applied [108-110]. Most of the assays reported involve the interaction of biotinylated LxxLL peptides and a tagged receptor LBD. The complex formation is detected using Eu-labelled antibody and APC-labelled streptavidin.

A large variety of Lance Eu- and APC-labelled reagents is commercially available which allow the capture of differently tagged receptors and coactivators [111]. A great advantage of applying the LANCE technology is the long signal stability, which can be more than 48 h.

4.4. Identification of NR modulators using in silico methods

Besides experimental approaches, computational methods have also been extensively applied in order to identify novel agonists or antagonists. The availability of LBD crystal structures allows employment of structure-based virtual screening techniques, for example molecular docking of virtual compound libraries. If the desired NR structure is not available, homology modeling techniques can be used to obtain structural data. Since the LBD structure is highly conserved this approach often results in high-quality protein models.

Once LBP-bound ligands have been co-crystallized, further methods such as pharmacophore-based searches can be applied that make use of specific protein-ligand interactions. The method is also often used as filtering step to reduce the number of compounds to be docked when applying structure-based virtual screening techniques. In any case, a virtual hit requires experimental investigation for validating its modulating effect on the nuclear receptor.

Many studies have reported the successful application of virtual screening approaches for the identification of NR agonists and antagonists, thereby confirming the suitability of these methods. Besides crystal structure data, also homology models have been utilized for the identification of NR agonists as described for the glucocorticoid receptor (GR) and the constitutive androstane receptor (CAR) that were modeled on the basis of the solved crystal structure of progesterone receptor (GR model) or PXR and VDR (CAR model), respectively [112, 113].

5. Final considerations

Nuclear receptors are an important protein family involved in many physiological processes. So far, several NRs have been successfully addressed by drugs in order to treat various diseases. Despite significant progress in the understanding of the physiological role of several NRs, the function of many receptors is not well understood which is mainly due to missing information of endogenous ligands. Since only a proportion of receptors are addressed by drugs, there is a tremendous potential for future drug discovery campaigns. The existence of a pronounced ligand-binding pocket renders many receptors addressable to drug-like molecules. The availability of alternative areas addressable by small molecules, for example protein-protein interaction sites on the NR surface, suggests further possibilities for modulating the function of NRs. In order to study NR function and to identify novel receptor modulators, a large set of experimental and computational methods has been developed and successfully applied in many research projects.

Acknowledgements

The authors would like to thank Fundação de Amparo à Pesquisa do Estado de São Paulo, FAPESP (grants 2013/10288-1, 2014/50255-8 and 2014/03644-9) as well as Conselho Nacional de Desenvolvimento Científico e Tecnológico, CNPq (grant no 202936/2014-7) for financial support.

Author details

Thales Kronenberger[1], Oliver Keminer[2], Carsten Wrenger[1*] and Björn Windshügel[2*]

*Address all correspondence to: bjoern.windshuegel@ime.fraunhofer.de or cwrenger@icb.usp.br

1 Unit for Drug Discovery, Department of Parasitology, Institute of Biomedical Sciences, University of São Paulo, São Paulo, Brazil

2 Fraunhofer Institute for Molecular Biology and Applied Ecology IME, Hamburg, Germany

References

[1] Zhang, Z., et al., Genomic analysis of the nuclear receptor family: new insights into structure, regulation, and evolution from the rat genome. Genome Res, 2004. 14(4): p. 580-90.

[2] Zhou, J. and J.A. Cidlowski, The human glucocorticoid receptor: one gene, multiple proteins and diverse responses. Steroids, 2005. 70(5-7): p. 407-17.

[3] Nuclear Receptors Nomenclature, C., A unified nomenclature system for the nuclear receptor superfamily. Cell, 1999. 97(2): p. 161-3.

[4] Sladek, F.M., What are nuclear receptor ligands? Mol Cell Endocrinol, 2011. 334(1-2): p. 3-13.

[5] Rask-Andersen, M., M.S. Almen, and H.B. Schioth, Trends in the exploitation of novel drug targets. Nat Rev Drug Discov, 2011. 10(8): p. 579-90.

[6] Tora, L., et al., The N-terminal region of the chicken progesterone receptor specifies target gene activation. Nature, 1988. 333(6169): p. 185-8.

[7] Shao, D. and M.A. Lazar, Modulating nuclear receptor function: may the phos be with you. J Clin Invest, 1999. 103(12): p. 1617-8.

[8]   Warnmark, A., et al., Activation functions 1 and 2 of nuclear receptors: molecular strategies for transcriptional activation. Mol Endocrinol, 2003. 17(10): p. 1901-9.

[9]   Khorasanizadeh, S. and F. Rastinejad, Nuclear-receptor interactions on DNA-response elements. Trends Biochem Sci, 2001. 26(6): p. 384-90.

[10] Naar, A.M., et al., The orientation and spacing of core DNA-binding motifs dictate selective transcriptional responses to three nuclear receptors. Cell, 1991. 65(7): p. 1267-79.

[11] Umesono, K., et al., Direct repeats as selective response elements for the thyroid hormone, retinoic acid, and vitamin D3 receptors. Cell, 1991. 65(7): p. 1255-66.

[12] Kishimoto, M., et al., Nuclear receptor mediated gene regulation through chromatin remodeling and histone modifications. Endocr J, 2006. 53(2): p. 157-72.

[13] Nolte, R.T., et al., Ligand binding and co-activator assembly of the peroxisome proliferator-activated receptor-gamma. Nature, 1998. 395(6698): p. 137-43.

[14] Greschik, H., et al., Structural and functional evidence for ligand-independent transcriptional activation by the estrogen-related receptor 3. Mol Cell, 2002. 9(2): p. 303-13.

[15] Heery, D.M., et al., A signature motif in transcriptional co-activators mediates binding to nuclear receptors. Nature, 1997. 387(6634): p. 733-6.

[16] Garcia-Becerra, R., et al., Mechanisms of Resistance to Endocrine Therapy in Breast Cancer: Focus on Signaling Pathways, miRNAs and Genetically Based Resistance. Int J Mol Sci, 2012. 14(1): p. 108-45.

[17] Wang, D.Y., et al., Identification of estrogen-responsive genes by complementary deoxyribonucleic acid microarray and characterization of a novel early estrogen-induced gene: EEIG1. Mol Endocrinol, 2004. 18(2): p. 402-11.

[18] Jordan, V.C., Fourteenth Gaddum Memorial Lecture. A current view of tamoxifen for the treatment and prevention of breast cancer. Br J Pharmacol, 1993. 110(2): p. 507-17.

[19] Shafi, A.A., A.E. Yen, and N.L. Weigel, Androgen receptors in hormone-dependent and castration-resistant prostate cancer. Pharmacol Ther, 2013. 140(3): p. 223-38.

[20] Gao, W., C.E. Bohl, and J.T. Dalton, Chemistry and structural biology of androgen receptor. Chem Rev, 2005. 105(9): p. 3352-70.

[21] Helsen, C., et al., Androgen receptor antagonists for prostate cancer therapy. Endocr Relat Cancer, 2014. 21(4): p. T105-18.

[22] Tran, C., et al., Development of a second-generation antiandrogen for treatment of advanced prostate cancer. Science, 2009. 324(5928): p. 787-90.

[23] Saad, F., Evidence for the efficacy of enzalutamide in postchemotherapy metastatic castrate-resistant prostate cancer. Ther Adv Urol, 2013. 5(4): p. 201-10.

[24] Korpal, M., et al., An F876L mutation in androgen receptor confers genetic and phenotypic resistance to MDV3100 (enzalutamide). Cancer Discov, 2013. 3(9): p. 1030-43.

[25] Li, H., et al., Discovery of Small-Molecule Inhibitors Selectively Targeting the DNA-Binding Domain of the Human Androgen Receptor. J Med Chem, 2014. 57(15): p. 6458-67.

[26] Dalal, K., et al., Selectively Targeting the DNA Binding Domain of the Androgen Receptor as a Prospective Therapy for Prostate Cancer. J Biol Chem, 2014.

[27] Rakhshandehroo, M., et al., Peroxisome proliferator-activated receptor alpha target genes. PPAR Res, 2010. 2010.

[28] Chang, T.K. and D.J. Waxman, Synthetic drugs and natural products as modulators of constitutive androstane receptor (CAR) and pregnane X receptor (PXR). Drug Metab Rev, 2006. 38(1-2): p. 51-73.

[29] Burk, O., et al., Antimalarial artemisinin drugs induce cytochrome P450 and MDR1 expression by activation of xenosensors pregnane X receptor and constitutive androstane receptor. Mol Pharmacol, 2005. 67(6): p. 1954-65.

[30] Handschin, C. and U.A. Meyer, Induction of drug metabolism: the role of nuclear receptors. Pharmacol Rev, 2003. 55(4): p. 649-73.

[31] Watkins, R.E., et al., Coactivator binding promotes the specific interaction between ligand and the pregnane X receptor. J Mol Biol, 2003. 331(4): p. 815-28.

[32] Chrencik, J.E., et al., Structural disorder in the complex of human pregnane X receptor and the macrolide antibiotic rifampicin. Mol Endocrinol, 2005. 19(5): p. 1125-34.

[33] Xu, R.X., et al., A structural basis for constitutive activity in the human CAR/RXRalpha heterodimer. Mol Cell, 2004. 16(6): p. 919-28.

[34] Baes, M., et al., A new orphan member of the nuclear hormone receptor superfamily that interacts with a subset of retinoic acid response elements. Mol Cell Biol, 1994. 14(3): p. 1544-52.

[35] Forman, B.M., et al., Unique response pathways are established by allosteric interactions among nuclear hormone receptors. Cell, 1995. 81(4): p. 541-50.

[36] Forman, B.M., et al., Androstane metabolites bind to and deactivate the nuclear receptor CAR-beta. Nature, 1998. 395(6702): p. 612-5.

[37] Huang, W., et al., Meclizine is an agonist ligand for mouse constitutive androstane receptor (CAR) and an inverse agonist for human CAR. Mol Endocrinol, 2004. 18(10): p. 2402-8.

[38] Honkakoski, P., S. Auriola, and M.A. Lang, Distinct induction profiles of three phenobarbital-responsive mouse liver cytochrome P450 isozymes. Biochem Pharmacol, 1992. 43(10): p. 2121-8.

[39] Yang, C., et al., Sterol intermediates from cholesterol biosynthetic pathway as liver X receptor ligands. J Biol Chem, 2006. 281(38): p. 27816-26.

[40] Hong, C. and P. Tontonoz, Liver X receptors in lipid metabolism: opportunities for drug discovery. Nat Rev Drug Discov, 2014. 13(6): p. 433-44.

[41] Xu, P., et al., LXR agonists: new potential therapeutic drug for neurodegenerative diseases. Mol Neurobiol, 2013. 48(3): p. 715-28.

[42] Loren, J., et al., Liver X receptor modulators: a review of recently patented compounds (2009 - 2012). Expert Opin Ther Pat, 2013. 23(10): p. 1317-35.

[43] Molteni, V., et al., N-Acylthiadiazolines, a new class of liver X receptor agonists with selectivity for LXRbeta. J Med Chem, 2007. 50(17): p. 4255-9.

[44] Hu, B., et al., Identification of phenylsulfone-substituted quinoxaline (WYE-672) as a tissue selective liver X-receptor (LXR) agonist. J Med Chem, 2010. 53(8): p. 3296-304.

[45] Temml, V., et al., Discovery of new liver X receptor agonists by pharmacophore modeling and shape-based virtual screening. J Chem Inf Model, 2014. 54(2): p. 367-71.

[46] Reilly, S.M. and C.H. Lee, PPAR delta as a therapeutic target in metabolic disease. FEBS Lett, 2008. 582(1): p. 26-31.

[47] Aleshin, S. and G. Reiser, Role of the peroxisome proliferator-activated receptors (PPAR)-alpha, beta/delta and gamma triad in regulation of reactive oxygen species signaling in brain. Biol Chem, 2013. 394(12): p. 1553-70.

[48] Miyachi, H., Design, synthesis, and structure-activity relationship study of peroxisome proliferator-activated receptor (PPAR) delta-selective ligands. Curr Med Chem, 2007. 14(22): p. 2335-43.

[49] Sakuma, S., et al., Synthesis of a novel human PPARdelta selective agonist and its stimulatory effect on oligodendrocyte differentiation. Bioorg Med Chem Lett, 2011. 21(1): p. 240-4.

[50] Oliver, W.R., Jr., et al., A selective peroxisome proliferator-activated receptor delta agonist promotes reverse cholesterol transport. Proc Natl Acad Sci U S A, 2001. 98(9): p. 5306-11.

[51] Huber, R.M., et al., Generation of multiple farnesoid-X-receptor isoforms through the use of alternative promoters. Gene, 2002. 290(1-2): p. 35-43.

[52] Lu, T.T., et al., Molecular basis for feedback regulation of bile acid synthesis by nuclear receptors. Mol Cell, 2000. 6(3): p. 507-15.

[53] Inagaki, T., et al., Regulation of antibacterial defense in the small intestine by the nuclear bile acid receptor. Proc Natl Acad Sci U S A, 2006. 103(10): p. 3920-5.

[54] Huang, W., et al., Nuclear receptor-dependent bile acid signaling is required for normal liver regeneration. Science, 2006. 312(5771): p. 233-6.

[55] Kim, I., et al., Spontaneous hepatocarcinogenesis in farnesoid X receptor-null mice. Carcinogenesis, 2007. 28(5): p. 940-6.

[56] Gadaleta, R.M., et al., Tissue-specific actions of FXR in metabolism and cancer. Biochim Biophys Acta, 2014.

[57] Pellicciari, R., et al., 6alpha-ethyl-chenodeoxycholic acid (6-ECDCA), a potent and selective FXR agonist endowed with anticholestatic activity. J Med Chem, 2002. 45(17): p. 3569-72.

[58] Jin, L., et al., The antiparasitic drug ivermectin is a novel FXR ligand that regulates metabolism. Nat Commun, 2013. 4.

[59] Huang, H., et al., Discovery and optimization of 1,3,4-trisubstituted-pyrazolone derivatives as novel, potent, and nonsteroidal farnesoid X receptor (FXR) selective antagonists. J Med Chem, 2012. 55(16): p. 7037-53.

[60] Renga, B., et al., Discovery that theonellasterol a marine sponge sterol is a highly selective FXR antagonist that protects against liver injury in cholestasis. PLoS One, 2012. 7(1): p. e30443.

[61] Caboni, L. and D.G. Lloyd, Beyond the ligand-binding pocket: targeting alternate sites in nuclear receptors. Med Res Rev, 2013. 33(5): p. 1081-118.

[62] Abnet, C.C., et al., Transactivation activity of human, zebrafish, and rainbow trout aryl hydrocarbon receptors expressed in COS-7 cells: greater insight into species differences in toxic potency of polychlorinated dibenzo-p-dioxin, dibenzofuran, and biphenyl congeners. Toxicol Appl Pharmacol, 1999. 159(1): p. 41-51.

[63] Chen, Y., C.L. Sawyers, and H.I. Scher, Targeting the androgen receptor pathway in prostate cancer. Curr Opin Pharmacol, 2008. 8(4): p. 440-8.

[64] Gunther, J.R., A.A. Parent, and J.A. Katzenellenbogen, Alternative inhibition of androgen receptor signaling: peptidomimetic pyrimidines as direct androgen receptor/coactivator disruptors. ACS Chem Biol, 2009. 4(6): p. 435-40.

[65] Axerio-Cilies, P., et al., Inhibitors of androgen receptor activation function-2 (AF2) site identified through virtual screening. J Med Chem, 2011. 54(18): p. 6197-205.

[66] Geistlinger, T.R. and R.K. Guy, An inhibitor of the interaction of thyroid hormone receptor beta and glucocorticoid interacting protein 1. J Am Chem Soc, 2001. 123(7): p. 1525-6.

[67] Estebanez-Perpina, E., et al., Structural insight into the mode of action of a direct inhibitor of coregulator binding to the thyroid hormone receptor. Mol Endocrinol, 2007. 21(12): p. 2919-28.

[68] Huang, H., et al., Inhibition of drug metabolism by blocking the activation of nuclear receptors by ketoconazole. Oncogene, 2007. 26(2): p. 258-68.

[69] Wang, H., et al., Activated pregnenolone X-receptor is a target for ketoconazole and its analogs. Clin Cancer Res, 2007. 13(8): p. 2488-95.

[70] Ekins, S., et al., Human pregnane X receptor antagonists and agonists define molecular requirements for different binding sites. Mol Pharmacol, 2007. 72(3): p. 592-603.

[71] Ekins, S., et al., Computational discovery of novel low micromolar human pregnane X receptor antagonists. Mol Pharmacol, 2008. 74(3): p. 662-72.

[72] Buzon, V., et al., A conserved surface on the ligand binding domain of nuclear receptors for allosteric control. Mol Cell Endocrinol, 2012. 348(2): p. 394-402.

[73] Grosdidier, S., et al., Allosteric conversation in the androgen receptor ligand-binding domain surfaces. Mol Endocrinol, 2012. 26(7): p. 1078-90.

[74] Munuganti, R.S., et al., Targeting the binding function 3 (BF3) site of the androgen receptor through virtual screening. 2. development of 2-((2-phenoxyethyl) thio)-1H-benzimidazole derivatives. J Med Chem, 2013. 56(3): p. 1136-48.

[75] McEwan, I.J., Nuclear Receptors: One Big Familiy, in Methods in Molecular Biology 2009. p. 3-18.

[76] Read, J.T., et al., Receptor-DNA interactions: EMSA and footprinting. Methods Mol Biol, 2009. 505: p. 97-122.

[77] Massie, C.E.a.M., I.G, Chromatin Immunoprecipitation (ChIP) Methodology and Readouts, in Methods in Molecular Biology 2009. p. 123-137.

[78] Goodson, M.L., B. Farboud, and M.L. Privalsky, High throughput analysis of nuclear receptor-cofactor interactions. Methods Mol Biol, 2009. 505: p. 157-69.

[79] Jones, S.A., et al., The pregnane X receptor: a promiscuous xenobiotic receptor that has diverged during evolution. Mol Endocrinol, 2000. 14(1): p. 27-39.

[80] Schulman, I.G. and R.A. Heyman, The flip side: Identifying small molecule regulators of nuclear receptors. Chem Biol, 2004. 11(5): p. 639-46.

[81] Lavery, D.N., Binding affinity and kinetic analysis of nuclear receptor/co-regulator interactions using surface plasmon resonance. Methods Mol Biol, 2009. 505: p. 171-86.

[82] Cheskis, B.J.a.F., L.P., Kinetic analysis of nuclear receptor interactions, in Nuclear Receptors – A Practical Approach, D. Picard, Editor. 1998. p. 95-117.

[83] Pelton, P.D., Nuclear Receptors as Drug Targets, in Minor: Handbook of Assay Development in Drug Discovery, L. K, Editor. 2006, CRC Taylor & Francis: New York. p. 173-181.

[84] Chu, V., et al., In vitro and in vivo induction of cytochrome p450: a survey of the current practices and recommendations: a pharmaceutical research and manufacturers of america perspective. Drug Metab Dispos, 2009. 37(7): p. 1339-54.

[85] Raucy, J.L. and J.M. Lasker, Cell-based systems to assess nuclear receptor activation and their use in drug development. Drug Metab Rev, 2013. 45(1): p. 101-9.

[86] Shukla, S.J., et al., Identification of clinically used drugs that activate pregnane X receptors. Drug Metab Dispos, 2011. 39(1): p. 151-9.

[87] Sinz, M., et al., Evaluation of 170 xenobiotics as transactivators of human pregnane X receptor (hPXR) and correlation to known CYP3A4 drug interactions. Curr Drug Metab, 2006. 7(4): p. 375-88.

[88] Dring, A.M., et al., Rational quantitative structure-activity relationship (RQSAR) screen for PXR and CAR isoform-specific nuclear receptor ligands. Chem Biol Interact, 2010. 188(3): p. 512-25.

[89] Willson, T.M. and S.A. Kliewer, PXR, CAR and drug metabolism. Nat Rev Drug Discov, 2002. 1(4): p. 259-66.

[90] Stanley, L.A., et al., PXR and CAR: nuclear receptors which play a pivotal role in drug disposition and chemical toxicity. Drug Metab Rev, 2006. 38(3): p. 515-97.

[91] Auerbach, S.S., et al., Retinoid X receptor-alpha-dependent transactivation by a naturally occurring structural variant of human constitutive androstane receptor (NR1I3). Mol Pharmacol, 2005. 68(5): p. 1239-53.

[92] Moore, L.B., et al., Pregnane X receptor (PXR), constitutive androstane receptor (CAR), and benzoate X receptor (BXR) define three pharmacologically distinct classes of nuclear receptors. Mol Endocrinol, 2002. 16(5): p. 977-86.

[93] Honkakoski, P., et al., A novel drug-regulated gene expression system based on the nuclear receptor constitutive androstane receptor (CAR). Pharm Res, 2001. 18(2): p. 146-50.

[94] Krey, G., et al., Fatty acids, eicosanoids, and hypolipidemic agents identified as ligands of peroxisome proliferator-activated receptors by coactivator-dependent receptor ligand assay. Mol Endocrinol, 1997. 11(6): p. 779-91.

[95] Inoue, I., et al., Fibrate and statin synergistically increase the transcriptional activities of PPARalpha/RXRalpha and decrease the transactivation of NFkappaB. Biochem Biophys Res Commun, 2002. 290(1): p. 131-9.

[96] Tien, E.S., J.W. Davis, and J.P. Vanden Heuvel, Identification of the CREB-binding protein/p300-interacting protein CITED2 as a peroxisome proliferator-activated receptor alpha coregulator. J Biol Chem, 2004. 279(23): p. 24053-63.

[97] Leo, C. and J.D. Chen, The SRC family of nuclear receptor coactivators. Gene, 2000. 245(1): p. 1-11.

[98] Treuter, E., et al., Competition between Thyroid Hormone Receptor-associated Protein (TRAP) 220 and Transcriptional Intermediary Factor (TIF) 2 for Binding to Nuclear Receptors: IMPLICATIONS FOR THE RECRUITMENT OF TRAP AND p160

COACTIVATOR COMPLEXES. Journal of Biological Chemistry, 1999. 274(10): p. 6667-6677.

[99]   Warnmark, A., et al., The N-terminal regions of estrogen receptor alpha and beta are unstructured in vitro and show different TBP binding properties. J Biol Chem, 2001. 276(49): p. 45939-44.

[100] Shatkina, L., et al., The cochaperone Bag-1L enhances androgen receptor action via interaction with the NH2-terminal region of the receptor. Mol Cell Biol, 2003. 23(20): p. 7189-97.

[101] Lavery, D.N. and I.J. McEwan, Functional characterization of the native NH2-terminal transactivation domain of the human androgen receptor: binding kinetics for interactions with TFIIF and SRC-1a. Biochemistry, 2008. 47(11): p. 3352-9.

[102] Rouleau, N.H., P., Bossé R. and Hemmilä, I., Development of Nuclear Receptor Homogeneous Assay Using the LanceTM Technology, in Minor: Handbook of Assay Development in Drug Discovery, L. K, Editor. 2006, CRC Taylor & Francis: New York. p. 209-219.

[103] Rouleau, N.a.B., R., Homogeneous Assay Development for Nuclear Receptor Using AlphaScreenTM Technology, in Handbook of Assay Development in Drug Discovery, L. K, Editor. 2006, CRC Taylor & Francis: New York. p. 193-207.

[104] Shukla, S.J., et al., Identification of pregnane X receptor ligands using time-resolved fluorescence resonance energy transfer and quantitative high-throughput screening. Assay Drug Dev Technol, 2009. 7(2): p. 143-69.

[105] Glickman, J.F., et al., A comparison of ALPHAScreen, TR-FRET, and TRF as assay methods for FXR nuclear receptors. J Biomol Screen, 2002. 7(1): p. 3-10.

[106] Wu, X., et al., Comparison of assay technologies for a nuclear receptor assay screen reveals differences in the sets of identified functional antagonists. J Biomol Screen, 2003. 8(4): p. 381-92.

[107] Rouleau, N., et al., Development of a versatile platform for nuclear receptor screening using AlphaScreen. J Biomol Screen, 2003. 8(2): p. 191-7.

[108] Tremblay, G.B., et al., Diethylstilbestrol regulates trophoblast stem cell differentiation as a ligand of orphan nuclear receptor ERR beta. Genes Dev, 2001. 15(7): p. 833-8.

[109] Drake, K.A., et al., Development of a homogeneous, fluorescence resonance energy transfer-based in vitro recruitment assay for peroxisome proliferator-activated receptor delta via selection of active LXXLL coactivator peptides. Anal Biochem, 2002. 304(1): p. 63-9.

[110] Liu, J., et al., A homogeneous in vitro functional assay for estrogen receptors: coactivator recruitment. Mol Endocrinol, 2003. 17(3): p. 346-55.

[111] Jones, S.A., D.J. Parks, and S.A. Kliewer, Cell-free ligand binding assays for nuclear receptors. Methods Enzymol, 2003. 364: p. 53-71.

[112] Schapira, M., R. Abagyan, and M. Totrov, Nuclear hormone receptor targeted virtual screening. J Med Chem, 2003. 46(14): p. 3045-59.

[113] Jyrkkarinne, J., et al., Insights into ligand-elicited activation of human constitutive androstane receptor based on novel agonists and three-dimensional quantitative structure-activity relationship. J Med Chem, 2008. 51(22): p. 7181-92.

4

Lipids and Liposomes in the Enhancement of Health and Treatment of Disease

Simon A. Young and Terry K. Smith

Additional information is available at the end of the chapter

1. Introduction

The discovery of liposomes initially came from studies by Bangham and Horne who observed by electron microscopy the self-association of the lipid phosphatidylcholine (mixed with or without cholesterol) in water formed 'spherulites' of varying sizes which had not a recognizable lamellar shell comprising a lipid bilayer [1]. The self-assembling 'spherulites', subsequently named liposomes from the greek *lipo* (fat) and *soma* (body), were recognised to be functionally analogous to studied biological membrane systems due to the similar rates of diffusion of ions [2]. However only when an ionophore, valinomycin, was utilised demonstrating selective diffusion of K^+ over Na^+ from liposomes containing equal concentrations of the ions, could liposomes be confirmed as entirely sealed membrane vesicles [3]. Furthermore Papahadjopoulos and Watkins showed the differential permeability to anions and cations could be significantly altered with liposomes of different phospholipid compositions [4]. Natural liposomes have bilayers composed of phospholipids and/or cholesterol and as such are poorly antigenic, typically non-toxic and physiologically inert. Liposomes can vary in size from 25 nm to 2.5 μm and are classified within three broad categories [5]: Multilamellar vesicles (MLV), which structurally resemble an onion with multiple concentric phospholipid bilayers separated by aqueous layers,large unilamellar vesicles (LUV) and small unilamellar vesicles (SUV) which have a single lipid bilayer surrounding the aqueous core. Typically multiple unilamellar vesicles of differing sizes can form inside of each other generating multilamellar structures.

The concept of liposomes as drug-carriers to aid in selectivity was explored in the early nineteen seventies predominantly through the work of drug-transport scientists such as Gregoriadis who initially looked at the fate of protein-containing liposomes delivered into animals [6]. The theory that liposomes stay intact and circulate in the bloodstream before accumulating in specific tissues where they release their molecules into cells was confirmed using radiolabelled proteins entrapped in liposomes. The radioactive signal from the proteins was barely detected in the bloodstream, but predominantly in the lysosomes of cells of the liver and spleen, showing the liposomes stayed intact prior to the radiolabelled proteins being taken up by the cells. This and related studies revealed the physiological behaviour of liposomes such as their integrity and long life span in the mammalian bloodstream. It was only through the use of cell culture it was confirmed that cargo carried by liposomes was directly delivered through endocytosis into the lysosomes and thus into the intracellular environment of cells [7]. These initial studies demonstrated the huge potential for liposomes as model systems, and a number of various applications were subsequently explored as listed here: The effect of surface charge on ion permeability [8]; their susceptibility to phospholipase hydrolysis [9]; the function of integral membrane ion transporters [10]; the delivery of active enzymes to functionally deficient cells [11]; their use as immunological adjuvants [12]; as stimulants of interferon production [13]; their interaction with polyene antibiotics [14]; their incorporation of local and general anaesthetics [15]; the inclusion and presentation of virus surface proteins [16]. Since those early experiments, there has been a continued interest in the use of liposomes and currently there are applications in a wide variety of scientific fields (Figure 1).

In this chapter we will focus on the use of lipids and liposomes in the enhancement of a number of health related areas and cover the development of new synthetic molecules, which have great potential in advancing improvements in health and the treatment of disease.

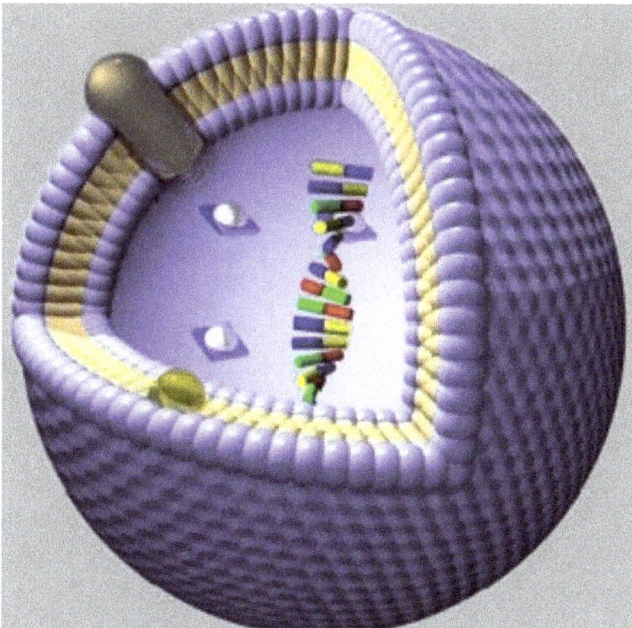

Figure 1. A schematic representation of a liposome. The liposome can facilitate the carrying of various cargo, water-soluble drugs, DNA or RNA, in the internal hydrophilic region, water-insoluble drugs within the hydrophobic region of the bilayer, or protein linked or incorporated into the phospholipid bilayer.

2. Current applications in treating disease

2.1. Non-communicable diseases

It is evident that with their physiological attributes, liposomes are an attractive means to deliver drugs to treat a variety of communicable and non-communicable diseases. Typically, drugs for the treatment of human diseases can often have a number of biochemical and pharmacological issues such as poor stability and solubility, rapid breakdown and lack of targeted delivery. As a result there are common problems in the use of such drugs, including the lack of a strong therapeutic cure and the necessity to consume high doses, which can result in unwanted side effects. If the disease is localised to a specific body tissue, the lack of selective targeting can result in poor bioavailability of the drug at the required site, potentially resulting in toxicity in other tissues, thus restricting the dose concentration. The use of natural phospholipid based liposome formulations having minimal toxicity, extended stability in the human body, tissue selectivity and a delayed release of the active compound at the site of action suggests clear benefits for drug development and treatment. In addition multiple compounds can be distributed by the same liposomes for added therapeutic impact. Equally, compounds of varying lipophilicities can transported, partitioning in the different hydrophobic and hydrophilic environments of the liposomes. Particle size is a critical factor both in the circulatory half-life of liposomes and also (along with the number of bilayers) dictates the amount of encapsulated drug [17]. In general, drug delivery systems are on the nanoscale, liposomes having diameters of 100 nm or less tend to have a good therapeutic index compared to conventional anticancer therapies. Typically liposomes for drug therapies approved for humans contain the neutrally charged phosphatidylcholine as the major membrane constituent, though occasionally cholesterol (up to a third of the total lipid content) is incorporated to reduce membrane instability due to serum protein binding. Thirty years ago, the application of liposomes to deliver an anti-cancer anthracycline drug doxorubicin trapped in negatively charged or neutral liposomes (called OLV-DOX) showed that it retained its antitumour activity in mice [18]. Importantly the use of the liposomal formulation reduced the accumulation of the drug in murine cardiac tissues, minimising toxicity and thus significantly improving their survival. When tested in humans however the OLV-DOX worked poorly, being rapidly cleared from the bloodstream with significant premature release of the drug, giving rise to potential cardiotoxicity [19]. These failings limited the application of liposomes in cancer treatment at that time, only resolved by the subsequent experimental trialling of polyethylene glycol (PEG) incorporation in phospholipid liposomes. The PEG was found to create a hydrophilic surface on the liposomes, reducing uptake by the reticuloendothelial system and thus increasing the circulation time of these so-called 'stealth' liposomes. This resulted in a revolution in liposome design and so in 1995 Doxil (PEGylated liposome-trapped doxorubicin) the first of the so-called 2nd generation was approved by the US Food and Drug Administration as the first liposome drug delivery system for human use [20]. Doxil was found to have extended stability in the bloodstream and reduced compound leakage resulting in increased accumulation in solid tumours (up to 22-fold) and reduced toxicity to non-target organs. Every year over 300,000 patients with ovarian cancer or Kaposi's sarcoma are now routinely intravenously treated with

Doxil [21] and it is occasionally utilised in cases of breast cancer and also in combination with bortezomib for multiple myeloma.

Alongside Doxil, to date five other liposomal formulations are approved for human cancer treatment (Table 1). Myocet, a related non-PEGylated liposome formulation of doxorubicin is used in combination with cyclophosphamide for breast cancer [22]. DaunoXome, a liposome formulation of daunorobicin is similarly used to treat Kaposi's sarcoma [23]. DepoCyt, a formulation of unusually large liposomes containing cytarabine is active against malignant lymphomatous meningitis [24], while Marqibo is a more typical nanoscale formulation of liposomes of vincristine utilised for acute lymphoblastic leukemia [25]. Recently, more success has come from the trial use of such liposome formulations in combination with standard anti-cancer drugs, one example being a Doxil and carboplatin composition which shows a better therapeutic index and less toxicity than the standard paclitaxel/carboplatin mixture used to treat ovarian cancer in the elderly [26]. Similarly in comparison to a standard treatment, a combination of Doxil, bortezomib and dexamethasone showed a strong therapeutic response and improved tolerability in patients with multiple myeloma [27].

Market Product	Drug used	Target diseases	Company
Doxil or Caelyx	Doxorubicin	Kaposi's sarcoma	SEQUUS, USA
DaunoXome	Daunorubicin	Kaposi's sarcoma, breast & lung cancer	NeXstar, USA
Amphotec	Amphotericin-B	Fungal infections, Leishmaniasis	SEQUUS, USA
Ventus	Prostaglandin-E1	Systemic inflammatory diseases	The liposome company, USA
Alec	Dry protein free powder of DPPC-PG	Expanding lung diseases in babies	Britannia Pharm, UK
Epaxal–Berna Vaccine	Inactivated hepatitis A virions	Hepatitis A	Swiss serum & vaccine institute, Switzerland
Avian retrovirus vaccine	Killed avian retrovirus	Chicken pox	Vineland lab, USA
Novasome	Smallpox vaccine	Smallpox	Novavax, USA
Depocyt	Cytarabine	Cancer therapy	Skye Pharm, USA
Topex-Br	Terbutaline sulphate	Asthma	Ozone, USA

Table 1. Current products utilising liposomes

A major issue in cancer treatments is the failure of many forms of chemotherapy due to the phenomenon of multidrug resistance. As a result, the tactic of using drug combinations has become widely adopted due to the greater therapeutic index and efficacy in reversing the multidrug resistant phenotype [28]. In a combination treatment drugs can have one of three effects, synergistic, additive or antagonistic and this can be shaped by their specific molar ratios in the formulation [29]. Unfortunately in an *in vivo* setting, the combinatorial effect can be weakened due to disrupted pharmacokinetics of the drugs in the system, leading to incorrect dose ratios at the site of action [30]. Based on prior research, it was clear that the pharmacokinetic issues of combination therapies can be eliminated by the use of liposome formulations, resulting in delivery of the drugs to their site of action at the correct effective ratio [31]. Equally important in the enhancement of health is the use of liposomes in the treatment of cardiovascular disease, the leading cause of deaths worldwide. Again relatively early in liposome research, it was observed that liposomes carrying the MRI contrast agent 99mTc-DTPA accumulated in regions of the heart experimentally induced to undergo myocardial infarction (MI), a common cause of death [32]. In MI, during the ischemic phase, the exhaustion of nucleotide pyrophosphates causes extensive myocardial cell damage [33]. The obvious solution, the infusion of adenosine triphosphate (ATP) intravenously to increase myocardial cell energy levels is sub-optimal due to the molecule's short circulatory half-life and strong charge. The relatively unstable ATP could however be protected and successfully delivered using liposomes and clearly accumulated in canine myocardia damaged by ischemia [34]. Subsequently it was discovered that targeted ATP-containing liposomes can significantly protect against the subsequent effects of ischemia in an *ex vivo* rat heart model [35]. When translated into an animal model, ATP-loaded liposomes reduced the amount of irreversible myocardial damage by greater than 50% compared to control treated rabbits [36].

Another significant agent in the prevention and treatment of ischemic injury and indeed heart failure, coronary artery disease and hypertension in general, is Coenzyme Q10 (CoQ10) [37]. Evaluation of CoQ10 loaded liposomes again in the aforementioned rabbit model revealed that only 30% of the affected myocardia was at risk of irreversible damage compared to the control, indicative of significant protection and great potential in this approach [38]. In humans, the use of large-scale trials of adenosine on clinical patients with acute MI has shown some promise but again is a poor compound with a short half-life and hypotensive and brachicardic inducing properties [39]. These issues may be overcome based on an experimental study using PEGylated liposomes of adenosine which generated non-toxic and cardioprotective effects against MI in rats [40]. In treating another common cause of ischemic damage, thrombus formation, a range of thrombolytic drugs have been developed. Due to its need for constant infusion and potential to cause haemorrhage, one of the first thrombolytic drugs, heparin was quickly assessed in a liposomal formulation [41]. Liposomal heparin was much more effective in its thrombolytic effects, being retained in the plasma longer and generated a prolonged activity due to a gradual release of the agent. Ultimately an inhalable formulation successfully replaced the intravenous version in rat models of deep vein thrombosis and pulmonary embolism giving promise to future clinical trials [42].

2.2. Communicable diseases

As significant as the development of liposomes in the treatment of non-communicable human diseases has been, the field of anti-parasitic drug development generated the first liposomal formulation to be mass marketed. With no vaccines effective against any of the primary parasitic infections, anti-parasitic drug treatment remains the main approach. Many current anti-parasitic compounds were developed over 50 years ago and though effective, are hardly comparable to the modern view of the biochemical and clinical properties of an ideal drug. Due to the fact that many anti-parasitic drugs have solubility issues, low bioavailability and poor absorption by the gastrointestinal tract, it was an obvious choice to test the potential of liposomes for anti-parasitic drug delivery. AmBisome, a natural liposome configuration of the potent anti-leishmanial amphotericin B was the first liposome drug based formulation to be commercialised in 1990 (Table 2) [43]. A sterol biosynthesis inhibitor, amphotericin B is the standard second-line treatment for visceral leishmaniasis (caused by *Leishmania donovani*) and is essential in endemic disease areas in India due to the extensive development of resistance against the standard pentavalent antimonial compounds [44]. AmBisome is particularly effective against *Leishmania* (2 to 5-fold more potent than the free drug) due to the fact that the parasite infects the very macrophages which clear the liposomes from the bloodstream, increasing the therapeutic effect and additionally reducing the nephrotoxicity of amphotericin B. Initially liposomes containing antimonial compounds were tested in a hamster model of visceral leishmaniasis and were greater than 700 fold more active than the free drug version showing the significant potential of liposome use [45]. Interestingly antimonial encapsulated liposomes were also shown to be potent against cutaneous leishmaniasis where the parasites alternatively reside in peripheral tissues [46].

Drug	Route of Administration	Targeted Diseases
Amphotericin-B	Oral	Mycotic infection, Leishmaniasis
Insulin	Oral, Ocular, Pulmonary and Transdermal	Diabetic mellitus
Ketoprofen	Ocular	Pain muscle condition
Pentoxifylline	Pulmonary	Asthma
Salbutamol	Pulmonary	Asthma
Tobramycin	Pulmonary	Pseudomonas infection, aeruginosa
Benzocain	Transdermal	Ulcer on mucous surface with pain
Ibuprofen	Oral	Rheumatoid arthritis
Adrenaline	Ocular	Glucoma, Conjectivitis
Penicillin G	Pulmonary	Meningococal, staphylococcal
Methotrexate	Transdermal	Cancer

Table 2. Therapeutic applications utilising liposomes

While AmBisome remains the only liposomal antiparasitic agent on the market, other liposome formulations have been developed showing potency against *Leishmania spp*. Liposomes modified with sugars improved the targeting of antileishmanial pentamidine to infected macrophages with increased potency as a result [47]. Similarly, delivery of the alkylphospho-lipid miltefosine (hexadecylphosphocholine) in a liposomal form proved twice as active against *L. donovani* and actually even increased the susceptibility of a miltefosine-resistant parasite line [48]. Far less exploration has been done to assess the value of liposomal agents against the causative agents of Human African Trypanosomiasis (HAT) and Chagas' disease,

Trypanosoma brucei and *Trypanosoma cruzi* respectively. Both species of parasite have disseminating infections and localise to tissues of the body where there is limited interaction with liposomes. However a number of *in vitro* and *in vivo* studies using liposomes have evaluated potential anti-trypanosomal effects. Two related investigations demonstrated that phosphatidylcholine/stearylamine only liposomes at low concentrations (100 µM) non-toxic to erythrocytes, rapidly killed both *T. cruzi* [49] and *T. brucei* [50] through destabilization of their plasma membranes. Notably this effect was not seen with identical concentrations of the individual lipid components, suggesting the vesicle structure was important for activity. The surprising failure of liposomes containing benznidazole to improve on the potency of this classical anti-*T. cruzi* treatment was hypothesised to be due to a lack of drug delivery [51], though the anti-leishmanial AmBisome demonstrated some success in supressing *T. cruzi* infections *in vivo* [52].

With so many anti-malarial drugs commercially available and in development, the focus of liposome development in this field is on the protection of drugs from premature metabolism, to generate a slow release to improve the therapeutic index and reduce toxicity. To this end, liposomes of Artesunate, a semi-synthetic derivate of artemisinin, were found to release only 30% of the drug in 24 h in an *in vitro* test, giving promise to this method as a means to reduce the dosing frequency of antimalarial drugs [53]. In a rabbit model, Arteether directed for chloroquine resistant *Plasmodium falciparum*, when trapped in dipalmitoylphosphatidylcholine, dibehynoylphophatidylcholine, cholesterol liposomes persisted longer with greater bioavailabilty in the gastrointestinal tract when compared to the aqueous suspension [54]. Similarly, liposomes of chloroquine, the widely used 4-aminoquinoline antimalarial, modified with an antibody to selectively deliver to infected erythrocytes were found to cure the majority of chloroquine-resistant *Plasmodium berghei*-malarial infections in mice [55], proving that targeted liposomes can be very efficient in overcoming drug resistance. In the treatment of systemic mycoses such as aspergillosis, there are few antifungal agents available, but due to its broad spectrum of action amphotericin-B is potent against a wide range of fungi. In the form of AmBisome and other related formulations (e.g. Abelcet and Amphocil) they are even more effective in treatment of infections [56]. These formulations have also proved valuable in treating *Candida albicans* infections in immunocompromised patients, eradicating an efficient pathogen that is able to form fungal biofilms [57].

Understandably as the second most lethal infectious disease, many therapeutic cures for tuberculosis (TB) have been available for over 50 years, but there are often patient issues with the length of treatment and dose burden. As a result, treatment failures are common and can promote the development of multi-drug resistant strains. Due to their potential to overcome these problems, the development of drug carrying liposomes has become an important focus in anti-tubercular studies. A ground-breaking study demonstrated that gentamicin loaded liposomes had significantly greater antibacterial activity than the free drug, reducing the bacterial load in the spleen and liver in a mouse model of *Mycobacterium avium* [58]. As well as similar results utilising second-line antibiotics, lung-targeted liposomes were created comprised of a mixture of phosphatidylcholine, cholesterol, dicetylphosphate, O-steroyl amylopectin and monosialogangliosides, distearylphosphatidylethanolamine-poly(ethylene glycol) 2000 to deliver with less toxic effects, isoniazid and rifampicin for more efficient chemotherapy [59]. As the predominant site of infection for TB is the respiratory system, many efforts are now being made to develop aerosolised liposome formulations to successfully deliver anti-tubercular drugs to the lungs by inhalation [60].

The strength of liposomes in supporting in the treatment of disease goes beyond purely as drug delivery vehicles as they can be powerful tools to deliver vaccines, notably against viral infections (Table 1). Significantly, liposomes can be engineered to deliver a variety of immunogenic molecules, whether protein, nucleic acid or carbohydrate to stimulate a strong protective response. A notable commercially available preparation, Epaxal is a vaccine based on inactivated intact Hepatitis A virus adsorbed on to liposomes (thus named virosomes) which in a single dose are well tolerated and highly immunogenic giving good seroprotection [61]. Marketed nearly twenty years ago, Inflexal V, a vaccine preparation against Influenza virus consists of the viral heamagglutinin and neuraminidase surface proteins displayed in phosphatidylcholine based liposomes [62]. In particular, Inflexal V mimicking a natural influenza infection is a paradigm for liposome based vaccines with its safe but strong immunogenicity covering a wide range of ages and health conditions.

2.3. Other medical conditions

In addition to the treatment of disease, liposomes have the capability to aid in many other medical-related conditions (Table 2). Notable examples of their use include in analgesia, alleviation of macular degeneration, and as surfactants for pulmonary diseases. A variety of liposome preparations have been marketed for use in analgesia or post-surgical pain-relief. DepoDur and EXPAREL are liposome preparations of morphine and bupivacaine respectively and when intravenously injected, demonstrate stability and extended release properties to give prolonged anaesthesia or analgesia [63,64]. The typical therapy for neovascular age-related macular degeneration requires repeated intravitreal injections of an anti-vascular endothelial growth factor drug, effective in stabilising vision but an encumbrance for patients. The creation of Visudyne, a liposome based formulation of the photosensitiser Verteporfin which requires only intravenous injection has simplified patient treatment with relative success [65]. A common problem in pulmonary diseases such as respiratory distress syndrome is a lack of pulmonary surfactant, the phospholipid-protein complex needed to contribute a functional respiratory surface at the mammalian lungs. Curosurf, a modified natural surfactant isolated from pig lungs contains the essential phospholipid-associated surfactant proteins B and C, and is widely used successfully in clinical treatment [66].

3. New approaches utilising synthetic lipids and fatty acids

3.1. Non-natural lipids and fatty acids

While having many advantages, natural liposomes utilised for the treatment of disease have some drawbacks. Typically they are difficult to produce and are inherently unstable reducing the potential storage time. In recent years a new generation of liposomes have been developed with altered biochemical properties designed to improve stability, functionalization and drug release in addition to altered immunogenic and selective targeting properties. Construction of these liposomes was only possible due to the use of non-natural fatty acids and lipids in the particles. As an alternative to the standard inclusion of cholesterol in liposomes for increased stability, a series of sterol-modified phospholipids were constructed [67]. These involved the covalent attachment of cholesterol to the glycerol backbone of phosphatidylcholine, replacing a fatty acid chain and resulting in sterol modified liposomes (SML). Other hydrophobic molecules such as porphyrins and photosensitive agents can similarly replace a fatty acid chain, [68]. In generating synthetic lipids, there are also many simple changes to the lipid headgroup possible, vastly changing their chemical and biophysical properties [69]. Common modifications can include the addition of a polymer, nucleic acid, carbohydrate, amino acid or an assortment of functional chemical moieties for the downstream covalent attachment of ligands.

3.2. Advantages of using synthetic lipids in liposomes

As mentioned above, liposomes incorporating synthetic lipids can have three main advantages, extended stability of the liposome, directed cell targeting and controlled release of the cargo and examples of the modifications are discussed here:

Sterol modified liposomes carrying doxorubicin had similar therapeutic efficacy to the standard Doxil in a colon carcinoma model, but with greater overall stability in circulation, improved uptake into the liver and spleen [70]. This and other studies show the potential of SMLs as drug delivery systems that are easy to synthesise from commercially available molecules. Similarly the use of synthetic lipids incorporating porphyrins or photosensitive agents to generate liposomes known as porphysomes which have applications in photodynamic therapy and diagnostics. Importantly these porphysomes demonstrate good pharmacokinetics in mice, are safe at high doses, accumulate in tumours and can be imaged for diagnostic purposes [68]. The use of the synthetic polyethylene glycol (PEG-2000) modified 1,2-distearoyl-*sn*-glycero-3-phosphoethanolamine in liposomes greatly altered the surface hydrophilicity and by decreasing cell uptake, extended the circulatory half-life as mentioned previously for Doxil [20].

Utilising liposomes constructed with synthetic lipids can create a number of novel functions. In addition to the aforementioned polymer coating, modified headgroups are useful for the attachment of cargo or specific ligand targeting. Often these modifications result in improved targeting and biodistribution of liposomes by interacting with ligands present on specific cells or tissue types. One notable example is nucleic acid modified lipids, which can result in the physical interaction of the liposomes with single-stranded nucleic acids via base pairing. This has proved biologically important in the efficient targeting of the nucleic acid binding drug cisplatin to its site of action overcoming previous limitations in drug delivery and showing potency against a number of sensitive and resistant cancer cell lines [71]. Liposomes have also been generated using lipids synthesised with a range of functional groups to bind a number of ligands. Most common is a maleimide lipid, although others with ester, ether, avidin, thiol, hydrazine and carboxylic acid moieties in the headgroup have also been constructed [72]. The maleimide group can react with a free thiol and thus can allow liposomes to couple to any exposed cysteine on a protein such as a single chain antibody. This approach has proved useful in the modification of amyloid-β-targeting liposomes, made of sphingomyelin/cholesterol/ phosphatidic acid and functionalised through a terminal maleimide group on PEG-phosphatidylethanolamine to display an anti-transferrin receptor antibody. This design gave the liposomes the ability to cross an *in vitro* blood brain barrier model of human brain capillary endothelial cells and thus hold huge potential for the successful delivery of therapeutics to the central nervous system targeting amyloid-β and other defective proteins in Alzheimer's disease [73].

In an ideal scenario in the liposomal drug delivery system, the liposomes should be stable in the circulation till they reach their destination and rapidly release their contents to have the desired effect. In optimising the release of cargo from liposomes, a number of methods are possible. Some such as altering the liposome formulation to destabilise the membrane or increasing the hydrophilicity of the cargo are applicable to natural liposomes. However, through the use of synthetic lipids, it is possible to control the release of liposome content with various environmental cues, either external such as heat, light or ultrasound; or internal e.g. pH or redox environment. This relies on the use of lipids to create liposomes that are sensitive to specific stimuli to trigger the delivery of material at the appropriate time and place. This is particularly useful in the delivery of small interfering RNAs (siRNA) where the use of pH responsive ionisable lipids containing amine headgroups means that liposomes release the nucleic acid only into the cytosol of the cell [74].

4. The use of lipids and liposomes as molecular tools

4.1. Molecules for imaging

The routine application of modified or synthetic lipids in liposomes and their subsequent biocompatibility *in vivo* or *ex vivo* demonstrated that such particles could also be visualised through the incorporation of fluorescently tagged lipids. This methodology effectively replaces the original inconsistent approach of using liposomes carrying fluorescein as cargo for imaging studies [75]. There are a number of commercially available synthetic lipid species which have a fluorophore replacing a lipid fatty acid chain or alternatively replacing or conjugated to a phospholipid headgroup. Common fluorophores attached to lipids include non-polar 4,4-difluoro-4-bora-3α,4α-diaza-s-indacene (BODIPY), polar nitrobenzo-2-oxa-1,3-diazole (NBD) and dansyl groups, hydrophobic pyrene and the highly fluorescent rhodamine dyes [76]. Importantly, in selecting a fluorophore to use in labelling lipids and liposomes, it is common to use dyes that emit light in the 650-1100nm far red/near infrared region to avoid the conflict with the UV responsive autofluorescence of most eukaryotic tissues. When fluorescent lipids are constructed into liposomes, the simple visualisation of the labelled particles has aided in the study of a number of areas of research such as drug delivery, disease diagnosis and membrane fusion events. A recent study using fluorescence microscopy specifically revealed that carbocyanine dye modified liposomes containing the antileishmanial agent meglumine antimoniate were taken up faster by *Leishmania major* infected macrophages compared with non-infected cells, most likely due to parasite-modified phagocytosis [77]. The attachment of the fluorescent curcumin molecule to 1,2-dipalmitoyl-3-(2-(1,7-bis(4-hydroxy-3-methoxyphenyl)-3,5-dioxohept-6-enylthio)ethyl phospho)-*sn*-glycerol (DPS) has a clinically relevant application for the diagnosis of Alzheimer's disease. As curcumin targets the Aβ peptide, injection of DPS-curcumin containing liposomes into the brains of mice revealed the nanoparticles could successfully target and stain the pathology causing Aβ deposits *in vivo* [78]. These types of imaging based studies may be further extended in a dual approach, for example in the efficient bimodal imaging of tumour angiogenesis through the use of rhodamine conjugated phosphatidylethanolamine and gadolinium-DTPA-bis(stearylamide) lipids for optical imaging and magnetic resonance imaging studies respectively [79]. These liposomes were additionally constructed with RGD cyclic peptide moieties conjugated to maleimide-PEG-DSPE, specifically to target the αvβ3 integrin highly expressed in angiogenesis. This and other studies [reviewed in 80] have strongly validated the use of these modified lipids in an effective streamlined approach for the *in vivo* visualisation and treatment of angiogenesis, a critical process in metastatic tumour biology.

4.2. Immune system modulators

Due to their biophysical properties, cell targeting and entering abilities, liposomes were candidate adjuvants to aid in the modulation of the human immune system. Initially it was observed that negatively charged liposomes of a certain composition of natural phospholipids carrying diphtheria toxin could induce an enhanced antibody response prior to release of the true antigen [81]. Subsequently this use was more deliberate, for example in the delivery of *Shigella flexneri* lipid A containing liposomes to stimulate an immune reaction [82]. To date, the wide use of liposomes containing monophosphoryl lipid A has proved highly effective in safely enhancing immune responses to candidate vaccines to HIV-1, malaria and a number of cancers [reviewed in 83]. Significantly, liposomes have been developed to act as primary adjuvants, incorporating lipids whose headgroup is covalently bound to antigens. Through the use of synthetic lipids like 1,2-dipalmitoyl-*sn*-glycero-3-phosphoethanolamine-N-[4-(*p*-maleimidophenyl)butyramide], a range of peptide, carbohydrate, lipid and even antibody-like molecules can be attached [84]. These modified liposomes can be administered via oral or nasal routes rather than injection and in addition to little or no toxicity have significant capability to be both prophylactic and therapeutic vaccines. One caveat however is that even early in liposome research it was clear that in certain circumstances any headgroup modified lipids could be adjuvants, and based on the evidence to date, it is likely that most synthetic lipids will induce some sort of immune response [69]. While the use of liposomes to stimulate the immune system to exert a seroprotective effect as discussed is desirable, there are situations where an immune suppressive effect may be desired. A directed suppression of the immune system is a desirable goal in the treatment of autoimmune disease, allergies and preventing the rejection of organ transplants. Administering liposomes coated in the bisphosphonate aldronate successfully caused an anti-inflammatory effect in a rabbit model through the systemic inactivation and depletion of macrophages and monocytes [85], similarly seen in models of tissue graft rejection [86] and arthritis [87]. These and other related liposomes based strategies have great potential to deliver therapeutic success in a safe manner for many immune-related conditions [88].

4.3. Nucleic acid carriers

It is clear liposomes have an enormous ability to transport an assortment of molecules to a variety of cells and tissue types and a rapidly expanding field is the delivery of nucleic acid into cells. In genetic modification, the delivery of genetic material to augment the existing genes or alternatively silence and/or remove genes has become essential. Some current approaches to deliver genetic material into cells and tissues include chemical-based and viral based methods and can be inefficient with membrane permeability issues and potentially cytotoxic effects. Particularly in exploring the concept of gene therapy, replacing a defective copy with a functional wild-type copy, the development of non-viral based vectors to deliver nucleic acid into cells has focused on liposomes due to their ability to carry large fragments of DNA and their low toxicity and immunogenicity. In the development of liposome based nucleic acid delivery systems, it was discovered that a cationic synthetic lipid N-[1-(2,3-dioleyloxy)propyl]-N,N,N-trimethylammonium chloride (DOTMA) would form liposomes that would readily interact with negatively charged DNA and stably hold it in the aqueous interior [89]. Typically cationic lipids have a positively charged polar amino head group on top of a lipid-like hydrophobic domain. In contrast, neutral or negatively charged lipid based liposomes can't form electrostatic interactions to bind and hold any negatively charged molecules. This ground-breaking research opened up the field of using cationic liposomes to deliver material and there are a now a wide range of synthetic phospholipid and cholesterol analogues that generally form positively charged liposomes [90]. Cationic liposomes have great promise as nucleic acid delivery agents as they are highly efficient, readily interacting with negatively charged membranes for uptake into cells to deliver their cargo. Since the initial discovery, many cationic liposomes have been used to deliver nucleic acids not just into cells in culture, but also animals and even in patients in phase I and II clinical trials though with some dose-dependent toxicity issues [90].

More recently, a revolution in the use of liposomes in nucleic acid delivery has come about through the discovery of small interfering RNAs (siRNA). These siRNA are molecules which are designed to bind the messenger RNA of a specific gene and thus silence its expression. This approach could potentially revolutionise the treatment of diseases such as cancer where suppression of gene expression is of paramount importance. However, the use of siRNA in a clinical setting has been restricted because the molecules have a short half-life, show poor uptake into cells and are rapidly cleared from the system. Again the application of liposome technology has resurrected this form of therapy with the potential of liposomes specifically targeting the siRNA to the appropriate tissue in high concentrations, preventing degradation of the molecule and therefore providing a safe non-toxic delivery system in humans and animals. Typically by using phosphatidylcholine based neutral liposomes, an efficient and stable targeted delivery of siRNAs into tumour tissues was observed in a variety of animal models, significantly with a concomitant inhibition of tumour growth [reviewed in 91].

4.4. Decoys for pathogens

Possibly the most unusual application for liposomes comes from the development of particles that when administered into an individual would impersonate the host cell type recognised by invading pathogens, trapping the infectious agent and thus reducing the potential for disease. A recent example is the use of liposomes bearing the glycan sialylneo-lacto-N-tetraose c (LSTc), an analogue of the influenza virus targeting sialic acid molecule found on the surface of respiratory tract cells. Decoy liposomes containing LSTc conjugated to 1,2-dioleoyl-*sn*-glycero-3-phosphoethanolamine successfully bind influenza virus particles in competition assays in culture and in a mouse model prevent virus spread and increase the survival time even under challenge of a lethal dose [92]. This is significantly better than using free sialic acid analogues, which have shown some success, but are not suitable due to toxicity and solubility issues. Importantly due to their mode of action, the decoy liposomes should have the ability to successfully target both newly emerging and established drug resistant influenza strains without discrimination. This approach has the possibility to become a key preventative treatment against a wide range of pathogens that target specific cell surface receptors.

5. Lipid analogues as cytotoxic molecules

5.1. Alkyllysophospholipids

Of all the lipid analogues that have be synthesised to date, the alkyllysophospholipids (ALPs) are probably the most studied for their toxicity to cells. This series of ether lipids was born out of the observation that the natural lipid lysophophatidylcholine (lysoPC) possessed potent immunomodulatory properties but was rapidly metabolised, reducing its effectiveness [93]. To increase the stability but retain the activity of this molecule, lysoPC analogues were synthesised that incidentally had inhibitory effects on tumour growth [94]. With a chemical structure containing a long alkyl chain, ALPs insert into the lipid bilayer of cell membranes and act similarly to a detergent at high concentrations causing cell lysis. At more physiologically relevant concentrations, ALPs have a number of biological effects relating to the disruption of cell membranes, including influencing membrane domains, phospholipid turnover and lipid associated signalling pathways [95]. The consequences of these diverse modes of action include growth inhibition, cell stress, cell cycle arrest and apoptosis. The most commonly studied ALPs are listed in table 3 showing the timeline of their development and primary publications. For their chemical structures see [95].

Alkyllysophospholipid	Year	Targeted disease	Ref.
Edelfosine (ET-O-CH$_3$)	1967	Cancer, Leishmaniasis, Human African Trypanosomiasis	96
Miltefosine (HePC)	1983	Cancer, Leishmaniasis, Human African Trypanosomiasis	97
Ilmofosine	1984	Cancer, Leishmaniasis, Human African Trypanosomiasis	98
Erucylphosphocholine (ErPC)	1992	Cancer	99
Perifosine (D-21266)	1997	Cancer, Leishmaniasis	100
Erufosine (ErPC3)	2002	Cancer	101

Table 3. Common alkyllysophospholipids used for disease treatment.

5.2. Anticancer

The first ALP to be studied in detail, edelfosine was demonstrated to have a cytotoxic effect on a wide range of cell types, both tumour derived and normal [96]. However it was apparent that edelfosine demonstrated a high selectivity towards tumour cells, strongly stimulating apoptosis by an unknown mechanism. Over the next forty years a number of analogues of edelfosine were similarly investigated for their cytotoxic anti-cancer properties. Although the most potent of the ALPs, the clinical use of edelfosine has remained limited to the treatment of acute leukaemia patients in the purging of bone marrow prior to autologous tissue transplantation [102]. Miltefosine, even though it is metabolised in cells unlike the other ALPs, still has potent anti-tumour activity in some animal models [103]. Unfortunately due to its haemolytic properties, its clinical use is restricted as a topical formulation, promising in phase II trials in the treatment of cutaneous metastases of breast cancer [104]. The most recent ALPs, the homologous erucylphosphocholine and erufosine are suitable for intravenous injection having longer 22 carbon chains and a double bond which causes them to associate in aqueous environments as non-haemolytic lamellar rather than micellar structures. They are valued ALPs in the development of cancer treatments as they have the ability to cross the blood-brain barrier, accumulate in the brain and show anti-tumour effects both in vitro [105] and in vivo [106]. Perhaps the ALP with the most therapeutic potential, perifosine, created by replacing the choline in miltefosine with a heterocyclic piperidine group, demonstrated good pharmacokinetics and strong cytotoxicity against a wide variety of tumours [107]. Its poor performance in single agent phase II trials however, has stimulated its use in successful application in combination with various anti-tumour treatments that affect other pathways in the cell. Perifosine has showed highly promising anticancer therapy in combination with inhibitors of the anti-apoptotic mTOR signalling network. Individually, drugs targeting mTOR are less effective as often the inhibition is overcome through induction of a positive feedback loop by the protein kinase Akt to upregulate mTOR [108]. The additive effect generated with the combinational approach is due to perifosine inhibition of Akt causing suppression of the positive feedback loop.

5.3. Antifungal

In the treatment of invasive mycoses, the use of miltefosine has demonstrated some broad spectrum fungicidal activity *in vitro* and in a mouse model of cryptococcosis [109]. In general however the application of ALPs to treat fungal infections in humans has been restricted by the limited therapeutic effect against cryptococcal infections in animals [110]. This may be in part due to their apparent mode of action in inhibiting cytochrome C oxidase in *Saccharomyces cerevisiae* and phospholipase B in *Cryptococcus neoformans*, two non-essential yeast proteins [109,111]. The use of ALPs as potent antifungal agents might be resurrected in part by two recent developments. The synthesis of new analogues based on existing structure–antifungal activity relationship (SAR) information of ALPs has given hope that this class of compounds can have benefit in the treatment of invasive or device-related fungal infections [112]. Furthermore, in a study of combinational therapeutics, some synergy was observed in a number of fungal strains with miltefosine and the broad-spectrum drug voriconazole which may develop with further research into clinical relevance [113].

5.4. Antiparasitic

It is in the field of parasitology where the ALPs have shown great promise. Initially, alongside their anti-cancer effects, a range of ALP analogues were found to have strong anti-protozoal activity against the free-living ciliate *Tetrahymena pyriformis* [114] and *Leishmania donovani*, the causative agent of visceral leishmaniasis [115]. Subsequent research demonstrated that different ALPs had varying potency against different protozoan species and lifecycle stage. In general however a range of *Leishmania* species, *Trypanosoma brucei* and *T. cruzi* parasites have showed significant susceptibility to these ALPs with effective dose killing responses in the low micromolar range [reviewed in 116]. The development of ALPs as potential anti-parasitic drugs in a clinical setting came from the discovery that miltefosine completely prevented *L. donovani* infection in mice with very little side effects [117]. Ultimately this research led to the development of a clinically approved formulation of miltefosine, Impavido in 2000, still to date the only approved oral drug for leishmaniasis [118]. Impavido is approved for the treatment of cutaneous and mucosal leishmaniasis but is particularly utilised for the first-line treatment of endemic visceral leishmaniasis in Asia. In addition, the use of miltefosine has been shown to be effective in curing patients infected with *L. donovani* parasites unresponsive or resistant to antimony treatment [119]. Similar to the anti-cancer effects of ALPs, the mode of action of miltefosine against *Leishmania spp.* is not entirely clear. There is a notable structural damage to the plasma membrane of most ALP treated parasites, suggestive of alterations to the lipid content [116]. Recent modern metabolomic approaches have defined cellular changes in miltefosine action against *Leishmania* and indicate disruption of the lipid metabolism of the cells as a primary target [120]. Issues with the development of resistance to miltefosine (partly due to weak therapeutics and rapid metabolism) have led to the development of ALP loaded liposomes. These have proven to be more active than the ALP alone in the treatment of animal models and as in other studies they have shown efficacy against the drug-resistant cell lines [121]. It is clear that the combined use of liposomes and ALPs is a powerful tool, giving a potential dual target approach to combat parasite infection and drug-resistance.

6. Lipids and liposomes in health and nutrition

6.1. Fatty acids and lipids

It is well documented that omega-3/omega-6 polyunsaturated fatty acids (PUFA) are essential for normal growth and development, especially for visual and neurological development in infants [122, 123]. These fatty acids have also been shown to have numerous beneficial effects on various aspects of human health, and as such the recommended minimal daily intake is set at 250 mg [124]. As humans we are unable to *de novo* synthesise omega-3 PUFA, as we do not have the necessary fatty acid desaturase enzyme(s) and thus rely solely upon dietary intake of these PUFA. Two crucial PUFAs are eicosapentaenoic acid (EPA) and docosahexaenoic acid (DHA), these are primarily accessed via marine sources, i.e. fish or krill oil, while α-linolenic acid (ALA), is found in numerous plant sources such as nuts and seeds. The biological activities of omega-3/omega-6 PUFA have been under extensive study for several decades and their beneficial effects on several diseases have been well documented, some of which will be now be discussed.

Dietary changes in fatty acid composition have been show to change the proportion of different types of PUFA in inflammatory and immune cells and thus influencing their function, this is thought to be because they can act as precursors to lipid mediators (eicosanoids/docosanoids) or as ligands for transcription factors [125]. Various omega-3 supplements also seem to boost the effectiveness of anti-inflammatory drugs, several clinical studies have reported that fish oil supplementation has beneficial effects in rheumatoid arthritis, inflammatory bowel disease, and among some asthmatics, supporting the idea that omega-3 PUFA trigger anti-inflammatory and immunomodulatory activities [126]. Along the same lines the PUFA arachidonic acid (AA) is a precursor for prostaglandins, leukotrienes, and related compounds acting as secondary messengers, modulating various roles in inflammation and immunity. Even gamma-linolenic acid a non-essential fatty acid, present in high levels in borage oil has been shown to have several beneficial effects in the treatment of rheumatoid arthritis, atopic eczema and diabetic neuropathy, as well as in the reduction of cholesterol levels [127].

The changing diet of Western societies since industrialisation has been argued to have promoted the pathogenesis of many inflammatory-related diseases, including depressive disorders. Researchers have found a correlation between cultures that eat foods with high levels of omega-3 PUFA also have lower levels of depression [128]. Several epidemiological studies have also shown a significant inverse correlation between intake of oily fish and depression and bipolar disorders [128, 129]. However it has been suggested that the preventive role of omega-3 PUFA may depend on other factors, such as overall diet quality and the social environment. Accordingly, some research suggests that omega-3 PUFAs may be effective in several ways in protecting people against Alzheimer's disease and dementia by reducing the rate of gradual memory loss linked to aging and enhancing the effectiveness of antidepressants [130].

It is common knowledge that fish and fish oil consumption (high in omega-3 PUFA) can significantly reduce the risk of cardiovascular diseases (CVDs) and slow the formation of plaque in the arteries [131]. It is now becoming clear that it is increasingly important to know which fatty acids especially EPA and DHA are attached to which lipid species. This has recently become apparent as no significant statistically correlation is observed between omega-3 PUFAs and the reduced risk of cardiovascular diseases (CVDs) when 20 studies on 68680 patients were re-evaluated. The latest evidence suggests the true biologically active component, or parent lipid species, has a direct influence on its delivery and subsequent usage/*in vivo* activity [132 and references therein]. Despite the various and numerous biological activities of omega-3 PUFA and their corresponding health benefits being extensively studied for several decades. However, the potential different forms in which these could be delivered via dietary intake such as triglycerides (TGs) versus ethyl esters or phospholipids (PLs), has largely been neglected. The fatty acid chain length and unsaturation on the lipids affects their intestinal absorption efficiency, whereas the chemical structure of the lipids (TGs *versus* PLs) determines their digestion products prior to absorption. The enrichment of essential fatty acids in particular phospholipids for increased dietary uptake and nutritional activity in the body is important. Several studies show evidence that dietary PLs have a positive impact in several diseases and potentially reduce side effects of some drugs [133, 134].

Modern diets are often depleted of complex and diverse mixtures of PLs due to increased use of refined oils and purified raw materials, which had led to an overall reduction in the uptake of PLs. Hence, the supplementation of marine PLs may serve three important functions within the functional food segment: (a) emulsifying properties, (b) supplementation of omega-3 PUFAs and (c) beneficial nutritional effects of the PLs themselves [135]. A better understanding of the impact of PL supplementation and its health benefits is required.

The potential anti-obesity effect of conjugated linoleic acid, and its mode of action lowering body fat mass has recently been reviewed by Kennedy *et al* [136]. Conjugated linoleic acid (CLA), a group of conjugated cis and trans isomers of octadecadienoic acid that have been converted from linoleic acid by microbes in the gastrointestinal tract of ruminant animals and often found in beef, dairy foods, and dietary supplements, reduces adiposity in several animal models of obesity and in some humans. CLA was discovered by Pariza and colleagues in 1987, and was first identified as an anti-carcinogen, but subsequently shown to exhibit anti-atherosclerotic and more recently anti-obesity properties [137]. Interest in CLA as an alternative treatment to conventional diabetic and weight loss therapies has increased over the past decade. Supplementation with a mixture of CLA isomers decreased the body fat mass in many animal and some human studies. The major 10,12 isomer of CLA, seems to be responsible for the antiobesity effects. Commercial preparations of CLA are now made from the linoleic acid of safflower or sunflower oils under alkaline conditions. Kennedy *et al* have summarised the recent *in vivo* and *in vitro* findings and propose potential mechanisms by which CLA reduces adiposity including its impact on energy metabolism, adipogenesis, inflammation, lipid metabolism, and apoptosis [136].

6.2. Liposomes

Liposomal encapsulation technology used by medical researchers to deliver drugs effectively to specific areas or organs in the body, as discussed earlier, is also being used to target delivery of a number of poorly soluble and high molecular weight bioactive dietary components including natural products such as carotenoids, phytosterol, omega-3 PUFAs, vitamins and other antioxidants to the body. The liposomes provide a number of advantages to other delivery systems and this is why a number of nutritional companies are now utilizing this technique in the oral delivery of dietary supplements and nutrients that are not prematurely decomposed and are pinpointed to specific tissues and organs. This approach has the added bonus that the doses can be reduced by 5 to 15 times less than normal supplement intake, i.e. tablets and capsules. The beneficial action of liposomes in oral delivery of nutrients is due to several modes of their action, including improved nutrient solubilisation and protection against environmental conditions such as moisture, oxygen and degradation by the presence of enzymes in oral and esophageal digestive juices prior to being absorbed into the body [138-140]. The phospholipids of the liposomes are able to repel undesirable activities of the digestive juices of the gastrointestinal tract, until the contents have reached the target tissue and are endocytosed, delivering their cargo into the intra-cellular space. It is important to note that more conventional delivery routes for nutrients, such as tablets, capsules etc., offer different and complementary forms of nutrient bio-availability, however the various food additives used in tablets and capsules, such as binders, fillers, gelatins and sugar affect the absorption process and may cause incomplete disintegration, hence reducing bioavailability of the active components.

More than 50 products and product combinations have been formulated using liposomal delivery systems, some of them are listed in Table 4. A key example of the full potential of using oral liposomal encapsulation is vitamin C, which causes a ~10-fold increase of vitamin C into cellular systems compared to oral tablet/capsule formulations, with no negative effects, such as gastric distress, urinary output or extra load on the liver [141].

Vitamin/herb/botanical	Active compound(s)	Health benefits
Vitamin A	Retinol	Retina function, Epithelial tissue growth, Bone growth, Embryonic development
Vitamin B2	Ribofiavin	Essential for metabolizing carbohydrates, fats, and lipids Necessary for the function of vitamins B6, folic acid, and niacin
Vitamin B12	Cyanocobalamine	Deficiency causes pernicious anemia, muscle and nerve paralysis
Vitamin C	Ascorbic acid	Antioxidant

Vitamin/herb/botanical	Active compound(s)	Health benefits
Vitamin E	alpha-Tocopherol	Detoxifies free radicals, Prevents damage to cell membranes. Enhances immune response, Antioxidant
CoEnzyme Q10	Ubiquinone-50	Increased mitochondria function, cofactor in oxidative respiration
DHEA	Dihydroepiandrosteindione	Increased libido, Feelings of well being Decreased viral load
Echinacea	Echinacosides	Immuno-stimulation
Gingko biloba extract	Gingolides	Dementia, Equilibrium disorders,Intermittent claudication
Glucosamine sulfate	Glucosamine	Osteoarthritis, Bone, cartilage, and Muscle growth
Grape seed extract	Procyanidines	Antioxidant, Inhibits tooth decay, Source of essential oils
IGF-1	Insulin, Growth Factor-1	Anti-aging
Kava kava	Kava lactones	Anxiolytic, insomnia
Ma huang	Ephedra	Cough, Bronchitis, Appetite suppression
Melatonin	Melatonin	Insomnia, Jet lag
Milk thistle	Silymarin	Hepatoprotection, Cirrhosis, Hepatitis, Immunomodulation
St. Johns wort	Hypericin, pseudohypercin	Anxiolytic, Depression, Topical inflammation, Wound healing
Zinc gluconate, zinc sulfate	Zinc ion	Essential part of more than 200 enzymes involved in digestion, metabolism, reproduction (sperm formation), and wound healing. Involved in sense of taste. Role in function and structure of cell membranes. Major part of the immune system. Component of insulin deficiency

Table 4. Liposomal nutritional products on the market

Dietary polyphenols, including flavonoids, have long been recognized as a source of important molecules involved in the prevention of several diseases, including cancer. However, due to their poor bioavailability, polyphenols remain difficult to be employed clinically. The recent use of liposomes, as a means of improving their pharmacokinetics and pharmacodynamics, hence their bioavailability means there is a renewed interest into the therapeutic benefits of wide range of polyphenols [142, 143].

7. Future perspectives

Liposomes are being used in a wide range of applications from drug and gene delivery to diagnostics, cosmetics and food nanotechnology being able to be administrated orally, parenterally or topically. Liposome formation and entrapment of various different types of cargo is now a well established methodology, allowing them to stabilise the encapsulated materials against a range of environmental and chemical changes, including enzymatic and chemical modification, as well as buffering against extreme pH and temperature [144].

There are a rapidly increasing number of new applications for liposomes in the drug and food industry, due to their biocompatibility and biodegradability. The natural composition of the liposomes, which helps in overcoming regulatory hurdles, and if required newly developed formulations can quickly be implemented. However, use of multiple lipid sources (e.g. animal, plant, synthetic sources) often requires additional characterisation and comparability studies. The quality and purity of the lipid starting materials for lipsome formulations are essential to maintain the quality of the later drug or encapsulated product. Therefore the appropriate characterization and specification of the lipid starting material is considered as vital as the product being delivered, as laid out by EU directive 2001/83/EC, along with guidance on process validation CHMP/QWP/848/99 and EMEA/CVMP/598/99 and marketing authorisation of a medicinal product (EMEA/CHMP/QWP/396951/2006).

The remarkable biocompatibility of liposomes probably stems from the fact that they are closely analogous to both naturally occurring endosomes that circulate in the bloodstream before accumulating in specific tissues, and lamellar bodies known to lubricate and protect tissue surfaces and serve in specialist functions, i.e. act a surfactant in the lungs to allow oxygen to pass from the air into the bloodstream. The depletion of lamellar bodies is also implicated in a range of diseases, including serious progressive respiratory conditions, including Cystic Fibrosis and Chronic Obstructive Pulmonary Disease [144]. These are obvious areas of research where liposome technology could be a game changer.

In order to extend and take full advantage of this highly biocompatible and safe biodegradable delivery system, future research should focus on the production of the lipid vesicles through safe, scalable methods, as well as accessing the required high quality/purity of lipids in a cheap and sustainable manner.

Acknowledgements

TKS research is supported in part by the Wellcome Trust, SUSLA, BBSRC and the European Community's Seventh Framework Programme under grant agreement No.602773 (Project KINDReD). TKS is also an academic consultant for Mylnefield Lipid analysis and Lamellar Biomedical Ltd.

Author details

Simon A. Young and Terry K. Smith*

*Address all correspondence to: tks1@st-andrews.ac.uk

Biomedical Sciences Research Complex, The North Haugh, The University, St. Andrews, Fife Scotland, U.K

References

[1] Bangham AD, Horne RW. Negative staining of phospholipids and their structural modification by surface-active agents as observed in the electron microscope. Journal of Molecular Biology 1964;8 660-8.

[2] Bangham AD, Standish MM, Watkins JC. Diffusion of univalent ions across the lamellae of swollen phospholipids. Journal of Molecular Biology 1965;13(1) 238-52.

[3] Bangham AD, Standish MM, Watkins JC, Weissmann G. The diffusion of ions from a phospholipid model membrane system. Protoplasma 1967;63(1) 183-7.

[4] Papahadjopoulos D, Watkins JC. Phospholipid model membranes. II. Permeability properties of hydrated liquid crystals. Biochimica et Biophysica Acta 1967;135(4) 639-52.

[5] Sharma A, Sharma US. Liposomes in drug delivery: progress and limitations. International Journal of Pharmaceutics 1997;154(2) 123–140.

[6] Gregoriadis G, Ryman BE. Liposomes as carriers of enzymes or drugs: a new approach to the treatment of storage diseases. Biochemistry Journal 1971;124(5) 58.

[7] Gregoriadis G, Buckland RA. Enzyme-containing liposomes alleviate a model for storage disease. Nature 1973;244(5412) 170-2.

[8] Nichols JW, Deamer DW. Net proton-hydroxyl permeability of large unilamellar liposomes measured by an acid-base titration technique. Proceedings of the National Academy of Sciences USA 1980;77(4) 2038-42.

[9] Dawson RM, Hemington NL, Miller NG, Bangham AD. On the question of an electrokinetic requirement for phospholipase C action. Journal of Membrane Biology 1976;29(1-2) 179-84.

[10] Guerrieri F, Nelson BD. Studies on the characteristics of a proton pump in phospholipid vesicles inlayed with purified complex III from beef heart mitochondria. FEBS Letters 1975;54(3) 339-42.

[11] Weissmann G, Bloomgarden D, Kaplan R, Cohen C, Hoffstein S, Collins T, Gotlieb A, Nagle D. A general method for the introduction of enzymes, by means of immunoglobulin-coated liposomes, into lysosomes of deficient cells. Proceedings of the National Academy of Sciences USA 1975;72(1) 88-92.

[12] Allison AG, Gregoriadis G. Liposomes as immunological adjuvants. Nature 1974;252(5480) 252.

[13] Straub SX, Garry RF, Magee WE. Interferon induction by poly (I): poly (C) enclosed in phospholipid particles. Infection and Immunity 1974;10(4) 783-92.

[14] Gent MP, Prestegard JH. Interaction of the polyene antibiotics with lipid bilayer vesicles containing cholesterol. Biochimica et Biophysica Acta 1976;426(1) 17-30.

[15] Papahadjopoulos D. Studies on the mechanism of action of local anesthetics with phospholipid model membranes. Biochimica et Biophysica Acta 1972;265(2) 169-86.

[16] Almeida JD, Edwards DC, Brand CM, Heath TD. Formation of virosomes from influenza subunits and liposomes. The Lancet 1975;2(7941) 899-901.

[17] Juliano RL. The role of drug delivery systems in cancer chemotherapy. Progress in clinical and biological research 1976;9 21-32.

[18] Gabizon A, Dagan A, Goren D, Barenholz Y, Fuks Z. Liposomes as in vivo carriers of adriamycin: reduced cardiac uptake and preserved antitumor activity in mice. Cancer Research 1982;42(11) 4734-9.

[19] Gabizon A, Chisin R, Amselem S, Druckmann S, Cohen R, Goren D, Fromer I, Peretz T, Sulkes A, Barenholz Y. Pharmacokinetic and imaging studies in patients receiving a formulation of liposome-associated adriamycin. British Journal of Cancer 1991;64(6) 1125-32.

[20] James JS. DOXIL approved for KS. AIDS Treatment News 1995;(no 236) 6.

[21] Safra T, Muggia F, Jeffers S, Tsao-Wei DD, Groshen S, Lyass O, Henderson R, Berry G, Gabizon A. Pegylated liposomal doxorubicin (doxil): reduced clinical cardiotoxicity in patients reaching or exceeding cumulative doses of 500 mg/m^2. Annals of Oncology 2000;11(8) 1029-33.

[22] Lorusso V, Giotta F, Bordonaro R, Maiello E, Del Prete S, Gebbia V, Filippelli G, Pisconti S, Cinieri S, Romito S, Riccardi F, Forcignanò R, Ciccarese M, Petrucelli L, Saracino V, Lupo LI, Gambino A, Leo S. Non-pegylated liposome-encapsulated doxorubicin citrate plus cyclophosphamide or vinorelbine in metastatic breast cancer not previously treated with chemotherapy: A multicenter phase III study. International Journal of Oncology 2014;45(5) 2137-42.

[23] Cabriales S, Bresnahan J, Testa D, Espina BM, Scadden DT, Ross M, Gill PS. Extravasation of liposomal daunorubicin in patients with AIDS-associated Kaposi's sarcoma: a report of four cases. Oncology Nursing Forum 1998;25(1) 67-70.

[24] Glantz MJ, LaFollette S, Jaeckle KA, Shapiro W, Swinnen L, Rozental JR, Phuphanich S, Rogers LR, Gutheil JC, Batchelor T, Lyter D, Chamberlain M, Maria BL, Schiffer C, Bashir R, Thomas D, Cowens W, Howell SB. Randomized trial of a slow-release versus a standard formulation of cytarabine for the intrathecal treatment of lymphomatous meningitis. Journal of Clinical Oncology 1999;17(10) 3110-6.

[25] Harrison TS, Lyseng-Williamson KA. Vincristine sulfate liposome injection: a guide to its use in refractory or relapsed acute lymphoblastic leukemia. BioDrugs 2013;27(1) 69-74.

[26] Kurtz JE, Kaminsky MC, Floquet A, Veillard AS, Kimmig R, Dorum A, Elit L, Buck M, Petru E, Reed N, Scambia G, Varsellona N, Brown C, Pujade-Lauraine E; Gynecologic Cancer Intergroup. Ovarian cancer in elderly patients: carboplatin and pegylated liposomal doxorubicin versus carboplatin and paclitaxel in late relapse: a Gynecologic Cancer Intergroup (GCIG) CALYPSO sub-study. Annals of Oncology 2011;22(11) 2417-23.

[27] Berenson JR, Yellin O, Chen CS, Patel R, Bessudo A, Boccia RV, Yang HH, Vescio R, Yung E, Mapes R, Eades B, Hilger JD, Wirtschafter E, Hilger J, Nassir Y, Swift RA. A modified regimen of pegylated liposomal doxorubicin, bortezomib and dexamethasone (DVD) is effective and well tolerated for previously untreated multiple myeloma patients. British Journal of Haematology 2011;155(5) 580-7.

[28] Pinto AC, Ângelo S, Moreira JN, Simões S. Schedule treatment design and quantitative in vitro evaluation of chemotherapeutic combinations for metastatic prostate cancer therapy. Cancer Chemotherapy and Pharmacology 2011;67(2) 275-84.

[29] Mayer LD, Harasym TO, Tardi PG, Harasym NL, Shew CR, Johnstone SA, Ramsay EC, Bally MB, Janoff AS. Ratiometric dosing of anticancer drug combinations: controlling drug ratios after systemic administration regulates therapeutic activity in tumor-bearing mice. Molecular Cancer Therapeutics 2006;5(7) 1854-63.

[30] Feldman EJ, Lancet JE, Kolitz JE, Ritchie EK, Roboz GJ, List AF, Allen SL, Asatiani E, Mayer LD, Swenson C, Louie AC. First-in-man study of CPX-351: a liposomal carrier containing cytarabine and daunorubicin in a fixed 5:1 molar ratio for the treatment of relapsed and refractory acute myeloid leukemia. Journal of Clinical Oncology 2011;29(8) 979-85.

[31] Tardi P, Johnstone S, Harasym N, Xie S, Harasym T, Zisman N, Harvie P, Bermudes D, Mayer L. In vivo maintenance of synergistic cytarabine:daunorubicin ratios greatly enhances therapeutic efficacy. Leukemia Research 2009;33(1) 129-39.

[32] Caride VJ, Zaret BL. Liposome accumulation in regions of experimental myocardial infarction. Science 1977;198(4318) 735-8.

[33] Freude B, Masters TN, Robicsek F, Fokin A, Kostin S, Zimmermann R, Ullmann C, Lorenz-Meyer S, Schaper J. Apoptosis is initiated by myocardial ischemia and executed during reperfusion. Journal of Molecular and Cellular Cardiology 2000;32(2) 197-208.

[34] Xu GX, Xie XH, Liu FY, Zang DL, Zheng DS, Huang DJ, Huang MX. Adenosine triphosphate liposomes: encapsulation and distribution studies. Pharmaceutical Research 1990;7(5) 553-7.

[35] Verma DD, Levchenko TS, Bernstein EA, Torchilin VP. ATP-loaded liposomes effectively protect mechanical functions of the myocardium from global ischemia in an isolated rat heart model. Journal of Controlled Release 2005;108(2-3) 460–71.

[36] Verma DD, Hartner WC, Levchenko TS, Bernstein EA, Torchilin VP. ATP-loaded liposomes effectively protect the myocardium in rabbits with an acute experimental myocardial infarction. Pharmaceutical Research 2005;22(12) 2115–20.

[37] Sarter B. Coenzyme Q10 and cardiovascular disease: a review. Journal of Cardiovascular Nursing 2002;16(4) 9–20.

[38] Verma DD, Hartner WC, Thakkar V, Levchenko TS, Torchilin VP. Protective effect of coenzyme Q10-loaded liposomes on the myocardium in rabbits with an acute experimental myocardial infarction. Pharmaceutical research 2007;24(11) 2131–7.

[39] Ross AM, Gibbons RJ, Stone GW, Kloner RA, Alexander RW. A randomized double-blinded, placebo-controlled multicenter trial of adenosine as an adjunct to reperfusion in the treatment of acute myocardial infarction (AMISTAD-II). Journal of the American College of Cardiology 2005;45(11) 1775–80.

[40] Takahama H, Minamino T, Asanuma H, Fujita M, Asai T, Wakeno M, et al. Prolonged targeting of ischemic/reperfused myocardium by liposomal adenosine augments cardioprotection in rats. Journal of the American College of Cardiology. 2009;53(8) 709–17.

[41] Kim TD, Kambayashi J, Sakon M, Tsujinaka T, Ohshiro T, Mori T. Metabolism of liposome-encapsulated heparin. Thrombosis Research. 1989;56(3) 369–76.

[42] Bai S, Gupta V, Ahsan F. Cationic liposomes as carriers for aerosolized formulations of an anionic drug: safety and efficacy study. European Journal of Pharmaceutical Sciences 2009;38(2) 165–71.

[43] Meyerhoff A. U S Food and Drug Administration approval of AmBiosome (liposomal amphotericin B) for treatment of visceral leishmaniasis. Clinical Infectious Diseases 1999;28(1) 42-8.

[44] Stauch A, Duerr HP, Dujardin JC, Vanaerschot M, Sundar S, Eichner M. Treatment of visceral leishmaniasis: model-based analyses on the spread of antimony-resistant *L. donovani* in Bihar, India. PLoS Neglected Tropical Diseases 2012;6(12) e1973.

[45] Alving C, Steck E, Chapman Jr W, Waits V, Hendricks L, Swartz Jr G, Hanson W. Therapy of leishmaniasis: superior efficacies of liposome encapsulated drugs. Proceedings of the National Academy of Sciences USA 1978;75(6) 2959–2963.

[46] New RR, Chance ML. Treatment of experimental cutaneous leishmaniasis by liposome-en-trapped Pentostam. Acta Tropica 1980;37(3) 253-6.

[47] Banerjee G, Nandi G, Mahato S, Pakrashi A, Basu M. Drug delivery system: targeting of pentamidines to specific sites using sugar-grafted liposomes. Journal of Antimicrobial Chemotherapy 1996;38(1) 145–150.

[48] Papagiannaros A, Bories C, Demetzos C, Loiseau P. Antileishmanial and trypanocidal activities of new miltefosine liposomal formulations. Biomedicine and Pharmacotherapy 2005;59(10) 545–550.

[49] Yoshihara E, Tachibana H, Nakae T. Trypanocidal activity of the stearylamine-bearing liposome *in vitro*. Life Sciences 1987;40(22) 2153-9.

[50] Tachibana H, Yoshihara E, Kaneda Y, Nakae T. In vitro lysis of the bloodstream forms of *Trypanosoma brucei gambiense* by stearylamine-bearing liposomes. Antimicrobial Agents and Chemotherapy 1988;32(7) 966-70.

[51] Morilla MJ, Montanari JA, Prieto MJ, Lopez MO, Petray PB, Romero EL. Intravenous liposomal benznidazole as trypanocidal agent: increasing drug delivery to liver is not enough. International Journal of Pharmaceutics 2004;278(2) 311-8.

[52] Yardley V, Croft SL. *In vitro* and *in vivo* activity of amphotericin B—lipid formulations against experimental *Trypanosoma cruzi* infections. American Journal of Tropical Medicine and Hygiene 1999;61(2) 193-7.

[53] Gabriëls M, Plaizier-Vercammen J. Physical and chemical evaluation of liposomes, containing Artesunate. Journal of Pharmaceutical and Biomedical Analaysis 2003;31(4) 655-67.

[54] Bayomi MA, Al-Angary AA, Al-Mehsal MA, Al-Dardiri MM. *In vivo* evaluation of arteether liposomes. International Journal of Pharmaceutics 1998;175 1–7.

[55] Owais M, Varshney GC, Choudhury A, Chandra S, Gupta CM. Chloroquine encapsulated in malaria-infected erythrocyte-specific antibody-bearing liposomes effectively controls chloroquine-resistant *Plasmodium berghei* infections in mice. Antimicrobial Agents and Chemotherapy 1995;39(1) 180-4.

[56] Maesaki S. Drug delivery system of anti-fungal and parasitic agents. Current Pharmaceutical Design 2002;8(6) 433-40.

[57] Klemens SP, Cynamon MH, Swenson CE, Ginsberg RS. Liposome-encapsulated-gentamicin therapy of *Mycobacterium avium* complex infection in beige mice. Antimicrobial Agents and Chemotherapy 1990;34(6) 967-70.

[58] Lacerda JF, Oliveira CM. Diagnosis and treatment of invasive fungal infections focus on liposomal amphotericin B. Clinical Drug Investigation 2013;33 Suppl 1 S5-14.

[59] Deol P, Khuller GK. Lung specific liposomes: stability, biodistribution and toxicity of liposomal antitubercular drugs in mice. Biochemica et Biophysica Acta, 1997;1334(2-3) 161-72.

[60] Vyas SP, Kannan ME, Jain S, Mishra V, Singh P. Design of liposomal aerosols for improved delivery of rifampicin to alveolar macrophages International Journal of Pharmaceutics 2004;269(1) 37-49.

[61] Bovier PA. Epaxal: a virosomal vaccine to prevent hepatitis A infection. Expert Review of Vaccines 2008;7(8) 1141-50.

[62] Herzog C, Hartmann K, Künzi V, Kürsteiner O, Mischler R, Lazar H, Glück R. Eleven years of Inflexal V-a virosomal adjuvanted influenza vaccine. Vaccine 2009;27(33) 4381-7.

[63] Kim T, Kim J, Kim S. Extended-release formulation of morphine for subcutaneous administration. Cancer Chemotherapy and Pharmacology 1993;33(3) 187-90.

[64] Cohen SM. Extended pain relief trial utilizing infiltration of Exparel, a long-acting multivesicular liposome formulation of bupivacaine: a Phase IV health economic trial in adult patients undergoing open colectomy. Journal of Pain Research 2012;5 567-72.

[65] Ebrahim S, Peyman GA, Lee PJ. Applications of liposomes in ophthalmology. Survey of Ophthalmology. 2005;50(2) 167-82.

[66] Bourbon JR, Chailley-Heu B, Gautier B. The exogenous surfactant Curosurf enhances phosphatidylcholine content in isolated type II cells. European Respiratory Journal 1997;10(4) 914-9.

[67] Huang Z, Jaafari MR, Szoka FC. Disterolphospholipids: nonexchangeable lipids and their application to liposomal drug delivery. Angewandte Chemie International Edition 2009;48(23) 4146-9.

[68] Lovell JF, Jin CS, Huynh E, Jin H, Kim C, Rubinstein JL, Chan WC, Cao W, Wang LV, Zheng G. Porphysome nanovesicles generated by porphyrin bilayers for use as multimodal biophotonic contrast agents Nature Materials 2011;10(4) 324-32.

[69] Kohli AG, Kierstead PH, Venditto VJ, Walsh CL, Szoka FC. Designer lipids for drug delivery: from heads to tails. Journal of Controlled Release 2014;190C 274-287.

[70] Huang Z, Szoka FC. Sterol-modified phospholipids: cholesterol and phospholipid chimeras with improved biomembrane properties. Journal of the American Chemical Society 2008;130(46) 15702-12.

[71] Khiati S, Luvino D, Oumzil K, Chauffert B, Camplo M, Barthélémy P. Nucleoside-lipid-based nanoparticles for cisplatin delivery. ACS Nano 2011;5(11) 8649-55.

[72] Nobs L, Buchegger F, Gurny R, Allémann E. Current methods for attaching targeting ligands to liposomes and nanoparticles. Journal of Pharmaceutical Sciences 2004;93(8) 1980-92.

[73] Salvati E, Re F, Sesana S, Cambianica I, Sancini G, Masserini M, Gregori M. Liposomes functionalized to overcome the blood-brain barrier and to target amyloid-β peptide: the chemical design affects the permeability across an *in vitro* model. International Journal of Nanomedicine. 2013;8 1749-58.

[74] Kanasty R, Dorkin JR, Vegas A, Anderson D. Delivery materials for siRNA therapeutics. Nature Materials 2013;12(11) 967-77.

[75] Leserman LD, Barbet J, Kourilsky F, Weinstein JN. Targeting to cells of fluorescent liposomes covalently coupled with monoclonal antibody or protein A. Nature 1980;288(5791) 602–604.

[76] Stocker BL, Timmer MS. Chemical tools for studying the biological function of glycolipids. Chembiochem 2013;14(10) 1164-84.

[77] Borborema SE, Schwendener RA, Osso JA Jr, de Andrade HF Jr, do Nascimento N. Uptake and antileishmanial activity of meglumine antimoniate-containing liposomes in *Leishmania* (*Leishmania*) *major*-infected macrophages. International Journal of Antimicrobial Agents 2011;38(4) 341-7.

[78] Lazar AN, Mourtas S, Youssef I, Parizot C, Dauphin A, Delatour B, Antimisiaris SG, Duyckaerts C. Curcumin-conjugated nanoliposomes with high affinity for Aβ deposits: possible applications to Alzheimer disease. Nanomedicine 2013;9(5) 712-21.

[79] Mulder WJ, Strijkers GJ, Habets JW, Bleeker EJ, van der Schaft DW, Storm G, Koning GA, Griffioen AW, Nicolay K. MR molecular imaging and fluorescence microscopy for identification of activated tumor endothelium using a bimodal lipidic nanoparticle. FASEB Journal 2005;19(14) 2008-10.

[80] Strijkers GJ, Kluza E, Van Tilborg GA, van der Schaft DW, Griffioen AW, Mulder WJ, Nicolay K. Paramagnetic and fluorescent liposomes for target-specific imaging and therapy of tumor angiogenesis. Angiogenesis 2010;13(2) 161-73.

[81] Allison AG, Gregoriadis G. Liposomes as immunological adjuvants. Nature 1974;252 252.

[82] Banerji B, Alving CR. Lipid A from endotoxin: antigenic activities of purified fractions in liposomes. Journal of Immunology 1979;123(6) 2558-62.

[83] Alving CR, Rao M, Steers NJ, Matyas GR, Mayorov AV. Liposomes containing lipid A: an effective, safe, generic adjuvant system for synthetic vaccines. Expert Review of Vaccines. 2012;11(6) 733-44.

[84] Liang MT, Davies NM, Blanchfield JT, Toth I. Particulate systems as adjuvants and carriers for peptide and protein antigens. Current Drug Delivery 2006;3(4) 379-88.

[85] Epstein H, Gutman D, Cohen-Sela E, Haber E, Elmalak O, Koroukhov N, Danenberg HD, Golomb G. Preparation of alendronate liposomes for enhanced stability and bioactivity: *in vitro* and *in vivo* characterization. AAPS Journal 2008;10(4) 505-15.

[86] Slegers TP, van Rooijen N, van Rij G, van der Gaag R. Delayed graft rejection in prevascularised corneas after subconjunctival injection of clodronate liposomes. Current Eye Research 2000;20(4) 322-4.

[87] Richards PJ, Williams BD, Williams AS. Suppression of chronic streptococcal cell wall-induced arthritis in Lewis rats by liposomal clodronate. Rheumatology 2001;40(9) 978-87.

[88] Landesman-Milo D, Peer D. Altering the immune response with lipid-based nano-particles. Journal of Controlled Release 2012;161(2) 600-8.

[89] Felgner PL, Gadek TR, Holm M, Roman R, Chan HW, Wenz M, Northrop JP, Ring-old GM, Danielsen M. Lipofection: a highly efficient, lipid-mediated DNA-transfection procedure Proceedings of the National Academy of Sciences USA 1987;84(21) 7413-7.

[90] Lonez C, Vandenbranden M, Ruysschaert JM. Cationic liposomal lipids: from gene carriers to cell signalling. Progress in Lipid Research 2008;47(5) 340-7.

[91] Ozpolat B1, Sood AK2, Lopez-Berestein G3. Liposomal siRNA nanocarriers for cancer therapy. Adv Drug Deliv Rev. 2014 Feb;66:110-6. doi: 10.1016. Epub 2013 Dec 30.

[92] Hendricks GL, Weirich KL, Viswanathan K, Li J, Shriver ZH, Ashour J, Ploegh HL, Kurt-Jones EA, Fygenson DK, Finberg RW, Comolli JC, Wang JP. Sialylneolacto-N-tetraose c (LSTc)-bearing liposomal decoys capture influenza A virus. Journal of Biological Chemistry 2013;288(12) 8061-73.

[93] Burdzy K, Munder PG, Fischer H, Westphal 0. Steigerung der Phagozytose von Peritonealmakrophagen durch Lysolecithin. Zeitung für Naturforschung 1964;19b 111X--l 120.

[94] Munder PG, Modolell M, Bausert W, Oettgen HF, Westphal 0. Alkyl-lysophospholipids in cancer therapy. In: Hersh EM. (ed.) Augmenting Agents in Cancer Therapy. New York; Raven Press; 1981. p441-458.

[95] van Blitterswijk WJ, Verheij M. Anticancer mechanisms and clinical application of alkylphospholipids. Biochimica et Biophysica Acta. 2013;1831(3) 663-74.

[96] Eibl H, Arnold D, Weltzien HU, Westphal O. On the synthesis of alpha and beta lecithins and their ether analogs. Justus Liebigs Annalen der Chemie 1967;709 226-30.

[97] Teshima K, Ikeda K, Hamaguchi K, Hayashi K. Bindings of cobra venom phospholipases A2 to micelles of n-hexadecylphosphorylcholine. Journal of Biochemistry 1983;94(1) 223-32.

[98] Heim ME, Swoboda M, Pahlke W, Edler L, Bicker U. Treatment of autochthonous rat colonic adenocarcinomas with a thioether-lysophospholipid derivative in mono-and combination chemotherapy. Journal of Cancer Research and Clinical Oncology 1984;108(3) 316-20.

[99] Reitz RC, Kötting J, Unger C, Eibl H. Comparison of the tissue distribution of hexadecylphosphocholine and erucylphosphocholine. Progress in Experimental Tumor Research 1992;34 143-52.

[100] Hilgard P, Klenner T, Stekar J, Nössner G, Kutscher B, Engel J. D-21266, a new heterocyclic alkylphospholipid with antitumour activity. European Journal of Cancer 1997;33(3) 442-6.

[101]   Konstantinov SM, Georgieva MC, Topashka-Ancheva M, Eibl H, Berger MR. Combi-
        nation with an antisense oligonucleotide synergistically improves the antileukemic
        efficacy of erucylphospho-N,N,N-trimethylpropylammonium in chronic myeloid
        leukemia cell lines. Molecular Cancer Therapeutics 2002;1(10) 877-84.

[102]   Vogler WR, Berdel WE, Olson AC, Winton EF, Heffner LT, Gordon DS. Autologous
        bone marrow transplantation in acute leukemia with marrow purged with alkyl-ly-
        sophospholipid. Blood 1992;80(6) 1423-9.

[103]   Hilgard P, Stekar J, Voegeli R, Harleman JH. Experimental therapeutic studies with
        miltefosine in rats and mice. Progress in Experimental Tumor Research 1992;34
        116-30.

[104]   Leonard R, Hardy J, van Tienhoven G, Houston S, Simmonds P, David M, Mansi J.
        Randomized, double-blind, placebo-controlled, multicenter trial of 6% miltefosine
        solution, a topical chemotherapy in cutaneous metastases from breast cancer. Journal
        of Clinical Oncology 2001;19(21) 4150-9.

[105]   Rübel A, Handrick R, Lindner LH, Steiger M, Eibl H, Budach W, Belka C, Jendrossek
        V. The membrane targeted apoptosis modulators erucylphosphocholine and erucyl-
        phosphohomocholine increase the radiation response of human glioblastoma cell
        lines in vitro. Radiation Oncology 2006;1 6.

[106]   Erdlenbruch B, Jendrossek V, Marx M, Hunold A, Eibl H, Lakomek M. Antitumor ef-
        fects of erucylphosphocholine on brain tumor cells *in vitro* and *in vivo*. Anticancer Re-
        search 1998;18(4A) 2551-7.

[107]   Vink SR, Schellens JH, van Blitterswijk WJ, Verheij M. Tumor and normal tissue
        pharmacokinetics of perifosine, an oral anti-cancer alkylphospholipid. Investigation-
        al New Drugs 2005;23(4) 279-86.

[108]   Cirstea D, Hideshima T, Rodig S, Santo L, Pozzi S, Vallet S, Ikeda H, Perrone G, Gor-
        gun G, Patel K, Desai N, Sportelli P, Kapoor S, Vali S, Mukherjee S, Munshi NC, An-
        derson KC, Raje N. Dual inhibition of akt/mammalian target of rapamycin pathway
        by nanoparticle albumin-bound-rapamycin and perifosine induces antitumor activity
        in multiple myeloma. Molecular Cancer Therapeutics 2010;9(4) 963-75.

[109]   Widmer F, Wright LC, Obando D, Handke R, Ganendren R, Ellis DH, Sorrell TC.
        Hexadecylphosphocholine (miltefosine) has broad-spectrum fungicidal activity and
        is efficacious in a mouse model of cryptococcosis. Antimicrobial Agents and Chemo-
        therapy. 2006;50(2) 414-21.

[110]   Ravu RR, Chen YL, Jacob MR, Pan X, Agarwal AK, Khan SI, Heitman J, Clark AM, Li
        XC. Synthesis and antifungal activities of miltefosine analogs. Bioorganic and Medic-
        inal Chemistry Letters 2013;23(17) 4828-31.

[111]   Wiederhold NP, Najvar LK, Bocanegra R, Kirkpatrick WR, Sorrell TC, Patterson TF.
        Limited activity of miltefosine in murine models of cryptococcal meningoencephali-

tis and disseminated cryptococcosis. Antimicrobial Agents and Chemotherapy 2013;57(2) 745-50.

[112] Zuo X, Djordjevic JT, Bijosono Oei J, Desmarini D, Schibeci SD, Jolliffe KA, Sorrell TC. Miltefosine induces apoptosis-like cell death in yeast via Cox9p in cytochrome c oxidase. Molecular Pharmacology 2011;80 476.

[113] Imbert S, Palous M, Meyer I, Dannaoui E, Mazier D, Datry A, Fekkar A. *In Vitro* Combination of Voriconazole and Miltefosine Against Clinically Relevant Molds. Antimicrobial Agents and Chemotherapy 2014;pii: AAC.03212-14.

[114] Tsushima S, Yoshioka Y, Tanida S, Nomura H, Nojima S, Hozumi M. Syntheses and antimicrobial activities of alkyl lysophospholipids. Chemical and Pharmaceutical Bulletin 1982;30(9) 3260-70.

[115] Herrmann HO, Gercken G. Metabolism of 1-O-[1'-14C]octadecyl-sn-glycerol in *Leishmania donovani* promastigotes. Ether-lipid synthesis and degradation of the ether bond. Molecular and Biochemical Parasitology 1982;5(2) 65-76.

[116] Croft SL, Seifert K, Duchêne M. Antiprotozoal activities of phospholipid analogues. Molecular and Biochemical Parasitology 2003;126(2) 165-72.

[117] Croft SL, Neal RA, Pendergast W, Chan JH. The activity of alkyl phosphorylcholines and related derivatives against *Leishmania donovani*. Biochemical Pharmacology 1987;36(16) 2633-6.

[118] Sindermann H, Croft SL, Engel KR, Bommer W, Eibl HJ, Unger C, Engel J. Miltefosine (Impavido): the first oral treatment against leishmaniasis. Medical Microbiology and Immunology 2004;193(4) 173-80.

[119] Sundar S, Gupta LB, Makharia MK, Singh MK, Voss A, Rosenkaimer F, Engel J, Murray HW. Oral treatment of visceral leishmaniasis with miltefosine. Annals of Tropical Medicine and Parasitology 1999;93(6) 589-97.

[120] Vincent IM, Weidt S, Rivas L, Burgess K, Smith TK, Ouellette M. Untargeted metabolomic analysis of miltefosine action in *Leishmania infantum* reveals changes to the internal lipid metabolism. International Journal of Parasitology: Drugs and Drug Resistance 2013;4(1) 20-7.

[121] Papagiannaros A, Bories C, Demetzos C, Loiseau PM. Antileishmanial and trypanocidal activities of new miltefosine liposomal formulations. Biomedicine and Pharmacotherapy 2005;59(10) 545-50.

[122] Burri L, Hoem N, Banni S, and Berge K Marine Omega-3 Phospholipids: Metabolism and Biological Activities Int. J. Mol. Sci. 2012, 13, 15401-15419

[123] Kitajka K, Sinclair AJ Weisinger RS, Weisinger HS, Mathai M, Jayasooriya AP, Halver JE and Puskás LG, Effects of dietary omega-3 polyunsaturated fatty acids on

brain gene expression Proceedings of the National Academy of Sciences USA 2014:101 10931-10936

[124] Küllenberg D, Taylor LA, Schneider M and Massing U. Health effects of dietary phospholipids Lipids in Health and Disease, 2012:11:3

[125] Murakami M. Lipid mediators in life science. Exp Anim 2011, 60(1):7-20.

[126] Calder PC Polyunsaturated fatty acids, inflammation, and immunity, Lipids 2001:36:1007-24

[127] Henz BM, Jablonska S, Van De Kerkhof PC, Stingl G, Blaszczyk M, Vandervalk PG, Veenhuizen R, Muggli R and Raederstorff D. Double-blind, multicentre analysis of the efficacy of borage oil in patients with atopic eczema. Br. J. Dermatol. 1999:140, 685-688.

[128] Grosso G, Galvano F, Marventano S, Malaguarnera M, Bucolo C, Drago F, Caraci F. Omega-3 fatty acids and depression: scientific evidence and biological mechanisms. Oxid Med Cell Longev. 2014:313570.

[129] Pepeu G, Pepeu IM, Amaducci L. A review of phosphatidylserine pharmacological and clinical effects. Is phosphatidylserine a drug for the ageing brain? Pharmacol Res 1996, 33(2):73-80.

[130] Kidd PM. Dietary phospholipids as anti-aging nutraceuticals. In Anti-Aging Medical Therapeutics. Volume IV. Edited by: Klatz RAGR. Chicago: American Academy of Anti-Aging Medicine; 2000:282-300.

[131] Wang C, Harris WS, Chung M, Lichtenstein AH, Balk EM, Kupelnick B, Jordan HS, Lau J. n-3 Fatty acids from fish or fish-oil supplements, but not alpha-linolenic acid, benefitcardiovascular disease outcomes in primary- and secondary-prevention studies: A systematic review. Am. J. Clin. Nutr. 2006: 84, 5–17.

[132] Nasopoulou C, Smith TK, Detopoulou M, Tsikrika C, Papaharisis L, Barkas D and Zabetaki I. Structural elucidation of olive pomace fed sea bass *Dicentrarchus labrax* polar lipids with cardioprotective activities Food chemistry 2014:145, 1097-1105

[133] Eros G, Ibrahim S, Siebert N, Boros M, Vollmar B: Oral phosphatidylcholine pretreatment alleviates the signs of experimental rheumatoid arthritis. Arthritis Res Ther 2009, 11(2):R43.

[134] Cohn JS, Wat E, Kamili A, Tandy S.Dietary phospholipids, hepatic lipid metabolism and cardiovascular disease. Curr Opin Lipidol 2008, 19(3):257-262.

[135] Cohn J, Kamili A, Wat E, Chung RW, Tandy S. Dietary Phospholipids and Intestinal Cholesterol Absorption. Nutrients 2010, 2(2):116-127.

[136] Kennedy A, Martinez K, Schmidt S, Mandrup S, LaPoint K and McIntosh M. Antiobesity Mechanisms of Action of Conjugated Linoleic Acid J Nutr Biochem. 2010: 21(3): 171–179.

[137] Ha YL, Grimm NK, Pariza MW. Anticarcinogens from fried ground beef: heat-altered derivatives of linoleic acid. Carcinogenesis 1987;8:1881–1887.

[138] Keller BC. Liposomes in nutrition Trends in Food Science & Technology. 2001:12 25–31.

[139] Gibbs BF, Kermasha S, Alii I, Mulligan CN.Encapsulation in the food industry: a review. Int J Food Sci Nut1999: 50:213–224.

[140] Kirby CJ, Whittle CJ, Rigby N, Coxon DT, Law BA. Stabilization of ascorbic acid by microencapsulation in liposomes. Int J Food Sci Technol 1991: 26:437–449.

[141] Tan C, Xue J, Lou X, Abbas S, Guan Y, Feng B, Zhanga X and Xia S. Liposomes as delivery systems for carotenoids: comparative studies of loading ability, storage stability and in vitro release. Food Funct. 2014:5, 1232

[142] Mignet N, Seguin J and Chabot GC Bioavailability of Polyphenol Liposomes: A Challenge Ahead Pharmaceutics 2013, 5, 457-471

[143] Lasic DD Novel applications of liposomes. TIBTECH 1998:16: 307-321

[144] Marcil PV, Drouin E and Levy E. Mechanisms of lipid malabsorption in Cystic Fibrosis: the impact of essential fatty acids deficiency Nutrition & Metabolism, 2005:2:11

5

The Small Molecule Inhibitor of Protein Kinase Revolution for the Treatment of Rheumatoid Arthritis

Charles J. Malemud

Additional information is available at the end of the chapter

1. Introduction

Targeted medical intervention for the treatment of rheumatoid arthritis (RA) has significantly revolutionized clinical outcomes for this autoimmune disease. Until the development of biological drugs which have the capacity to block the activity of most of the critical pro-inflammatory cytokines involved in RA as well as a host of immune cell-mediated events, the medical therapy of RA was limited to the use of first-line treatments including, non-steroidal anti-inflammatory drugs, sulphasalazine, and several immunosuppressive agents, such as glucocorticoids, prednisone and dexamethasone, methotrexate, and anti-malarial drugs (e.g. hydroxychloroquine) [1-5]. Agents that blocked the proliferation of T-lymphocytes, such as leflunomide, abatacept and/or B-lymphocytes (e.g. rituximab) were also employed, but mainly as second-line therapies [6-9].

The momentous development of additional biological drugs for RA arose through the identification of those pro-inflammatory cytokines that were intimately involved in initiating and perpetuating the RA process. Thus, blocking tumor necrosis factor-α/tumor necrosis factor-α receptor, interleukin-1β (IL-1β) IL-1β receptor and IL-6/IL-6 Receptor/gp130 signaling pathways with either monoclonal antibodies or engineered fusion proteins prominently entered into the armamentarium for the medical therapy of RA [10-15].

However, what does all of this mean for the future development of additional novel therapies for this chronic and debilitating synovial joint disease? For one thing the revolution in new drug development implies that although additional cellular targets including vascular endothelial growth factor (VEGF), adhesion molecules (e.g. vascular cell adhesion molecule-1; VCAM-1; CD106) and chemokines (e.g. CXC, C, CX3C and their corresponding receptors, CXCR, CCCR, CR and CX3CR) [16-26] which fit securely into a system of well-orchestrated RA pathophysiologic processes in man have been validated through *in vitro* studies as well as from impressive clinical results and *ex vivo* cell analyses with rodent models of human RA. Although none of the CC chemokine receptor antagonists have thus far yielded drugs effective in a rheumatology clinical practice, there are CXCR4 small drug antagonists in clinical trials for cancer, human immunodeficiency virus and the rare WHIM immunodeficiency condition [27].

One aspect in the study of human RA progression revolves around successfully translating from "hypothesis" to experimental validation and then going forward to drug development. This advancement has occurred by recognizing the crucial role played by signal transduction pathways in perpetuating the inflammatory state of RA. Thus, signal transduction has also been identified as the crucial cellular pathway that can cause "apoptosis-resistance" resulting in the aberrant survival of activated T-lymphocytes, B-lymphocytes and synoviocytes in RA synovial tissue [28, 29]. Signal transduction has also been identified as playing a role in the elevated frequency of apoptotic chondrocytes in RA articular cartilage [30, 31]. In that regard, blocking the phosphorylation of specific protein kinases involved signal transduction was explored as a mechanism to not only restore the appropriate balance between cell survival and cell death, which is skewed towards cell survival in RA, but also for blocking those protein kinases involved in up-regulating pro-inflammatory cytokine and matrix metalloproteinase (MMP) gene expression that is so integral to perpetuating inflammation and therefore, the destruction of synovial joints in RA [32-36].

Over the past 8 years or so, we have extensively detailed the genesis of interest in, and the extent to which, kinase activity of mitogen-activated protein kinases (MAPK) and the phosphatidylinositide-3-kinase/AKT/mammalian target of rapamycin (mTOR) (PI3K/AKT/mTOR) pathways influence MMP gene expression and cell survival, respectively [37-41]. We and others have also focused attention on the Janus Kinase/Signal Transducers and Activators of Transcription (JAK/STAT) pathway which was identified and targeted for drug development in RA because JAK/STAT signaling was found to play a major role in RA by promoting pro-inflammatory cytokine gene expression and abnormal cell survival [42-48]. Thus, this latter research focus resulted in the first JAK3-selective small molecule inhibitor (SMI), tofactinib, for use in the treatment of RA [reviewed in 49, 50].

This chapter will critically analyze the current state of drug development for novel protein kinase SMIs for RA, including a brief update and perspective on newer JAK SMI, besides tofacitinib, which are likely to be the targets for future drug development as well as additional protein kinase targets for RA.

2. Newer JAK SMIs

There are 4 members of the JAK family: JAK1, JAK2, JAK3 and Tyk2 [51]. JAK1 and JAK3 bind constitutively to the cytoplasmic region of the common gamma chain of cytokine receptors. This domain is the common subunit for many cytokines involved in T-cell and natural killer cell development in addition to B-cell activation making JAK1/JAK3 pertinent targets for intervention in RA [47, 52]. In addition to the JAK3-selective SMI, tofacitinib [54], several other

JAK SMIs, with activity towards JAK 1 and JAK2, including baricitinib [55], CEP-33779 [55], INCB028050, PF-956980 [56, 57], filgotinib (INCB-039110), decernotinib, ruxolitinib, pefcitinib, ABT-494, INCB 047986 and AC-410 [58] are currently in various stages of preclinical testing and/or clinical assessment for altering the clinical course of RA, organ transplant rejection and psoriasis [59].

It has been widely held that JAK1 and JAK3 are essentially regulated by specific tyrosine sites within their respective activation loops [60], including the NH_2-terminal kinase domain [45]. As such the activity of both JAK1 and JAK3 need be blocked to ensure inhibition of IL-2-induced STAT5 activation [47]. This assertion is bolstered by evidence that JAK1 has a dominant role over JAK3 [61] likely making selective ATP-competitive JAK3 inhibitors less effective by themselves at the cellular level. Thus, the targeting of suppressor of cytokine signaling as a means to suppress JAK/STAT signaling [45, 62, 63] is also being investigated for its potential to block cytokine-mediated STAT activation.

3. Update on tofacitinib — 2014

The approval of tofacitinib by the United States Food & Drug Administration in 2012 for the treatment of moderate-severe RA has paved the way for the development of other JAK inhibitor compounds [64, 65]. The clinical data emerging from 4 Phase II and 4 Phase III RA clinical trials involving tofacitinib was recently summarized [Malemud CJ: Submitted]. In the Phase III RA trials where tofacitinib was compared to placebo a significant American College of Rheumatology-20 (ACR20) response was consistently demonstrated in the tofacitinib arm together with an improvement in the Health Assessment Questionnaire Disability Index and ACR50 response after 3 months of treatment with tofacitinib [66]. Most critically, these Phase III trials demonstrated that the clinical efficacy of tofacitinib was similar to the clinical responses achieved with the TNF inhibitor, adalimumab. Several common adverse events observed in these clinical trials were associated with the tofacitinib group and raised some concerns. This included an increase in the incidence of infections, infestations and creatinine along with an increase in the LDL-cholesterol/HDL-cholesterol ratio and decreased neutrophil counts. However, a recent meta-analysis of various RA clinical trials involving tofacitinib concluded that the frequency of adverse events was not increased by tofacitinib [67].

In another clinical trial where the clinical efficacy of tofacitinib was compared to methotrexate [68], 3 cases of confirmed lymphoma in 5 patients receiving tofacitinib compared to 1 subject in the methotrexate arm was reported. However, the ACR70 response was greater in the tofacitinib group compared to methotrexate, but the mean change in number of bone erosions in both the tofacitinib and methotrexate groups was modest. Importantly the subjects receiving tofacitinib had less cartilage loss at 6, 12 and 24 months of treatment.

Malemud and Blumenthal [50] recently reviewed the variety of cellular mechanisms that have been shown to be altered by tofacitinib which likely contributed to the clinical efficacy of the drug in human RA clinical trials, including the relative selectivity of tofacitinib for JAK1 and JAK3 over JAK2 in ameliorating the severity of arthritis in the rat-adjuvant model [69] as well as data showing that multiple cytokines and signaling pathways in addition to JAK/STAT were inhibited by tofacitinib at effective clinical doses which was distinct from conventional disease-modifying antirheumatic drugs [70].

Although it is expected that the efficacy of tofacitinib in rheumatology clinical practice will have to be continuously monitored, tofacitinib will likely emerge as an important option for RA patients who inadequately respond to low-dose glucocorticoids, methotrexate and the several biologic drugs that are now routinely prescribed for the management of moderate-to-severe RA [50, 71, 72].

4. Selective JAK inhibitors in development

4.1. Baricitinib

Baricitinib (alternatively known as 1187594-09-7; INCB028050; UNII-ISP444213Y; LY3009104; LY-3009104 (Figure 1) [72] is a novel orally administered JAK inhibitor compound with relative selectivity for JAK1 and JAK2 [74]. In a study conducted among normal volunteers, baricitinib showed a dose-linear and time variant pharmacokinetics with low oral-dose clearance (i.e. 17L/h) and minimal systematic accumulation. Baricitinib also inhibited STAT3 phosphorylation in whole blood *ex vivo*, the results of which correlated with plasma concentrations of the drug. Although baricitinib was well-tolerated with negligible adverse events, the expected reduction in neutrophil counts was also recorded [75].

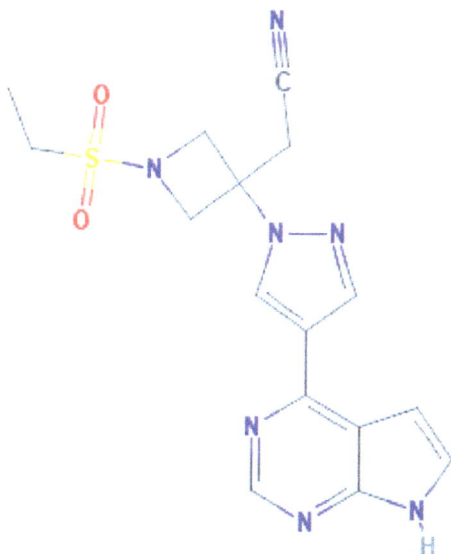

Figure 1. The chemical structure (IUPAC Name) of 2-[1-ethylsulfonyl-3-[4-(7H-pyrrolo[2,3-d]pyrimidin-4-yl)pyrazol-1-yl]azetidin-3-yl]acetonitrile (Baricitinib) [73]

4.2. Decernotinib

Decernotinib (Figure 2) alternatively known as VX-509, is an orally administered selective JAK3 inhibitor compound which is being evaluated for the possible medical management of RA [58, 76]. In a recently completed study the results of which were reported at the 2014 European League Against Rheumatism (EULAR) annual meeting, the pharmacologic activity of decernotinib was compared to tofacitinib, filgotinib (GLPG 0634) and baricitinib with reference to the blockade of several cytokine signaling pathways in whole blood cell cultures from normal subjects. The cytokine pathways evaluated were the type I and type II interferon (i.e. INFα and INFγ) pathways, the common γ chain cytokine pathways involving IL-15 and IL-21, and the IL-6 and IL-27-mediated signaling [77]. Although the results of this study showed that each of the JAK inhibitor compounds were relatively similar to each other in terms of their ability to block INFα and INFγ, IL-15, IL-21, IL-6 and IL-27 signaling, tofacitinib and baricitinib were more potent than decernotinib and filgotinib. Of note, these JAK inhibitor compounds exhibited lesser activity towards IL-10, IL-12, IL-23 and erythropoietin, which also signal via JAK/STAT [45]. Moreover, the results of the *ex vivo* studies evaluating the effect of these JAK inhibitor compounds on inhibition of cytokine signaling showed that they had markedly similar activities at clinically relevant doses.

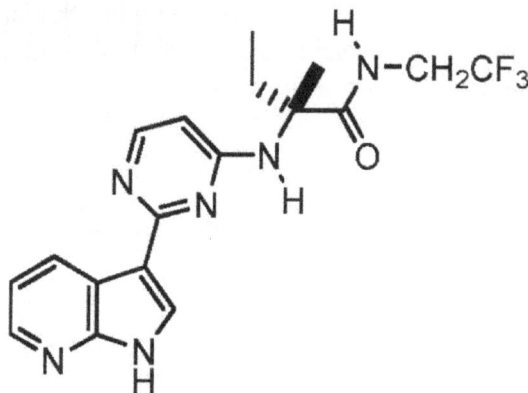

Figure 2. The chemical structure (IUPAC Name) of disodium N2-[2-(1H-Pyrrolo[2,3-pyridin-3-yl)pyrimidin-4-yl]-N-(2,2,2-trifluoroethyl)-D-isovalinamide (Decernotinib) [76]

A recently completed 24-week randomized, placebo-controlled, double-blind, phase II study compared 4 dosing regimens of orally administered decernotinib given to 358 active RA patients, measured by increased C-reactive protein levels and in RA patients with at least 6 swollen and 6 tender joints who had an inadequate clinical response to methotrexate [78]. After 24 weeks, the clinical response to decernotinib was statistically significant by ACR20, ACR50 and ACR70 criteria and by positive changes in the Disease Activity Score-28 outcomes measure. However, the percentage of patients with any adverse event was higher in the decernotinib arm relative to placebo (i.e. a stable dose of methotrexate) which led to 9.1% of patients in the decernotinib group and 8.5 patients in the placebo group, respectively, to discontinue treatment. Of note, safety profiles were comparable across all dosage levels of decernotinib.

5. Compounds that inhibit TyK2

Tyrosine kinase-2 (TyK2) is the fourth member of the Janus kinase family. However, the development of TyK2-selective SMIs has lagged significantly behind the development of SMIs with activity against the other 3 members of the JAK family [79, 80]. Thus, this remains an ongoing controversy for developing additional small compounds for RA despite the purported critical importance of TyK2 in driving IL-12-related cytokine IL-23 signaling which plays a key role in RA [81, 82].

In RA IL-23 is widely recognized as a key cytokine because of its role in perpetuating the inflammatory response as well as its involvement in the development of the IL-17-produc- ing T_H17 T-cell subset, the latter developing as a distinct T-cell lineage apart from the cytokine-producing T_H1 and T_H2 T-cells [82]. Although the IL-23 receptor was the initial potential target for intervention in RA, inflammatory bowel disease, psoriasis and multi- ple sclerosis [83], a few laboratories focused on designing and synthesizing diamino 1, 2, 4 triazole compounds which could potentially demonstrate differential inhibition of TyK2 and JAKs 1-3 [81] or small molecule compounds such as APY0201 which was reported to directly inhibit IL-23 production [84].

Until recently, there were no patents filed for the design or production of selective TyK2 inhibitors. In that regard, both tofacitinib and one other small molecule compound, CMP6, failed to markedly inhibit TyK2. However, results with another small molecule compound, Cmpd1, showed some promise in preclinical analyses [85, 86]. For example, Qi et al. [87] recently demonstrated in human cervical cancer HeLa cells that apoptosis was enhanced after incubation of these cells with TNF-α but only if TNF-α-induced heat shock protein (HSP)27 phosphorylation was suppressed by Cmpd1, or by MAPKAPK2 knockdown or by overex- pression of a non-phosphorylatable HSP27 mutant, HSP27-3A. Thus, these results reported for Cmpd1 could indicate a role for TyK2 inhibition as influencing apoptosis in HeLa which may be useful to "cure" the apoptosis-resistance characteristic of RA synovial tissue [88]. However, in that study, HSP27 phosphorylation also facilitated TNF-α ubiquitination and phosphorylation of TAK1 as well as activation of p38 MAPK and ERK, the TAK1 pro-survival pathway downstream of p38 MAPK and ERK. Therefore, the extent to which further devel- opment of TyK2 small molecule inhibitor compounds such as Cmpd1 go forward will likely depend on its capacity to alter arthritis severity in rodent animal models of RA which will be solely dependent on the design and successful synthesis of selective TyK2 SMIs.

6. The spleen tyrosine Kinase (SyK) inhibitor, fostamatinib

SyK and the ζ-chain associated protein-70 (ZAP-70) are non-receptor kinases which are preferentially produced by hemopoietic cells of the spleen, mast cells, polymorphonuclear leukocytes and macrophages [89]. In the context of adaptive immunity relevant to RA, Syk and ZAP-70 are major components in T-cell and B-cell receptor signaling [90]. Based on those findings, Syk was considered to be a promising target for RA primarily because of its involvement in regulating, not only T-cell and B-cell proliferation as well as those proliferating cells with the Fγ-activating receptor, but also in mediating immunoreceptor signaling by inflammatory cells and in signaling pathways regulated by immune complexes [91, 92].

Several years ago, Pine et al [93] showed that R788, which is the prodrug of the novel SyK SMI, R406, suppressed the severity of arthritis in collagen-induced arthritis (CIA), a well-validated mouse model of human RA. In addition to the finding that R788 showed significant clinical efficacy in mouse CIA, several surrogate molecules known to play important roles in inflammatory arthritis, namely the CXCR2 ligand KC-GRO-α, macrophage chemoattractant protein-1, IL-1 and IL-6 were also reduced in mice with CIA treated with R788 compared to the vehicle control. Of note, the release of cartilage oligomeric matrix protein (COMP), a biomarker of extracellular matrix degradation in articular cartilage, was also suppressed by R788 suggesting a possible chondroprotective effect of R788.

More recent studies have been conducted to assess the pharmacokinetic/pharmacodynamic (PKPD) of R788, alternatively known as Fostamatinib disodium; R935788; R 935788 sodium; FosD, tamatinib fosdium (Figure 3) [94]. Results of these studies revealed that the converted form of the drug, R406, exhibited a PKPD relationship with changes in blood pressure [95]. Thus, the PKPD analysis revealed a concentration-dependent increase in blood pressure with increasing concentrations of R406. Nevertheless Baloum et al. [96] showed that R406 was rapidly absorbed with a terminal $t_{1/2}$ of 12-21 hrs. Furthermore, the solid dosage forms of fostamatinib provided a drug administration regimen whereby fostamatinib could be administered once daily or twice daily to achieve therapeutic levels of the drug.

What additional parameters of adaptive immunity were found to be altered by fostamatinib? Although R406 reduced the responsiveness of dendritic cells to immune complexes administered to mice, R406 did not reduce specific CD4+T-cell proliferation in these mice after immunization with these immune complexes [97]. However, R406 did reduce the interactions that occur between dendritic cells and antigen-specific CD4+T-cells. This resulted in reduced proliferation of these antigen-specific CD4+T-cells compared mice treated with the vehicle control. This change in antigen-specific CD4+T-cell proliferation in response to R406 was also characterized by a reduction in the level of several T-cell co-stimulatory biomarkers, namely, inducible T-cell co-stimulator and PD-1 as well as diminished production of the pro-inflammatory cytokines, INF-γ and IL-17. Taken together, these *ex vivo* results provided additional support for the indication that inhibiting SyK activity with fostamatinib could be an effective drug therapy to eliminate FcR-driven CD4+T-cells responses in RA.

So how did fostamatinib fare in RA clinical trials? The results of several RA clinical trials assessed the clinical efficacy of fostamatinib [98, 99]. Thus, Taylor et al. [98] reported that treatment of moderate-severe RA subjects with fostamatinib improved the DAS-28/C-reactive protein (CRP) score from baseline versus placebo injection at 6 wks at 2 dosage regimens: 100 mg twice daily for 24 wks plus placebo injection every 2 wks and 100 mg twice daily for 4 wks, followed by 150 mg once daily up to wk 24. However, DAS-28/CRP failed to improve when

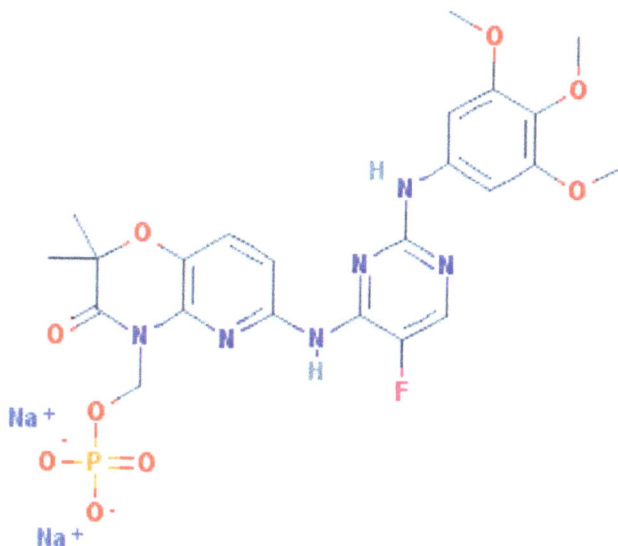

Figure 3. The chemical structure (IUPAC Name) of [6-[[5-fluoro-2-(3,4,5-trimethoxyanilino)pyrimidin-4-yl]amino]-2,2-dimethyl-3-oxopyrido[3,2-b][1,4]oxazin-4-yl]methyl phosphate (Fostamatinib Sodium) [94]

fostamatinib was administered at 100 mg twice daily for 4 wks, then 100 mg once daily up to wk 24. Most critically, in a comparator analysis, fostamatinib was less effective than the TNF-α blocker, adalimumab, at wk 24 based on the DAS-28/CRP criteria. The most common adverse effects of fostamatinib in this clinical trial were similar to those previously reported which included increased hypertension and diarrhea. Thus, although fostamatinib demonstrated significant clinical efficacy when employed as a monotherapy using DAS-28/CRP criteria at 6 wks, fostamatinib was inferior to adalimumab at wk 24.

Three additional RA clinical trials measured the effectiveness of fostamatinib on subchondral bone erosions using the modified total Sharp score as an indicator of whether inhibition of SyK retarded the destruction of subchondral bone over a period of 6 months. ACR response criteria were also measured [99]. Once again, hypertension was the most relevant adverse event affecting 40% of fostamatinib-treated subjects with other common negative responses, including, diarrhea, neutropenia and increased hepatic enzyme levels. Some of the fostamatinib-treated RA subjects also developed infections. Most critically, although RA subjects treated with fostamatinib showed a positive clinical response by ACR criteria, none of the 3 clinical trials revealed any significant effects on erosive bone damage over the 6 months of treatment.

Although SyK was shown to play an influential role in regulating the aberrant proliferation of several immune cell types critical to the RA process *in vitro* and *ex vivo*, the results of several RA clinical trials with fostamatinib were not impressive enough to warrant further development of this SyK SMI for RA.

7. A perspective on the future development of protein kinase SMIs for RA

The current state of affairs regarding the future development of additional protein kinase small molecule compounds for the treatment of RA should arise from the paradigm employed that ultimately led to the US FDA approving tofacitinib for moderate-to-severe RA. An assessment of the extent to which tofacitinib would be regularly prescribed for the treatment of RA recently concluded that most-marketing surveillance data will ultimately determine the extent to which tofacitinib will only be used to treat RA patients with inadequate responses to conventional DMARDs and/or the several types of biologic drugs now available to treat RA or whether tofacitinib will be employed as a first-line therapy for RA [50]. Although this assertion appears to have some validity based on the current thinking by rheumatologists regarding the use of tofacitinib, decisions must be made by the biopharmaceutical industry as to whether to develop other JAK SMIs for future therapy of autoimmune diseases. Some of these newer small molecule compounds were shown to inhibit JAK1 and JAK3, whereas others may be designed to selectively inhibit JAK2. In that respect, the structure of the JAK3 enzyme may be instructive (Figure 4). It was recently pointed out that tofacitinib was originally introduced as a JAK3-selective SMI, but in reality tofacitinib also inhibits JAK1 and JAK2 [100]. In addition, Chrencik et al. [101] indicated that computational analysis comparing tofacitinib with the TyK2 SMI, CMP-6, showed that kinome-selectivity will be a challenge as a consequence of the overall similarities in structure between JAKs 1-3 and TyK2, as well as the fact that the JAK3 SMI binds to the ATP-binding cavities in an orientation which is similar to JAK1 and JAK2. Therefore, the jury is still out, so to speak, as to whether or not immune-mediated inflammation and other pathophysiologic abnormalities associated with aberrant JAK/STAT signaling in RA can be regulated by focusing on developing a JAK SMI specific for a single member of the JAK family or whether small molecule compounds which are designed to inhibit more than one JAK form would be a more effective RA therapy.

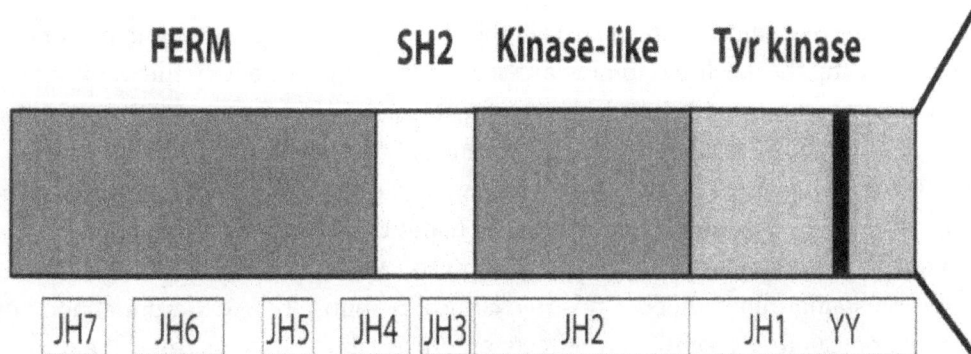

Figure 4. The JH domains and phosphorylation sites of JAK3 [45]

The drug armamentarium for treating RA now include, immunosupressants such as metho-trexate, as well as immunomodulatory drugs which block TNF-α, anti-IL-1, and T-and B-cell activation among other pathways. Therefore the extent to which JAK and/or SyK inhibitors will be employed with equal footing to these well-established drugs with clinical efficacy for RA remains to be determined.

Then there is a host of data that supports a role for other protein kinases in the RA process. However, it can be stated at this time that the results of preclinical and RA clinical trials analyses are more compelling for developing small molecule compounds to inhibit TyK2 than SyK.

Recently, we pointed out that in addition to JAK, TyK2 and SyK, it may be prudent for investigators to consider the role that abnormalities play in other signal transduction pathways associated with RA as future targets for therapeutic intervention [40]. The data supporting a robust level of "cross-talk" between several signaling pathways that contribute to cytokine, matrix metalloproteinase, pro-apoptosis and anti-apoptosis gene expression is well-proven [28, 29, 35, 40, 41] and should be taken into account. In that regard, aberrations found in RA in the PI3K/Akt/mTOR pathway, transforming growth factor kinase-1, bone marrow kinase, nuclear factor κB-inducing kinase and Bruton's tyrosine kinase could become a focus of future small molecule inhibitor drug development.

Author details

Charles J. Malemud*

Address all correspondence to: cjm4@cwru.edu

Department of Medicine, Division of Rheumatic Diseases, Case Western Reserve University, School of Medicine, Cleveland, Ohio, USA

References

[1] Feely MG, Erickson A, O'Dell JR. Therapeutic options for rheumatoid arthritis. Expert Opin Pharmacother 2009 10(13) 2095-2106.

[2] Upchurch KS, Kay J. Evolution of treatment for rheumatoid arthritis. Rheumatology (Oxford) 2012; 51 Suppl 6 vi28-vi36.

[3] Taherian E, Rao A, Malemud CJ, Askari A. The biological and clinical activity of anti-malarial drugs in autoimmune disorders. Curr Rheum Rev 2013 9(1) 45-62.

[4] Braun J. Methotrexate: optimizing the efficacy in rheumatoid arthritis. Ther Adv Musculoskelet Dis 2011; 3(3) 151-158.

[5] Kumar P, Banik S. Pharmacotherapy options in rheumatoid arthritis. Clin Med Insights Arthritis Musculoskelet Disord 2013; 6 35-43.

[6]   Finckh A, Dehler S, Gabay C. The effectiveness of leflunomide as a co-therapy of tumor necrosis factor inhibitors in rheumatoid arthritis; a population-based study. Ann Rheum Dis 2009; 68(1) 33-39.

[7]   Meier FM, Frerix M, Hermann W, Müller-Ladner U. Current immunotherapy in rheumatoid arthritis. Immunotherapy 2013; 5(9): 955-974.

[8]   Gibbons LJ, Hyrich KL. Biologic therapy for rheumatoid arthritis; clinical efficacy and predictors of response. Biodrugs 2009; 23(2) 111-124.

[9]   Östör AJ. Abatacept: a T-cell co-stimulation modulator for the treatment of rheumatoid arthritis. Clin Rheumatol 2008; 27 (11) 1343-1353.

[10] Astry B, Harberts E, Moudgil KD. A cytokine-centric view of the pathogenesis and treatment of autoimmune arthritis. J Interferon Cytokine Res 2011; 31(12) 927-940.

[11] Mertens M, Singh JA. Anakinra for rheumatoid arthritis: a systematic review. J Rheumatol 2009; 36(6) 1118-1125.

[12] Tanaka T, Kishimoto T. Immunotherapy of tocilizumab for rheumatoid arthritis. J Clin Cell Immunol 2013; S6 001

[13] Malemud CJ. Targeted drug development for rheumatoid arthritis. Future Med Chem 2012; 4(6) 701-703

[14] Taylor PC. Pharmacology of TNF blockade in rheumatoid arthritis and other chronic inflammatory diseases. Curr Opin Pharmacol 2010; 10(3) 308-315.

[15] Geyer M, Müller-Ladner U. Actual status of antiinterleukin-1 therapies in rheumatic diseases. Curr Opin Rheumatol 2010; 22(3) 246-251.

[16] Giatromanolaki A, Sivridis E, Athanassou N et al. The angiogenic pathway 'vascular endothelial growth factor/flk-1(KDR)-receptor' in rheumatoid arthritis. J Pathol 2001; 194(1) 101-108.

[17] Malemud CJ, Reddy SK. Targeting cytokines, chemokines and adhesion molecules in rheumatoid arthritis. Curr Rheum Rev 2008; 4 219-234.

[18] Agawal SK, Brenner MB. Role of adhesion molecules in human synovial inflammation. Curr Opin Rheumatol 2006; 18(3) 268-276.

[19] Szekanecz Z, Koch AE. Vascular endothelium and immune responses: implications for inflammation and angiogenesis. Rheum Dis Clin North Am 2004; 30(1) 97-114.

[20] Lee DM, Kiener HP, Agarwal SK et al. Cadherin-11 in synovial lining formation and pathology in arthritis. Science 2007; 315(5814) 1006-1010.

[21] Haringman JJ, Kraan MC, Smeets TJM, Zwinderman KH, Tak PP. Chemokine blockade and chronic inflammatory disease: proof of concept in patients with rheumatoid arthritis. Ann Rheum Dis 2003; 62(8) 715-721.

[22] Haringman JJ, Gerlag DM, Smeets TJM et al. A randomized controlled trial with anti-CCL2 (anti-monocyte chemotactic protein-1) monoclonal antibody in patients with rheumatoid arthritis. Arthritis Rheum 2006; 54(8) 2387-2392.

[23] Liu J, Merritt JR. CC chemokine receptor small molecule antagonists in the treatment of rheumatoid arthritis and other diseases: a current view. Curr Top Med Chem 201; 10(13) 1250-1267.

[24] White GE, Iqbal AJ, Greaves DR. CC chemokine receptors and chronic inflammation —therapeutic opportunities and pharmacological challenges. Pharmacol Rev 2013; 65(1) 47-89.

[25] Ellingsen T, Hansen I, Thorsen J et al. Upregulated baseline plasma CCL19 and CCR7 cell-surface expression on monocytes in early rheumatoid arthritis normalized during treatment and CCL19 correlated with radiographic progression. Scand J Rheumatol 2014; 43(2) 91-100

[26] Antonelli A, Ferrari SM, Giuggioli D, Ferrannini E, Ferri C, Fallahi P. Chemokine (C-X-C motif) ligand (CXCL) 10 in autoimmune diseases. Autoimmun Rev 2014; 13(3) 272-280.

[27] Debnath B, Xu S, Grande S, Garofalo A, Neamati N. Small molecule inhibitors of CXCR4. Theranostics 2013; 3(1) 47-75.

[28] Wylie MA, Malemud CJ. Perspective: Deregulation of apoptosis in arthritis by altered signal transduction. Int J Clin Rheumatol 2013; 8(4) 483-490.

[29] Malemud CJ. Intracellular signaling pathways in rheumatoid arthritis. J Clin Cell Immunol 2013; 4 160.

[30] Korb A, Pavenstädt H, Pap T. Cell death in rheumatoid arthritis. Apoptosis 2009; 14(4) 447-454.

[31] Malemud CJ, Sun Y, Pearlman E, Ginley NM, Awadallah A, Wisler BA et al. Monosodium urate and tumor necrosis factor-α increase apoptosis in human chondrocyte cultures. Rheumatology (Sunnyvale) 2012; 2 113.

[32] Chang L, Karin M. Mammalian MAP kinase signaling cascades. Nature 2001; 410(6824) 37-40.

[33] Burrage PS, Mix KS, Brinckerhoff CE. Matrix metalloproteinases : role in arthritis. Front Biosci 2006; 11 529-543.

[34] Wu T, Mohan C. The AKT axis as a therapeutic target in autoimmune diseases. Endocr Metab Immune Disord Drug Targets 2009; 9(2) 145-150.

[35] Malemud CJ. The discovery of novel experimental therapies for inflammatory arthritis. Mediators Inflamm 2009; 698769.

[36] Malemud CJ. Regulation of chondrocyte matrix metalloproteinase gene expression. 2014; In: Dhalia NS, Chakraborti S (Editors) Role of Proteases in Health and Disease. Springer Science, UK.

[37] Malemud CJ. Small molecular weight inhibitors of stress-activated and mitogen-activated protein kinases. Mini Rev Med Chem 2006; 6(6) 689-698.

[38] Malemud CJ: Inhibitors of stress-activated/mitogen-activated protein kinase pathways. Curr Opin Pharmacol 2007; 7(3) 339-343.

[39] Malemud CJ. Defining novel targets for intervention in rheumatoid arthritis: An overview. Curr Rheum Rev 2008; 4 214-218.

[40] Malemud CJ. Dysfunctional immune-mediated inflammation in rheumatoid arthritis dictates that development of anti-rheumatic disease drugs target multiple intracellular signaling pathways. Anti-Inflammatory Anti-Allergy Agents Med Chem 2011; 10(2) 78-84.

[41] Wisler BA, Dennis JE, Malemud CJ. New organ-specific pharmacological strategies interfering with signaling pathways in inflammatory disorders/autoimmune disorders. Curr Signal Transduct Ther 2011; 6 279-291.

[42] Yokota A, Narazaki N, Shima Y et al. Preferential and persistent activation of the STAT1 pathway in rheumatoid synovial fluid cells. J Rheumatol 2001; 28(9) 1952-1959.

[43] Kasperkovitz PV, Verbeet NL, Smeets TJ et al. Activation of the STAT1 pathway in rheumatoid arthritis. Ann Rheum Dis 2004; 63(3) 233-239.

[44] Walker JG, Ahern MG, Coleman M et al. Characterisation of a dendritic cell subset in synovial tissue which strongly expresses Jak/STAT transcription factors from patients with rheumatoid arthritis. Ann Rheum Dis 2007; 66(8) 992-999.

[45] Malemud CJ, Pearlman E. Targeting JAK/STAT signaling pathway in inflammatory diseases. Curr Signal Transduct Ther 2009; 4 201-221.

[46] Malemud CJ. Differential activation of JAK enzymes in rheumatoid arthritis and autoimmune disorders by proinflammatory cytokines – potential drug targets. Int J Interferon Cytokine Mediator Res 2010; 2 97-111.

[47] Malemud CJ. Suppression of pro-inflammatory cytokines via targeting of STAT-responsive genes. 2013; In: El-Shemy H (Editor), Drug Discovery. InTech, Croatia.

[48] Laurence A, Pesu M, Silvennoinen O, O'Shea J. JAK kinases in health and disease. An update. Open Rheumatol J 2012; 6 232-244.

[49] Malemud CJ. Inhibitors of JAK for the treatment of rheumatoid arthritis: Rationale and clinical data. Clin Invest 2012; 2 39-47.

[50] Malemud CJ, Blumenthal DE: Protein kinase small molecule inhibitors for rheumatoid arthritis: Medicinal chemistry/Clinical perspectives. World J Orthopedics: 2014; 5(4) 496-503.

[51] Cutulo M, Meroni M. Clinical utility of the oral JAK inhibitor tofacitinib in the treatment of rheumatoid arthritis. J Inflamm Res 2013; 6: 129-136.

[52] Thoma G, Nuninger F, Falchetto R, Hermes E, Tavares GA, Vangrevelinghe E et al. Identification of a potent Janus kinase 3 inhibitor with high selectivity within the Janus kinase family. J Med Chem 2011; 54(1) 284-288.

[53] Smolen JS, van der Heijde D, Machold KP, Aletaha D, Landewé R. Proposal for a new nomenclature of disease-modifying antirheumatic drugs. Ann Rheum Dis 2014; 73(1) 3-5.

[54] Vafadari R, Weimar W, Baan CC. Phosphospecific flow cytometry for pharmacodynamic drug monitoring: analysis iof the JAK-STAT signaling pathway. Clin Chim Acta 2012; 413(17-18) 1398-1405.

[55] Stump KL, Lu LD, Dobrzanski P, Serdikoff C, Gingrich DE, Dugan BJ et al. A highly selective, orally active inhibitor of Janus kinase 2, CEP-33779, ablates disease in 2 mouse models of rheumatoid arthritis. Arthritis Res Ther 2011; 13(2) R68.

[56] Fridman JS, Scherle PA, Collins R, Burn TC, Li Y, Covington MB et al. Selective inhibition of JAK1 and JAK2 is efficacious in rodent models of arthritis: preclinical characterization of INCB028050. J Immunol 2010; 184(9) 5298-5307.

[57] Migita K, Izumi Y, Torigoshi T, Satomura K, Izumi M, Nishino Y et al. Inhibition of Janus kinase/signal transducer and activator of transcription (JAK/STAT) signalling pathway in rheumatoid synovial fibroblasts using small molecule compounds. Clin Exp Immunol 2013 174(3) 356-363.

[58] Norman P. Selective JAK inhibitors in development for rheumatoid arthritis. Expert Opin Investig Drugs 2014; 23(8) 1067-1077.

[59] Hsu L, Armstrong AW. JAK inhibitors: treatment efficacy and safety profile in patients with psoriasis. J Immunol Res 2014; 2014 283617.

[60] Liu KD, Gaffen SL, Goldsmith MA, Greene WC. Janus kinases in interleukin-2 mediated signaling: JAK1 and JAK3 are differentially regulated by tyrosine phosphorylation. Curr Biol 1997; 7(11) 817-826.

[61] Haan C, Rolvering C, Raulf F, Kapp M, Drückes P, Thomas G et al. Jak1 has a dominant role over Jak3 in signal transduction through γc-containing cytokine receptors. Chem Biol 2011; 18(3) 314-323.

[62] O'Sullivan LA, Liongue C, Lewis RS, Stephenson SE, Ward AC. Cytokine receptor signaling through the Jak-Stat-Socs pathway in disease. Mol Immunol 2007; 44(10) 2497-2506.

[63]   Himpe E, Kooijman R. Insulin-like growth factor-1 receptor signal transduction and the Janus Kinase/Signal Transducer and Activator of Transcription (JAK-STAT) pathway. Biofactors 2009; 35(1) 76-81.

[64]   Vaddi K, Luchi M. JAK inhibition for the treatment of rheumatoid arthritis: a new era in oral DMARD therapy. Expert Opin Investig Drugs 2012; 21(7) 961-973.

[65]   Dymock BW, See CS. Inhibitors of JAK2 and JAK3: an update on the patent literature 2010-2012. Expert Opin Ther Pat 2013; 23(4) 449-501.

[66]   Kaur K, Kalra S, Kaushal S. Systematic review of tofacitinib: a new drug for the management of rheumatoid arthritis. Clin Ther 2014; 36(7) 1074-1086.

[67]   Kawalec P, Mikrut A, Wiśniewska N, Pilic A. The effectiveness of tofacitinib: a novel Janus kinase inhibitor, in the treatment of rheumatoid arthritis: a systematic review and meta-analysis. Clin Rheumatol 2013; 32(10) 1415-1424.

[68]   Lee FB, Fleischmann R, Hall S, Wilkinson B, Bradley JD, Gruben D et al. Tofacitinib versus methotrexate in rheumatoid arthritis. N Engl J Med 2014; 370(25) 2377-2386.

[69]   Meyer DM, Jesson MI, Li X, Elrick MM, Funckes-Shippy CL, Warner JD et al. Anti-inflammatory activity and neutrophil reductions mediated by the JAK1/JAK3 inhibitor, CP690,550 in rat adjuvant-induced arthritis. J Inflamm (London) 2010; 7 41.

[70]   Yamaoka K, Tanaka Y. Targeting the Janus kinases in rheumatoid arthritis: focus on tofacitinib. Expert Opin Pharmacother 2014; 15(1) 103-113.

[71]   Vyas D, O'Dell KM, Bandy JL, Boyce EG. Tofacitinib: the First Janus kinase (JAK) inhibitor for the treatment of rheumatoid arthritis. Ann Pharmacother 2013; 47(11) 1524-1531.

[72]   Gaujoux-Viala C, Nam J, Ramiro S, Landewé B, Buch MH, Smolen JS et al. Efficacy of conventional synthetic disease-modifying antirheumatic drugs, glucocorticoids and tofacitinib: a systematic literature review informing the 2013 update of the EULAR recommendations for management of rheumatoid arthritis. Ann Rheum Dis 2014; 73(3) 510-515.

[73]   http://pubchem.ncbi.nlm.nih.gov/summary/summary.cgi?cid=44205240   (Accessed 10/17/14)

[74]   van Vollenhoven RF. Small molecular compounds in development for rheumatoid arthritis. Curr Opin Rheumatol 2013; 25(3) 391-397.

[75]   Shi JG, Chen X, Lee F, Emm T, Scherle PA, Lo Y et al. The pharmacokinetics, pharmacodynamics and safety of baricitinib, an oral JAK1/2 inhibitor, in healthy volunteers. J Clin Pharmacol 2014 ; 54(12) 1354-1361.

[76]   http://newdrugapprovals.org/2014/07/21/decernotinib-jak-inhibitor-for the treatment of autoimmune and inflammatory disease/ Accessed 8/20/14

[77] https://b-com.mci-group.com/AbstractList/EULAR2014.aspx Lack of differentiation of Janus kinase inhibitors in rheumatoid arthritis based on Janus kinase pharmacology and clinically meaningful concentrations. Accessed 8/20/14

[78] EULAR Meeting-Van Vollenhoven R et al. Ann Rheum Dis 2014; 73 Suppl 2 Accessed 8/20/14

[79] Malemud CJ. Suppression of autoimmune arthritis by small molecule inhibitors of the JAK/STAT pathway. Pharmaceuticals 2010; 3 1446-1455.

[80] Norman P. Selective JAK 1 inhibitor and selective Tyk2 inhibitor patents. Expert Opin Ther Pat 2012; 22(10) 1233-1249.

[81] Malerich JP, Lam JS, Hart B, Fine RM, Klebansky B, Tanga MJ et al. Diamino-1,2,4-triazole derivatives are selective inhibitors of TYK2 and JAK1 over JAK2 and JAK3. Bioorg Med Chem Lett 2010; 20(24) 7454-7457.

[82] Dalila AS, Mohd Said MS, Shaharir SS, Asrul AW, Low SF, Shamsul AS et al. Interleukin-23 and its correlation with disease activity, joint damage, and functional disability in rheumatoid arthritis. Kaohsiung J Med Sci 2014; 30(7) 337-342.

[83] Boniface K, Blom B, Liu YJ, de Waal Malefyt R. From interleukin-23 to T-helper 17 cells: human T helper cell differentiation revisited. Immunol Rev 2008; 226 132-146.

[84] Hayakawa N, Noguchi M, Takeshita S, Eviryanti A, Seki Y, Nishio H et al. Structure-activity relationship study, target identification, and pharmacological characterization of a small molecular IL-12/IL-23 inhibitor, APY0201. Bioorg Med Chem 2014; 22(11) 3021-3029.

[85] Tang C, Chen S, Qian H, Huang W. Interleukin-23: as a drug target for autoimmune inflammatory diseases. Immunology 2012; 135(2) 112-124.

[86] Liang Y, Zhu Y, Xia Y, Peng H, Yang XK, Liu YY et al. Therapeutic potential of tyrosine kinase 2 in autoimmunity. Expert Opin Ther Targets 2014; 18(5) 571-580.

[87] Qi Z, Shen L, Zhou H, Jiang Y, Lan L, Luo L et al. Phosphorylation of heat shock protein 27 antagonizes TNF-α induced HeLa cell apoptosis via regulating TAK1 ubiquitination and activation of p38 and ERK signaling. Cell Signal 2014; 26(7) 1616-1625.

[88] Malemud CJ, Haque A, Louis NA, Wang J: Immune response and apoptosis – Introduction. J Clin Cell Immunol 2012; S3: e001.

[89] Malemud CJ. Role of nonreceptor tyrosine and threonine kinase inhibitors. 2009; In. Gracia-Foncillas J. (Editor) Molecular Biology of Cancer: Toward New Therapies. Prous Science, Barcelona.

[90] Wong BR, Grossbard D, Payan G, Masuda ES. Targeting Syk as a treatment for allergic and autoimmune disorders. Expert Opin Investig Drugs 2004; 13(7) 743-762.

[91]   Scott DL. Role of spleen tyrosine kinase inhibitors in the management of rheumatoid arthritis. Drugs 2011; 71(9) 1121-1132.

[92]   Gomez-Puerta JA, Mócsai A. Tyrosine kinase inhibitors for the management of rheumatoid arthritis. Curr Top Med Chem 2013; 13(6) 760-773.

[93]   Pine RR, Chang B, Schoettler N, Banquerigo ML, Wang S, Lau A et al. Inflammation and bone erosion are suppressed in models of rheumatoid arthritis following treatment with a novel SyK inhibitor. Clin Immunol 2007; 124(3) 244-257.

[94]   http://pubchem.ncbi.nlm.nih.gov/summary/summary.cgi?cid=25008120   (accessed 10/17/14)

[95]   Boström E, Ohrn F, Hanze E, Sandström M, Martin P, Wählby-Hamrén U. Exposure vs. response of blood pressure in patients with rheumatoid arthritis following treatment with fostamatinib. J Clin Pharmacol 2014 ; 54(12) 1337-1346 doi: 10.1002/jcph. 341

[96]   Baloum M, Grossbard EB, Mant T, Lau DT. Pharmacokinetics of fostamatinib, a spleen tyrosine kinase (SYK) inhibitor, in healthy human subjects following a single and multiple oral dosing in three phase I subjects. Br J Clin Pharmacol 2013; 76(1) 78-88.

[97]   Platt AM, Benson RA, Mc Queenie R, Butcher JP, Braddock M, Brewer JM et al. The active metabolite of spleen tyrosine kinase inhibitor fostamatinib abrogates the CD4+T cell-priming capacity of dendritic cells. Rheumatology (Oxford) 2014 Jul 26 pii.keu273 [Epub ahead of print]

[98]   Taylor PC, Genovese MC, Greenwood M, Ho M, Nasonov E, Oemar B et al. OSKIRA-4: a phase IIb randomised, placebo-controlled study of the efficacy and safety of fostamatinib monotherapy. Ann Rheum Dis 2014 Jul 29 pii:annrheumdis-2014205361. doi: 10.1136/annrheumdis-2014-205361 [Epub ahead of print]

[99]   Scott IC, Scott DL. Spleen tyrosine kinase inhibitors for rheumatoid arthritis: where are we now? Drugs 2014; 74(4) 415-422.

[100] Thoma G, Drückes P, Zerwes G. Selective inhibitors of the Janus kinase Jak3-Are they effective? Bioorg Med Chem Lett 2014; 24(19) 4617-4621 pii:S9060-894X(14)00890-7. doi: 10.1016/j.bmcl.2014.08.046

[101] Chrencik JE, Patny A, Leung IK, Korniski B, Emmons TL, Hall T et al. Structural and thermodynamic characterization of the TYK2 and JAK3 kinase domains in complex with CP690550 and CMP-6. J Mol Biol 2010; 400(3) 413-433.

6

Clinical Trials in Paediatrics — Regulatory and Methodological Aspects

Adriana Ceci, Viviana Giannuzzi, Donato Bonifazi,
Mariagrazia Felisi, Fedele Bonifazi and
Lucia Ruggieri

Additional information is available at the end of the chapter

1. Introduction

Until very recently, decisions about the medical treatment of children with acute or chronic health conditions were based on the results of research conducted almost exclusively in adults. Although differences in treatment effects between young and adult patients are well known (e.g. regarding mechanism of action and metabolism), there were less clinical trials (CTs) than needed to adequately evaluate the effects of new medicines in children. This was mainly due to:

- the lack of appropriate rules for the conduct of paediatric CTs, especially with regard to ethical considerations;

- the lack of an adequate methodology enabling to provide powered evidences while taking into account the paediatric specificities [1];

- the lack of economic interest of the industrial developers due to the limited market offered by children.

Starting from 1994, Food and Drug Administration (FDA) adopts different measures to promote, incentive or oblige to conduct paediatric trials. More recently, for effect of the Paediatric Regulation (EC) No 1901/2006 [2] requiring a sound scientific evidence for treatment benefits in children and adolescents, the conduct of CTs testing medications for their use in children and adolescents becomes mandatory in the European Union (EU).

Despite the high number,,(more than 1000) of Paediatric Investigation Plans (PIPs) applied to receive an opinion by the Paediatric Committee (PDCO) at the European Medicines Agency

(EMA) since the Regulation entry into force very few advancements have been done in terms of new studies, new trials and new paediatric approved medicines on the market. [3]. At the same time, looking at the American side, we can observe that the implementation of the existing rules has been and are still strongly problematic and under debate, allowing to recent modifications of rules and guidelines.

The aim of this chapter is to describe the requisites for implementing paediatric CTs in compliance with the principles of good clinical practice (Good Clinical Practice, GCP), and with the regulatory standards in order to be part of an agreed PIP in EU or of a Pediatric Study Plan (PSP) in the United States (U.S.).

It will include the following topics:

1. Paediatric trial regulatory aspects

Currently covered by the CTs Directive 2001/20/EC [4], rules on paediatric trials are changing for effect of the recently approved CT Regulation that will enter into force by 2016 [5]. The transition phase and the new context deriving by this transition will be considered in this chapter mainly in terms of a) trial authorisation, b) rules and competencies of Ethics Committees, c) consent and assent from parents and children, d) children privacy and confidentiality.

2. Paediatric Plans and paediatric trials methodology

The traditional drug development approaches do not satisfy the requirements of research in the paediatric population. In particular, in paediatrics the following issues are challenging: large population needed for Randomised Controlled Trials (RCTs), randomisation procedure, placebo use, validate paediatric endpoint, appropriate outcomes, long-term effects evaluations, etc.

In the last years, the main activities performed at scientific and regulatory levels to cover these gaps have been aimed to identify innovative methods of research to overcome the existing paediatric limitations.

3. Paediatric trial incentives and main results of the existing legislation

By many years the U.S. legislation provides financial incentives to study medicines in children. This has produced a significant increase in the number of paediatric trials conducted since 1997. The EU paediatric medicines Regulation, which was adopted in 2007 [2] is also based on a series of incentives and requirements and will lead to a further stimulation of paediatric drug development. This chapter explores the distribution and other characteristics of recently conducted paediatric trials in EU and US also providing a comparison between the two areas.

2. Paediatric trial regulatory aspects

2.1. The legislative framework to promote paediatric medicines and research

To overcome the lack of paediatric trials, many initiatives have been promoted both in U.S. and in Europe.

The first rule came from FDA in 1994 [1]. It was an attempt to use existing data (may be extrapolated from adults) and additional pharmacokinetic (PK), pharmacodynamic (PD), and safety studies, if the course of the disease and the response to the drug are similar in children and adults. The 1994 law did not impose a general requirement to the manufacturers to carry out studies when existing information was not sufficient and was not successful to obtain its aim.

In 1997, for the first time, the FDA Modernisation Act [6] introduced incentives for conducting paediatric studies on drugs for which exclusivity or patent protection exists, while off-patent drugs were excluded. At that time it was not accepted that FDA would mandate timing and other paediatric studies provisions to the manufacturers.

Today, the current U.S. regulatory framework includes:

- The Best Pharmaceuticals for Children Act **(BPCA)** [7], that provides incentives for drug companies to conduct (after FDA Written Request) paediatric studies by granting additional six months of marketing exclusivity.

- The Paediatric Research Equity Act **(PREA)** [8] that requires drug companies to study their products in children under certain circumstances. When paediatric studies are required, they must be conducted with the same drug and for the same use for which they were approved in adults.[1]

Noticeably, BPCA provided mechanisms for studying on- and off-patent drugs and to test off-patent drugs by:

- Identifying and prioritising drugs which need to be studied;

- Developing study requests in collaboration with experts at National Institutes of Health (NIH), FDA and other organisations;

- Conducting studies on priority drugs after manufacturers decline to do so.

On the other hand, under the **PREA** as originally enacted, a proposed timeline and plan for the submission of paediatric studies were not required to be submitted during the New Drug Application (NDA).By July 9th 2012, for the first time PREA includes a provision that requires manufacturers to submit a Pediatric Study Plan **(PSP)** early in the drug development process. Pediatric Review Committee (PeRC) is a consultative body which reviews all activities under PREA (the same committee is in charge for the activities foreseen under BPCA).

A similar intervention in the EU arrived almost 10 years later. In fact, the EU Paediatric Regulation [2] entered into force in January 2007. After the Paediatric Regulation approval, relevant changes have been implemented not only in Europe but also in the U.S.

The main pillars of the EU Paediatric Regulation are:

- to set up a new Committee at EMA named the Paediatric Committee (PDCO);

---

1 More details at: Drugs/DevelopmentApprovalProcess/DevelopmentResources/ucm049867.htm

- to rule a new type of Marketing Authorisation, the Paediatric Use Marketing Authorisation (PUMA) only accessible to off-patent drugs;

- to introduce the obligation for the manufacturers to apply for a PIP early in the drug developmental process;

- the obligation to conduct the paediatric studies in compliance with an approved PIP that can also include waiver (exemption to conduct any paediatric studies) or deferral (the right for the manufacturer to delay the paediatric study respect to the adults MA);

- to state that dedicated incentives should be provided under the European Research Framework to develop off-patent drugs if included in a 'Priority List' published by the PDCO-EMA

2.2. The current regulatory framework for approving clinical trials

The introduction of specific rules devoted to implement the paediatric research in the paediatric population allowed an increased attention to the CT approval and conduct.

For many years, the traditional approach to diagnosis and treatment has been based on symptoms and signs, which reflect, in the majority of the cases, the patient phenotype. Accordingly, trials have been conducted by grouping patients into broad groups with similar symptoms. Pharmaceutical and biotechnology companies have developed medicines for these broad populations, and the regulatory assessment of risk and benefit has been based on the average clinical response across these groups. This model has been strongly regulated with the aim of performing ethically and methodologically well-conducted CTs.

In Europe several guidelines, directives and regulations have been released, including Directives 2005/28/EC [9] and 2001/20/EC [4], GCP Guidelines (CPMP/ICH/135/95) [10], Reg. (EC) No 726/2004 [11]. In particular, Directive 2001/20/EC has established specific provisions regarding the conduct of CTs on human subjects involving medicinal products and recognises GCP principles. As internationally agreed and in accordance with GCP [10], a CT may not commence in EU if an Ethics Committee has not approved the study. The Directive 2001/20/EC also introduced the concept of "Competent Authority", adding the legal obligation to obtain an "authorisation" in addition to the positive opinion of the Ethic Committee.

However, the above mentioned provisions in Europe have never considered the paediatric specificity until the approval of the CT Directive. In fact, the main novelty of the Directive has been represented by the introduction of a dedicated article (art. 4) that refers to differences in the ethical and methodological approaches between paediatric and adult trials and provides the basis for including paediatric trials in the developmental process of adult drugs. Moreover, following the approval of the Paediatric Regulation, destined to increase the number of paediatric trials, the art. 4 of Directive 2001/20/EC was considered insufficient to protect children involved in a trial [12]. The 'Ethical Recommendations on paediatric trials' issued in 2008 by the EU Commission [13], represent the more advanced regulatory framework for paediatric research in Europe.

In U.S. the ethics framework for approval of CTs is quite similar. Every CT must be approved and monitored by an **Institutional Review Board** (IRB) to make sure the risks are as low as possible and potential benefits are valuable. An IRB is an independent committee of physicians, statisticians, community advocates, and others people ensuring that a clinical trial is ethical and the rights of study participants are protected. All institutions that conduct or support biomedical research involving people must, have an IRB that initially approves and periodically reviews the research.

In the U.S. legislation, details on how to conduct trials in the paediatric population are included into Subpart D (401-409) of the '*Code of Federal Regulations TITLE 45 PUBLIC WELFARE, PART 46 PROTECTION OF HUMAN SUBJECTS'*: Additional Protections for Children Involved as Subjects in Research [14]. In the code different provisions are identified on the basis of the risk level of the trial such as: 1- Research not involving greater than minimal risk; 2- Research involving greater than minimal risk but presenting the prospect of direct benefit to the individual subjects; 3- Research involving greater than minimal risk and no prospect of direct benefit to individual subjects, but likely to yield general knowledge about the subject's disorder or condition.

In addition, research that presents a reasonable opportunity to advance the understanding, prevention, or alleviation of a serious problem affecting the health or welfare of children can be also approved under special conditions.

A great relevance is given to the procedures to obtain the children assent. The permission to include a child in the trial is given by both parents in case of researches involving greater than minimal risk, and by only one parent if only a minimal risk is concerned.

2.2.1. What is changing in the regulatory framework

After its entry into force, the EU Directive 2001/20/EC has been the object of many concerns and debates leading to a new legislative process aimed to change and consolidate a EU framework by the means of a *Regulation*[2] instead of a *Directive*. In line with different reports and publications [15] the main problems dealing with the Directive were:

1. *The need for harmonisation of aspects and procedures aimed at providing ethical protection*

In contrast with the U.S. where only one Federal rule applies, in Europe Directive 2001/20/EC, given its 'non-binding' nature, needed to be implemented by all the different Member States (MSs). Therefore, the harmonisation of ethical issues and the authorisation procedures in different countries were faced but not solved in the context of Directive 2001/20/EC, and this holds true in the case of paediatric trials [16]. In addition, Directive 2001/20/EC does not provide information on how competent authorities and Ethics Committees of each MS should act in case of multi-centre and multi-national studies, while these studies prevail among the trials aimed to a MA approval.

2. *The increased burden of administrative and authoritative procedures causing delay in conducting clinical trials in Europe*

2*Regulation, unlike Directive, supersedes national laws and it is directly implemented throughout Europe without the need for transposition into national laws.*

The main cause for the decreasing number of trials conducted in Europe and for the increasing of costs is due to the double obligation to obtain an "authorisation" from the Ethic Committees and the Concerned Authorities to be repeated in all the concerned member states. As reported in the EC Explanatory Memorandum preparing a new Regulation [15]: *'The number of applications for clinical trials fell by 25% from 2007 to 2011. For non-commercial sponsors, the increase in administrative requirements due to the Directive 2001/20/EC has led to a 98% increase in administrative costs; the insurance fees have increased by 800% for industry sponsors; the average delay for launching a clinical trial has increased by 90%, to 152 days'.*

From 2016, with the application of the new EU Regulation on CTs (Regulation 536/2014) [5], a unique central procedure will be applied to be carried out through a single EU CT portal, where an homogeneous submission package (valid for all MSs) will be submitted in order to obtain the CT authorisation. The centralised submission will include also the ethical assessment, both for adults and paediatric trials.

Noticeable, the principal duty of the centralised assessment will consist in confirming or not the nature of trial that could be 'interventional' 'low-risk interventional' or 'non-interventional'.

The category of 'non-interventional trial is a novelty in the EU context and is based on a recognised 'minimal risk' of the trial (e.g. only limited procedures added to the current therapy) to which a lower level of requirements (including insurance coverage) is needed.

A "Reporting Member State", in charge to draw up an "assessment report" and the release of the authorisation, will be proposed by the sponsor corresponding to the country where it intends to carry out the Clinical Trial Application (CTA) at first. In case of multi-national trials, the other involved MSs follow a simplified procedure of assessment focused on national and ethical aspects (e.g. informed consent, recruitment of subjects, data protection, suitability of investigators and trial sites, mechanisms of insurance compensation collection of biological samples, submission fees, arrangements for rewarding/compensating investigators and subjects) for their own territory compliance.

In case of paediatric trials, for effect of a large consultation process and after relevant amendments provided by different stakeholders, in particular by the Paediatric Research Networks (such as EnPREMA[3], TEDDY[4] and GRiP[5]), the new Regulation represents a potential positive step in the process to increase the number and the quality of paediatric trials.

In more details, the Regulation states that:

• The application should refer to the PDCO opinions and related approved PIPs: The Reporting MS shall assess the application with regard to the relevance of the CT, including PDCO' opinions on PIPs.

---

3 EnPREMA is the Network of the existing Paediatric Network, stated in the Paediatric Regulation and set up at EMA

4 TEDDY is a European Network of Excellence for Paediatric Clinical Research. For more information, http://www.teddyoung.net/

5 GRiP amendments are available here http://www.grip-network.org/index.php/sfPropelFileStorage/download/name/GRiP+on+CT+regulation.pdf

- As stated in the Paediatric Regulation [2], all paediatric studies should be registered in the EU register of CTs, including studies that are part of an agreed PIP and carried out in third countries.

With regards to the preparation of submission documents, besides the rules applying for every type of trials, issues specifically dealing with paediatrics have been established as follow:

- the cover letter shall indicate the reference to trial population (minors), and a statement that the trial is part of an agreed PIP.

- the link to the Decision of the Agency on its website must be indicated in order to demonstrate that at the time of the Ethic Committee application, the Agency will have already issued the Decision about the PIP;

- the protocol shall include a justification for including minors and detail the procedures for inclusion of single subjects;

- the summary of the results of the CT shall include paediatric regulatory details (information whether the CT is a part of a PIP).

Finally, some important requirements, already stated in previous non-mandatory documents, such as the need for paediatric expertise or advice in Ethics Committees, become mandatory, such as the involvement of minors in the informed consent procedure according to their age and mental maturity. The table below shows the comparison between EU and U.S. rules on specific key topics of paediatric trials.

TOPICS	Europe (Regulation 536/2014)	U.S. (Subpart D (401-409) - Code of Federal Regulations title 45-46)
Trial authorisation/ approval	The Reporting Member State and other MSs involved authorise the trial. The assessment includes the Ethics Committees review. The reporting Member State shall assess the application with regard to the relevance of the clinical trial, including PDCO' opinions on PIPs.	An Institutional Review Board (IRB) approves and monitors the trial.
Ethics Committee rules and competencies	Experts in paediatric research are members of Ethics Committees reviewing the protocol. Alternatively the Ethics Committees take advice from external experts on clinical, ethical and psychosocial issues in the field of paediatrics.	IRBs are also allowed to invite individuals with special expertise or knowledge to provide consultation and information on individual protocols, where needed.

TOPICS	Europe (Regulation 536/2014)	U.S. (Subpart D (401-409) - Code of Federal Regulations title 45-46)
Research involving neonates	No specific rules. All rules intended to paediatric research apply. Research on non viable or of uncertain viability neonates are not cited.	Specific rules apply to neonates: a) non viable, b) of uncertain viability, c) viable (general rules apply).
Risk/Benefit	No specific rules for paediatric population.	Each IRB shall approve only Paediatric Research not involving greater than minimal risk or involving greater than minimal risk if: - presenting the prospect of direct benefit to the individual subjects - likely to yield general knowledge about the subject's disorder or condition (if minimal risk increase) - research not otherwise approvable which presents an opportunity to understand, prevent, or alleviate a serious problem affecting the health or welfare of children (under special conditions).
Minimal Risk definition	Minimal risk could be defined as the probability of harm or discomfort not greater than that ordinarily encountered in daily life or during the performance of routine physical or psychological examinations or tests.	Minimal risk means that the probability and magnitude of harm or discomfort anticipated in the research are not greater than those ordinarily encountered in daily life or during the performance of routine physical or psychological examinations or tests (this rule is not a specific paediatric rule).
Consent and assent from parents and children	Informed consent of the parents or legal representative. Assent of the children, that are entitled to receive information according their age and maturity. No minimum age is defined for providing assent. Need to obtain the consent if the subject reaches the age of legal competence during the trial	Parents (both or only one, according the level of risk) or guardians provide permission before children can be enrolled in research. Researchers must seek a child's assent unless the IRB determines that the children to be involved are not capable of providing assent, given their age, maturity, and psychological state. The regulations do not describe the information that must be provided to children but rely on IRBs to use their discretion in judging assent provisions.
Children privacy and confidentiality	No specific rules for children issued in Reg. 536/2014 (as well as in the Privacy Directive 95/46/EC)	Children confidentiality and privacy is not mentioned in FDA code.

TOPICS	Europe (Regulation 536/2014)	U.S. (Subpart D (401-409) - Code of Federal Regulations title 45-46)
	The only reference is present in the EC Ethical Recommendation,2008	FDA regulation (50.25(a)(5)) states that in seeking parents' informed consent, (5) a statement describing the extent, if any, to which confidentiality of records identifying the subject will be maintained (including the possibility of FDA inspection) must be provided. However, this point is not cited with reference to children's assent.

Table 1. EU and U.S. regulations on paediatric research

3. Paediatric plans and paediatric trials methodology

3.1. Paediatric plans

As detailed before, both EU and U.S. legislation currently require that a developmental plan (i.e. the PIP in EU and the PSP in U.S.) is approved by the responsible Official Bodies before the paediatric studies will start.

PSP is required for each drug or biological product that includes a new active ingredient, new indication, new dosage form, new dosing regimen, or new route of administration (including a biosimilar product that has not been determined to be interchangeable with the reference product).

FDA strongly regulates the timing to which the **PSP** should be presented (not later than 60 calendar days after the date of the end-of-phase 2 meeting or equivalent timing if the meeting would not have place. A PSP should include;"(i) an outline of the paediatric study or studies that the sponsor plans to conduct (including, to the extent practicable study objectives and design, age groups, relevant endpoints, and statistical approach); (ii) any request for a deferral, partial waiver, or waiver if applicable, along with any supporting information; and (iii) other information specified in the regulations"

In EU the Paediatric Regulation [2] requires **PIPs** to be submitted to the Agency early, wherever possible and the PIPs should:

- include a description of the studies and of the measures to adapt the medicineformulation to make its use more acceptable in children, such as use of a liquid formulation rather than large tablets;

- cover the needs of all age groups of children, from birth to adolescence;

- define the timing of studies in children compared to adults[6].

The table below describes the main measures included in the EMA-PDCO and FDA guidance.

TOPICS	EMA provisions (PIP)[17]	FDA provisions (PSP) [18]
WHO	The sponsor of a 'product not yet authorised' (that NOT includes variations) (art.7). The sponsor of a marketed patented drug willing to introduce variations (art. 8). The sponsor (even different from the MAH) willing to develop a paediatric study on an old off-patent drug (art. 30. This is voluntary and lead to a PUMA).	The sponsor of a 'new active ingredient' (that includes variations) (this is an obligation under PREA).
WHEN	Early, wherever possible (in time for studies to be conducted in the paediatric population, where appropriate, before MAAs are submitted). PDCO requires: "not later than upon completion of the human PK studies and initial tolerability studies, or the initiation of the adult phase-II studies (proof-of-concept studies), but before pivotal trials or confirmatory (phase-III) trials are initiated. Applications during confirmatory or phase-III trials in adults, or after starting CTs in children, are likely to be considered unjustified.	Not later than 60 calendar days after the date of the end-of-phase 2 meeting (special rules apply according with the FDA meetings timing). For products for life-threatening diseases, at the end-of-phase 1 meetings.
which AGE TO COVER	All the paediatric population's groups (birth to 18 years).	All relevant paediatric populations (birth to 16 years).
CONTENTS	**Administrative and product information** also including: - A.5: Regulatory information on CTs related to the condition (EAA). A.6: Marketing authorisation status of the medicinal product. A.7: Advice from any regulatory authorities. A.8: Orphan drug status in the EEA.	n.a.
	Overview of the **Disease Condition** in the Paediatric Population: - pathophysiology of the disease,	Overview of the **Disease Condition** in the Pediatric Population: - pathophysiology of the disease,

6 EMA website: http://www.ema.europa.eu/ema/index.jsp?curl=pages/regulation/document_listing/document_list-ing_000293.jsp&mid=WC0b01ac0580025b91

TOPICS	EMA provisions (PIP)[17]	FDA provisions (PSP) [18]
	- diagnosis, - currently available treatments and/or prevention - incidence and prevalence of the disease.	- diagnosis, -currently available treatments and/or prevention - incidence and prevalence of the disease.
	Overview of the **Drug or Biological Product:** - mechanism of action - potential therapeutic benefits - Other possible therapeutic uses of the drug	Overview of the **Drug or Biological Product:** - mechanism of action - potential therapeutic benefits - Other possible therapeutic uses of the drug
	Extrapolation could include: - efficacy from adults to children or from older to younger children, - safety information from adults to children can also be included, - modelling of PK and/or PD if used for decision-making.	Overview of Planned **extrapolation** to Specific Paediatric Populations: - any plans to extrapolate efficacy from adult or from one paediatric age group to another including neonates, - extrapolation for other drugs in the same class, can be considered as supportive information,
	Request for Drug-specific waivers (global or partial): The requirement to submit a PIP shall be waived for specific medicinal products or classes of medicinal products that: are likely to be ineffective or unsafe in part or all of the paediatric population; are intended for conditions that occur only in adult populations; do not represent a significant therapeutic benefit over existing treatments for paediatric patients.	**Request for Drug-Specific Waiver(s):** (a) Necessary studies are impossible or highly impracticable (because, for example, the number of patients is so small or the patients are geographically dispersed). (b) There is evidence strongly suggesting that the drug or biological product would be ineffective or unsafe in all paediatric age groups. (c) The drug or biological product (1) does not represent a meaningful therapeutic benefit and (2) is not likely to be used in a substantial number of paediatric patients Partial waiver provision also apply: -if attempts to produce a paediatric formulation failed - for a specific age group.
	Planned **Nonclinical and Clinical Studies and timeline**	Planned **Nonclinical and Clinical Studies and timeline**
	Paediatric Formulation Development	**Pediatric Formulation Development**

Table 2. Main provision to apply for PIP and PSP

Considering the two described systems, we noted some interesting differences. In particular, while the EU Paediatric Regulation covers all the paediatric medicines (in-patent, off-patent, under development) and deserves incentives only to the off-patent drugs, in U.S. two different regimens apply for: a) medicines to be granted a paediatric exclusivity after a solicited request (Written Request) as stated in BPCA, and b) medicines for which a PSP is mandatory under PREA. Noticeably, the medicines that are under PREA can also be granted a Written Request, allowing to receive a paediatric exclusivity (see also Fig.1).

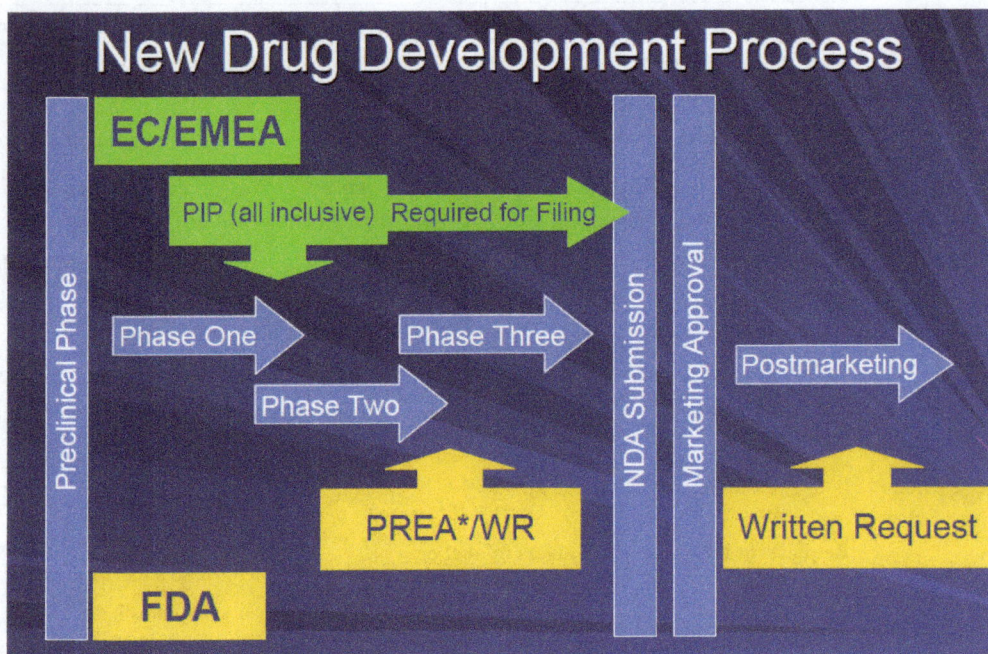

Figure 1. Paediatric drug regulatory process in EU and U.S. (source: FDA and EMA Paediatric Regulatory Process: J Temek, MD, FDA website)

Moreover, the paediatric developmental plan procedures of the two Agencies are not completely aligned mainly due to the different regulatory status provided by the different regulations and the different approaches of the two Committees. In particular:

- In EU, unlike in the U.S., a MAA (Marketing Authorisation Application) (equivalent to NDA in U.S.) must contain the results of the paediatric studies conducted in compliance with the agreed PIP (or waiver or deferral). In lack of this, the MA cannot be granted.

- In EU, the paediatric product development is requested earlier in the regulatory process than in U.S.

- In EU, the PDCO, the counter part to the PeRC in the U.S, unlike the PeRC, makes binding decisions.

- FDA "feasibility " criteria for waivers do not exist in the EU legislation. Thus, a study may be required in EU but waived in the U.S. under PREA.

- FDA may request or grant paediatric studies under BPCA, using the voluntary financial incentive, even during the PSP process, while in Europe patented drugs do not have access to financial incentives.

- Finally, unlike the U.S., the EU does not have a public process whereby paediatric focused post-marketing safety reviews are presented to an Advisory Committee.

These differences still represent an obstacle to a prompt development of paediatric drugs in a global context. An intensive work aimed at merging the paediatric efforts at the two levels is highly required and desirable. To this aim, currently a process of 'Information Exchange' is in place to discuss product-specific paediatric development issues and general scientific/ regulatory/safety issues. The Japan Pharmaceuticals and Medical Devices Act (PMDA) has recently joined this initiative as observer.

3.2. Paediatric trials methodology

3.2.1. The ICH-E11 guideline

Before specific paediatric legislations were in place, regulators, companies and clinicians were well aware that the current methodological approach, based on well-designed RCTs, could result difficult to apply in selected cases such as the paediatric population.

In particular, in paediatrics the following issues are challenging large population available for RCTs, randomisation procedure, placebo use, availability of validate paediatric endpoints, appropriate outcomes, long-term effects evaluations, etc.

The ICH-E11 Guideline, issued in 2000 at international level [19], has represented the main international reference for paediatric CTs and the methodological standard to perform paediatric CTs scientifically correct, and ethical in the same time. It still represents the only standard acceptable by the Regulatory Authorities.

The guideline milestones are:

- Paediatric patients should be given medicines that are properly evaluated for their use in the intended population.

- Product development programs should include paediatric studies when paediatric use is anticipated.

- Development of appropriated products in paediatric patients should be timely and, often requires the development of paediatric formulations.

- The rights of paediatric participants should be protected and they should be shielded from undue risks.

- Responsibility should be shared among companies, regulatory authorities, health professionals and society as a whole.

- Marketing Authorisation Holders (MAHs), and competent authorities/medicine regulatory agencies are the two major stakeholders responsible for medicine safety at the time of authorisation.

The approach to the clinical programme needs to be clearly addressed with the regulatory authorities at an early stage and then periodically during the development process. To this aim, the guideline has provided specific indications on trial characteristics, including:

- when initiating a paediatric program for a medicinal product (need of a medicinal products, therapeutic benefits, lack of alternatives);

- timing of initiation of paediatric studies during medicinal product development (need that preliminary safety/tolerability data are known in adults);

- types of studies (PK, PK/PD, efficacy, safety); according to the principle to avoid unnecessary studies in all paediatric age groups, large efficacy studies should be considered only when extrapolation of results from adults (or from older children to younger) is not feasible; on the contrary, PK studies and short and long term safety evaluations are always required.

- age categories: five paediatric ages have been identified from neonates to adolescents and each paediatric group should be given medicines that have been appropriately evaluated for their use;

- special rules for ethic approval of paediatric clinical investigation (including children right to be informed and privacy).

3.2.2. The ICH-E11 modification process

Currently, a revision of the ICH-E11 guideline is ongoing. It derives by the relevant changes occurred in the last years, both at scientific and regulatory levels. **Innovative methods of research are in progress** to overcome the existing paediatric studies limitations and are having a profound impact on the assessment procedures at the regulatory agencies level. The main novelties in the field are:

- use of innovative PK/PD methodologies for dosing and efficacy extrapolation exercises [20];

- use of population PK PD (pop PKPD) models to assess different clinical scenarios without exposing children to any risk to explore new drug [21];

- use of alternative statistical approaches to reduce the size of the experimental population and the number of the trials needed in the clinical phase [22].

The updated E11 Guideline as proposed in August 2014, aims to include the new scientific and technical knowledge advances in paediatric drug development in a new regulatory guidance. To this aim, an addendum to the ICH Topic E11 guideline will be finalised by November 2015 with the following revised topics:

- Timing of paediatric development: need for more harmonisation and clarity to guide the developers of paediatric medicines; it is proposed to focus on the multi-national/multi-regional status of many paediatric trials for which the requirements of multiple regulatory authorities should be satisfied.

- Age classification and paediatric subsets including neonates: there is the need for better understanding the developmental process in paediatric subsets, especially neonates and infants.

- Ethical considerations in paediatric studies: there is the need for enhance the ethical considerations in paediatric studies.

- Types of studies and methodology of CTs: the advances in paediatric CTs design and conduct should be incorporated in the ICH-E11 guidance including: innovative study designs, development of clinical outcome assessments, development of validated age-appropriate clinical endpoints and surrogate markers (biomarkers), specific scales for measuring outcomes particularly in case of younger age groups,

- Common rules to apply appropriate principles for extrapolation of data (from adult to paediatric populations or older children or different indication). This last point could possibly lead both the Agencies to agree a Paediatric Algorithm firstly proposed at FDA level and still now not regularly adopted at EMA level.

- Formulation challenges in paediatric drug development: need for developing specific comprehensive guidance on formulation development for children.

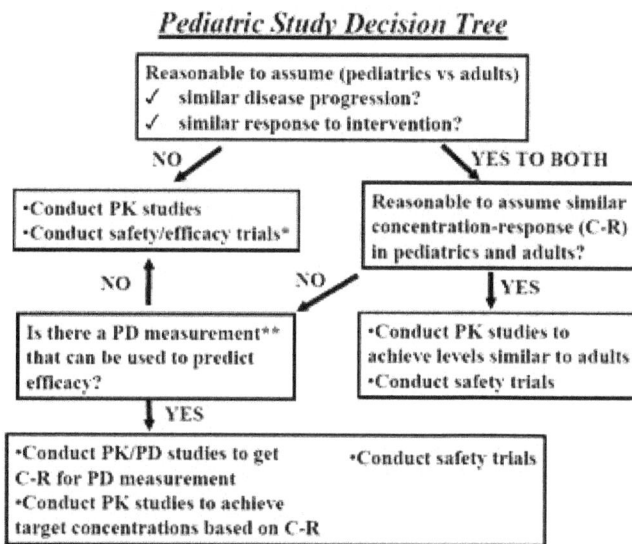

Figure 2. Paediatric Study decision tree for bridging efficacy data in an adult population to a paediatric population (source: FDA)

4. Paediatric trial incentives and main results of the existing legislation

As stated before, important changes both in U.S. and EU legislations both imposed the pharmaceutical industry to study medicines in children, with the aim to increase the number of paediatric trials to be conducted, to reduce the existing gap. A comparison between the two regulations in terms of impact on paediatric trials is difficult, because of the existing differences on requirements and incentives provided in the two contexts, as well as the very limited amount of published data on the regulations results. As a general finding, it seems that public funding provisions and active strategies both in Europe and US have a strong relevance in improving the current situation through the conduction of studies in children and adolescent in the world.

4.1. Impact of paediatric regulation on paediatric trials

In Europe, the most recent available document summarising the main results of the Paediatric Regulation has been released by the EC covering the period 2007-2012. It provides relevant information on PIPs and paediatric trials approved in Europe. It states that:

By the end of 2012, the Agency had agreed 600 PIPs (more than 1.000 presented). Of these, 453 were for medicines that were not yet authorised in the EU (Article 7), while the remaining ones are related to new indications for patent-protected products (Article 8) or PUMA (Article 30).These plans cover a broad range of therapeutic areas, as shown in the figure below and all the paediatric ages including neonates.

Therapeutic areas addressed by the paediatric investigation plans (2007-2011)

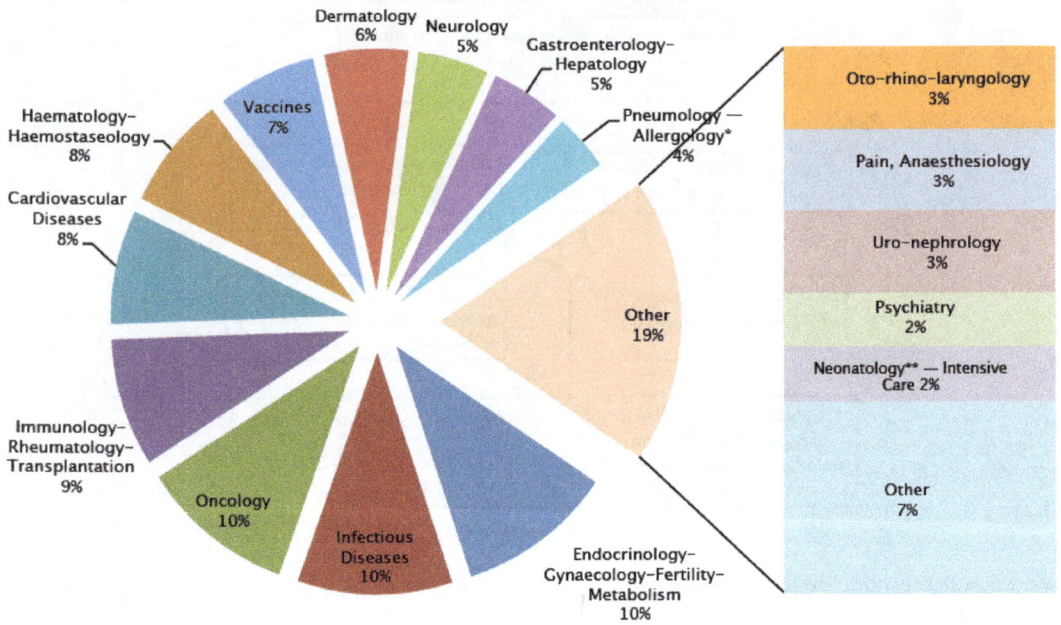

Source: EMA Paediatric database.

Figure 3. Therapeutic areas addressed by the PIPs (2007-2011).[7]

Regarding the number of paediatric trials, the reference derived by the official source Eu-draCT[8] demonstrates that the number of trials in children did not increase after the approval of the Regulation but remained stable between 2006 and 2012, corresponding to an average of 350 trials per year. However, until recently EudraCT was limited to paediatric trials com-

---

7 Progress Report on the Paediatric Regulation COM (2013) 443 Final

8 EUDRACT is the EU register of all (ongoing, completed, prematurely terminated) trials with medicinal products taking place in the European Union and those studying medicines for paediatric use contained in an agreed PIP carried out in third countries.

mencing in the EU, while data on paediatric trials that are part of a PIP and conducted outside the EU have only become available since spring 2011.

	2005	2006	2007	2008	2009	2010	2011	2012
Paediatric trials (number)	254	316	355	342	404	379	334	332
Paediatric trials that are part of an agreed PIP*	2	1	2	6	16	30	76	76
Proportion of paediatric trials that are part of an agreed PIP among paediatric trials*	1 %	0 %	1 %	2 %	4 %	8 %	23 %	23 %
Total number of trials (adults and / or children)	3 350	3 979	4 749	4 512	4 445	4 026	3 809	3 698
Proportion of paediatric trials of all trials	8 %	8 %	7 %	8 %	9 %	10 %	9 %	9 %

Source: EudraCT Data Warehouse using a predefined query on 6 March 2013 and counting the first authorised trial only, in the case of more than one Member State.

Table 3. Paediatric Clinical Trials by year of authorisation.

Of the total number of trials conducted in the last years after the approval of the Paediatric Regulation, only a few have been included in the Marketing Authorisation documentation, in order to obtain a paediatric indication.

In particular, data from TEDDY-EPMD[9], a database including information on the paediatric medicines approved by EMA, demonstrate that, after the implementation of the Paediatric Regulation, on a total of almost 70 new active substances approved for children by EMA, 33 applications include a paediatric plan (all available in 'COM (2013) 443 Final' at www.ema.europa.eu). Additional 12 medicines received a paediatric indication using results of the existing studies after reviewing all the studies at central level (art.45-46 of the Paediatric Regulation) (26).

4.2. Impact of FDA rules on paediatric trials

Between the 1998 and 2011 the FDA issued ~340 Written Requests for new paediatric studies, today 533 labelling changes associated with BPCA and PREA acts have been approved (BPCA only = 161; BPCA + PREA = 73; PREA only = 249; Rule = 49; None = 1), which is significantly higher if compared to the number of labelling changes approved in Europe.

On the basis of these data, according to Lynn Yao it is possible to affirm that: 'Before BPCA and PREA became law, more than 80% of the drugs approved for adult use were being used

---

9 www.teddyoung.net

in children, even though their safety and effectiveness had not been established in children. Today that number has been reduced to about 50%. (http://blogs.fda.gov/fdavoice/index).

With New Pediatric Studies	N°484
PK	122
Efficacy	133
Safety	281
With no New Pediatric Studies	N°49
TOTAL	N°533

Table 4. FDA- New Pediatric Labelling Information Database (1998-2014)

An analysis performed on 174 CTs completed for Pediatric Exclusivity published in May 2010 [23], demonstrated that the U.S. is the most frequent site for conducting CTs, followed by Europe. However, 65% of paediatric trials were conducted in at least 1 country outside the U.S. and 11% did not include any sites in the U.S. Fifty-four countries were represented, and 38% of trials enrolled patients in more than 1 site located in a developing/transition country.

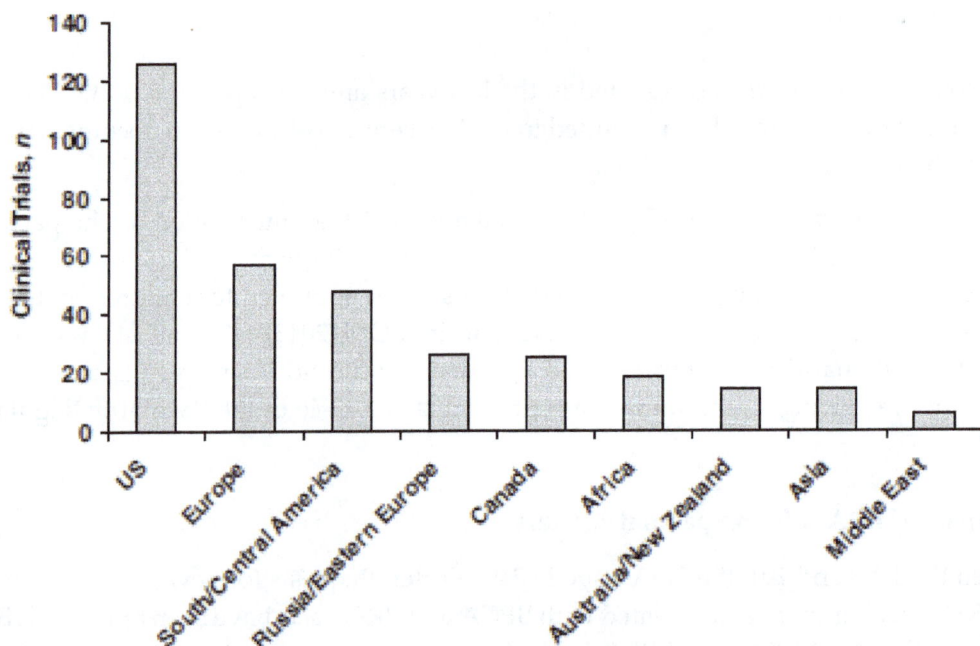

Figure 4. Location of 174 trials included in BPCA act.

Under these programs, ~436 separate studies that enrolled ~56,000 children were performed over a 5-years period. An example of results achieved by public incentives to paediatric research is provided by an extensive study evaluating outcomes of BPCA procedures granted from 2002 to 2007 [24]. This study, analysing 99 Written Request[10] applications submitted to FDA, reports that:

- 257 paediatric CTs (average 2.6 trials per application) have been conducted, covering approximately 60 indications. The most commonly studied indications were bacterial infections;

- the paediatric trials enrolled at least 46,000 subjects in 5,850 clinical centres;

- all paediatric ages have been addressed, but most of patients were aged 12-17 years old;

- in contrast with the sponsors' trend to shift the location of adult trials away from the country, the U.S. remains the dominant location for paediatric trials (54%), although most paediatric drug programmes are global;

- The trials were distributed across more than 60 countries and the EU contributed 11% of the centres and 7% of patients

4.3. Funded studies for paediatric medicines in EU and US

Both in EU and in U.S., funding is devoted to better support paediatric drugs development. Initiatives in this direction are justified under many points of view such as:

Relatively few trials specifically studying the younger age groups, (neonates, infants and toddlers) were approved. In fact it has been demonstrated [23] that from 1998 through 2010, only 23 (6 percent) of the 365 labelling changes, after the submission of new paediatric studies, included the addition of information from studies with neonates.

The most commonly studied indications do not necessarily reflect greatest paediatric thera-peutic needs but closely matched the distribution of these drugs over the adult market, and not the drug utilization by children [23].

Off-label drugs are poorly studied. Neither the financial benefit for the pharmaceutical companies in USA, neither the new MA, the PUMA, ad hoc created in EU, demonstrated to be attractive for the commercial sponsors.

Strategies have put in place to overcome this limitation mainly based on funding ad hoc studies and promoting non-commercial, research-driven paediatric trial. Positive examples of these strategies in EU and in US are described below.

1.   *FP7 Research Framework provisions to develop off-patent drugs currently used off-label in children*

The EU supports research into paediatric medicinal products through its multi-annual Framework Programme for Research and Technological Development.

According to article 40 of the Regulation, the European Research Framework Programs should reserve funds to support PUMAs in case of off-patent drugs recognised as of high therapeutic interest for children and included in a 'Priority List' (PL) adopted, on annual basis, by the EMA (European Medicines Agency) through its Paediatric Committee.

---

10 A Written Request may be initiated by FDA or in response to a Proposed Pediatric Study Request (PPSR).

In the last 6 years such EC funds have been delivered through the Seventh Framework Programme for Research (FP7-FRP). In particular, with reference to HEALTH-(2007-2013) Programme area, five calls for proposal have been released with reference to the topic 4.2-1 'to develop off-patent medicinal products for the paediatric population'.

From 2007 to 2013, 20 projects were granted with funds. The total amount awarded to these projects is 98.6 million Euros.

The twenty approved projects are investigating a total of 24 active substances, in 10 therapeutic areas (see tab. 5). In particular a total of 71 studies have been funded, involving almost 400 investigational sites in EU and non-EU countries, 246 partners of whom 51 are private companies and around 7000 children (representing 23% of all the paediatric patients included in clinical trials in Europe from 2007 to 2011) were recruited. Eighty percent of the projects include studies to develop new age-appropriate formulations or dosage form and all paediatric subgroups are represented in the clinical trials with particular reference to preterm and/or term newborns.

Project	Active Substance(S)	Addressed paediatric indication(s)	Therapeutic area
TINN	Ciprofloxacin* / Fluconazole	treatment of infections in preterm and term newborns	Infections
TINN2	Azithromycin	treatment of infections in preterm and term newborns	
NeoMero	Meropenem	treatment of late-onset sepsis in neonates and infants aged <3 months treatment of bacterial meningitis in neonates and infants aged <3 months	
NeoVanc	Vancomycin	treatment of late onset bacterial sepsis caused by vancomycin susceptible bacteria in neonates and infants aged under three months	
NeoOpioid	Morphine / Fentanyl	treatment of acute pain	Pain
GAPP	Gabapentin	treatment of chronic pain	
Loulla & Philla	Methotrexate* / 6-Mercaptopurine*	treatment of Acute Lymphoblastic Leukemia	Malignant neoplasms
03K	Cyclophosphamide / Temozolomide	treatment of paediatric malignancies	
EPOC	Doxorubicin*	treatment of childhood cancer	
HIP trial	Dopamine	management of hypotension in preterm newborns	Cardiology
NeoCirc	Dobutamine	treatment of systemic hypotension in infants	
LENA	Enalapril	cardiac failure in children	

Project	Active Substance(S)	Addressed paediatric indication(s)	Therapeutic area
NEMO	Bumetanide	treatment of neonatal seizures in babies with hypoxic ischemic encephalopathy	Neurology
KIEKIDS	Ethosuximide	treatment of absence and myoclonic epilepsy	
TAIN	Hydrocortisone*	treatment of adrenal insufficiency in neonates and infants	Endocrinology
METFIZZ	Metformin	treatment of polycystic ovary syndrome	
CloSed	Clonidine*	Sedation in intensive care	Intensive care/ anaesthesiology
DEEP	Deferiprone*	treatment of chronic iron overload	Haematology
PERS	Risperidone	treatment of conduct disorder treatment of schizophrenia	Child & adolescent psychiatry
NEuroSIS	Budesonide*	prevention of bronchopulmonary dysplasia	Respiratory and cardiovascular disorders

* received an Orphan Drug designation (four in the same indication addressed by the project)

Table 5. FP7 approved projects in Europe ([25]

These data demonstrated that paediatric studies receiving support from the EU institutions are attractive even outside Europe and also for the private companies engaged in view of the final PUMA approval.

Furthermore, to date, 22% of the planned enrolment for these trials is completed, that is in contrast with the reported low recruitment capacity and difficulties with the conduct of paediatric trials in Europe.

2.   *The Pediatric Trials Network (PTN)*

Sponsored by the Eunice Kennedy Shriver National Institute of Child Health and by the Human Development (NICHD), the Pediatric Trials Network (PTN) is an alliance of clinical research sites located around the United States that are cooperating in the design and conduct of paediatric CTs. PTN relates to BPCA since funds are devoted to develop research driven studies in the area where the investments of private companies are very limited and the FDA incentives resulted insufficient.

As European Consortia, the PTN is studying the formulation, dosing, efficacy, and safety of drugs used in paediatric patients. In keeping with the goals of the Best Pharmaceuticals for Children Act, data collected from PTN trials will help regulators to revise drug labels for safer and more effective use in infants and children.

Currently 20 PTN trials are in progress, the results of 4 of them have been published. Noticeably, 3 active substances funded within PTN are also funded under EU FP7 projects. The list of the projects is available on the FDA website and results are continuously updated.

Trial	Status
Metronidazole	Enrolment and analysis completed, clinical study report submitted to FDA, results published
TAPE	Enrolment completed in less than 2 months, results published
Acyclovir	Enrolment complete, analysis in progress, results published
Hydroxyurea	Enrolment completed
POPS	Enrolment ongoing
Lisinopril PK	Database locked; analyses in progress
Midazolam	Data analysis in progress
Ampicillin	Results published
Obesity informatics	Analysis in progress
Anti-staph trio	Enrolment ongoing
Sildenafil	Enrolment ongoing, interim PK analysis
Clindamycin obesity	Enrolment ongoing
Fluconazole safety	Meta-analysis ongoing
Midazolam obesity	Protocol in development
Acyclovir phase II	Protocol complete, opening sites
Pantoprazole	Enrolment ongoing
Pediatrix meta-analysis	Protocol complete, analysis ongoing
Antibiotic safety (SCAMP)	Protocol complete, selecting sites
Diuretic safety	Protocol complete, opening sites
Methadone pharmacokinetics	Enrolment ongoing

Table 6. PTN trials

Taking into account these results, we consider that the problems issued by paediatric drug development are only partially solved. Regulations are now quite similar both with reference to the requirements and the incentives provided but profound differences still exist in the practical application.

The U.S. remains the dominant location for paediatric trials but the balance may change in the future. EU results in increasing the numbers of paediatric approved drugs are still disappointing but in EU the number of studies in specific categories (neonates) and of projects responding to real therapeutic need (off-label) is higher than in US. However the approved drugs in this category still remain very few (on a total of 533 labelling changes in U.S. only 19 off-patent drugs have been the object of a FDA Written Request while in EU only 2 PUMA have been granted till now).

5. Conclusive remarks

Despite many regulatory provisions have globally focused, in EU and in US, the attention on the paediatric themes, some significant issues have to be further improved in order to fill in the existing gaps. Some of the most relevant criticisms are summarised below.

1. Especially in EU, it has been recognised that paediatric development strategy is still often perceived as a regulatory obligation, more than an integral part of the whole medicinal development process [26].

2. Paediatric provisions demonstrated not to be able to specifically address the paediatric needs. For example, in Europe most of the therapeutic needs periodically identified by expert groups at EMA/PDCO are still uncovered by PIPs and/or PUMAs. In the U.S. there is a discrepancy between the drug prescription pattern in children and the drugs granted paediatric exclusivity. Actually, the majority of drugs granted paediatric exclusivity is rarely used by children and drugs frequently used by children are underrepresented in the paediatric studies aimed to obtain exclusivity [27].

3. The field of neonatology is quite critical. In Europe, the number of neonates included in clinical trials substantially increasedafter the Paed. Reg. entered into force [3]. However many neonatal therapeutic needs recognised by EMA/PDCO are still unmet [28]. Similarly, in the U.S. only a small percentage (6%) of the labelling changes involving the submission of new paediatric studies included the addition of information from studies with neonates [29].

4. With reference to the availability of drug formulations suitable for children, a lack of age-appropriate formulations, in terms of safety of excipients, palatability, acceptability, dosing flexibility, accuracy and practical handling still exists [3]. In U.S., a public-funded Pediatric Formulations Platform[11] is trying to fill this gap but no similar initiatives have been identified in Europe.

5. Deferral measures have been introduced in both regions to avoid delays, provoked by paediatric development, to the availability of drugs for adults. As a negative counterpart, deferrals are deeply impairing paediatric drug development: 63% of new medicines intended for both adults and children have a deferral in the agreed PIP [3]. In the U.S, despite nearly all (98%) of the rationales for deferrals were consistent with the law, the amount of deferred studies delayed and/or pending is relevant (78%). It has been estimated that the number of pending studies grew by 50%, while the number of delayed studied increased by more than 80% [30].

6. Another example of criticism in paediatric drugs availability deals with rare diseases: both in EU and in the U.S, very few medicinal products for rare diseases affecting children have a paediatric indication[12]. As a consequence, in the U.S. (but not in EU), specific orphan

11 http://bpca.nichd.nih.gov/collaborativeefforts/initiatives/pages/index.aspx

12 data deriving from EuOrphan, a database of EU and U.S. orphan drugs hosted by Gianni Benzi Foundation

programs for paediatrics have been recently proposed (Rare Pediatric Disease Priority Review Voucher Program). The first voucher was awarded under this program in February 2014, but it is still too early to measure the impact.

7. Finally, a lack of appropriate measures to incentive paediatric research has been observed especially in EU. As already mentioned, the PUMA has been unsuccessful until now and, despite the positive results achieved by the projects for the development of off-patent drugs, the specific funding programme set up from 2007 to 2013 under the EU Seventh Framework Programme has not been renewed in Horizon 2020.

On the basis of these few considerations, EU and U.S. regulators should continue to discuss coordinated approaches and to share results.

In particular, these efforts should be concentrate to minimize unnecessary paediatric trials and to optimize trial design, so that the limited paediatric populations available are enrolled only in ethically implemented, scientifically important trials.

Acknowledgements

This project has received funding from the European Union's Seventh Framework Programme for research, technological development and demonstration under grant agreement n° 261060 - GRiP (Global Research in Paediatrics).

Author details

Adriana Ceci[1*], Viviana Giannuzzi[1], Donato Bonifazi[2], Mariagrazia Felisi[2], Fedele Bonifazi[2] and Lucia Ruggieri[3]

*Address all correspondence to: adriceci.uni@gmail.com

1 Fondazione per la Ricerca Farmacologica Gianni Benzi onlus, Valenzano, Italy

2 Consorzio per Valutazioni Biologiche e Farmacologiche, Pavia, Italy

3 Gruppo Italiano per gli Studi di Farmacoeconomia, Pavia, Italy

References

[1] U.S. Code 21 CFR Part 201, Specific Requirements on Content and Format of Labeling for Human Prescription Drugs; Revision of "Pediatric Use" Subsection in the Labeling; Final Rule, December 13, 1994 (FR 59 64240).

[2] European Parliament and Council of the European Union. Regulation (EC) No 1901/2006 of 12 December 2006 on medicinal products for paediatric use and amending Regulation (EEC) No 1768/92, Directive 2001/20/EC, Directive 2001/83/EC and Regulation (EC) No 726/2004. Official Journal of the European Union, 2006,L 378/1.

[3] EMA/PDCO 5-year Report to the European Commission General report on the experience acquired as a result of the application of the Paediatric Regulation (2012) EMA/428172/2012.

[4] European Parliament and the Council of the European Union. Directive 2001/20/EC of 4 April 2001 on the approximation of the laws, regulations and administrative provisions of the Member States relating to the implementation of good clinical practice in the conduct of clinical trials on medicinal products for human use. Official Journal L121, 01/05/2001.

[5] European Parliament and Council of the European Union. Regulation (Eu) No 536/2014 Of The European Parliament And Of The Council of 16 April 2014 on clinical trials on medicinal products for human use, and repealing Directive 2001/20/EC. Official Journal of the European Union, 2014, L158.

[6] Food and Drugs Administration, Food Safety Modernization Act (FSMA) of 1997 P.L. 105-115 111 Stat. 2296

[7] Food and Drugs Administration, Best Pharmaceuticals for Children Act (BPCA) of 2002 P. L. 107-109. Stat. 1789

[8] Food and Drugs Administration, Paediatric Research Equity Act (PREA) of 2003 P. L. 108-155. Stat. S 650

[9] European Parliament and Council of the European Union. Directive 2005/28/EC of 8 April 2005 laying down principles and detailed guidelines for good clinical practice as regards investigational medicinal products for human use, as well as the requirements for authorisation of the manufacturing or importation of such products. Official Journal of the European Union, 2005, L91.

[10] European Medicines Agency. ICH Topic E 6 (R1): Guideline for Good Clinical Practice. CPMP/ICH/135/95. July 2002.

[11] European Parliament and Council of the European Union. Regulation (EC) No 726/2004 of 31 March 2004 laying down Community procedures for the authorisation and supervision of medicinal products for human and veterinary use and establishing a European Medicines Agency. Official Journal of the European Union, 2006,L 136/1.

[12] Altavilla A, Giaquinto C, Giocanti D, Manfredi C, Aboulker JP, Bartoloni F, et al. Activity of ethics committees in Europe on issues related to clinical trials in paediatrics: Results of a survey. Pharmaceuticals Policy and Law. 2009; 11(1.2):79-87.

[13] European Commission. Ethical Considerations for Clinical Trials on medicinal products conducted with the paediatric population - Recommendations of the Ad Hoc

Group for the development of implementing guidelines for Directive 2001/20/EC relating to good clinical practice in the conduct of clinical trials on medicinal products
for human use, 2008.

[14] Code of Federal Regulations, Title 45 Public Welfare Department of Health and Human Services Part 46 Protection of Human Subjects, 2009.

[15] European Commission, Proposal for a Regulation of the European Parliament and of
the Council on clinical trials on medicinal products for human use, and repealing Directive 2001/20/EC (COM(2012) 369 final), 17.7.2012

[16] Altavilla A, Giaquinto C, Ceci A. European survey on ethical and legal framework of
clinical trials in paediatrics: results and perspectives. J Int Bioethique. 2008; 19(3): p.
17-48.

[17] European Commission. Communication from the Commission — Guideline on the
format and content of applications for agreement or modification of a paediatric investigation plan and requests for waivers or deferrals and concerning the operation
of the compliance check and on criteria for assessing significant studies (2014/C
338/01).

[18] Food and Drugs Administration, Guidance for Industry Pediatric Study Plans: FDA,
July 2013.

[19] European Medicines Agency. ICH Topic E 11. Clinical Investigation of Medicinal
Products in the Paediatric Population Note for guidance on clinical investigation of
medicinal products in the paediatric population (CPMP/ICH/2711/99).

[20] De Cock RF, Piana C, Krekels EH, Danhof M, Allegaert K, Knibbe CA. The role of
population PK-PD modelling in paediatric clinical research. Eur J Clin Pharmacol.
2011 May;67 Suppl 1:5-16.

[21] Knibbe C, Della Pasqua O, Danhof M. Personal communication: Introduction to population PKPD modelling in paediatric paediatric clinical pharmacology. Available at:
http://www.ema.europa.eu/docs/en_GB/document_library/Presentation/2009/11/
WC500009645.pdf

[22] Ceci A, Catapano M, Manfredi C, Wong I et al. Drug Development – A Case Study
Based Insight into Modern Strategies, edited by Chris Rundfeldt, p.cm. ISBN
978-953-307-257-9.

[23] Dunne J. et al. Globalization Facilitates Pediatric Drug Development in the 21st Century, Drug Information Journal, Vol. 44, pp. 757–765, 2010.

[24] Pasquali S. et al. Globalization of Paediatric Research, Paediatrics Vol 126: September
2010.

[25] Ruggieri L, Giannuzzi V, Baiardi P, Bonifazi F, Davies EH, Giaquinto C, Bonifazi D,
Felisi M, Chiron C, Pressler R, Rabe H, Whitaker MJ, Neubert A, Jacqz-Aigrain E,
Eichler I, Turner MA, Ceci A; on behalf of the GRiP Consortium. Successful private-

public funding of paediatric medicines research: lessons from the EU programme to fund research into off-patent medicines. Eur J Pediatr. 2014 Sep 23.

[26] General report on experience acquired as a result of the application of the Paediatric Regulation, summary of the replies to the public consultation, Brussels, SANCO/D5/FS/ci D(2013) 27105

[27] Boots I, Sukhai RN, Klein RH, Holl RA, Wit JM, Cohen AF, Burggraaf J.Stimulation programs for pediatric drug research – do children really benefit? Eur J Pediatr. 2007 Aug;166(8):849-55. Epub 2007 Jan 17.

[28] European Medicines Agency/Paediatric Committee (2007-2013) priority list for studies on off-patent paediatric medicinal products

[29] Institute of Medicine. Safe and Effective Medicines for Children: Studies Conducted Under the Best Pharmaceuticals for Children Act and the Pediatric Research Equity Act. Washington, DC: National Academies Press; 2012.

[30] Outcomes of Written Requests, Requirements, Studies, and Labeling Changes Cover of Safe and Effective Medicines for Children in "Safe and Effective Medicines for Children: Pediatric Studies Conducted Under the Best Pharmaceuticals for Children Act and the Pediatric Research Equity Act." Committee on Pediatric Studies Conducted Under the Best Pharmaceuticals for Children Act (BPCA) and the Pediatric Research Equity Act (PREA); Board on Health Sciences Policy; Institute of Medicine; Field MJ, Boat TF, editors. Washington (DC): National Academies Press (US); 2012 Feb 29

7

Current Management and Novel Therapeutic Strategies to Combat Chronic Delta Hepatitis

Hrvoje Roguljic, Sonja Sarcevic, Robert Smolic,
Nikola Raguz Lucic, Aleksandar Vcev and
Martina Smolic

Additional information is available at the end of the chapter

1. Introduction

Forty years ago Mario Rizzeto's group identified a new antigen-antibody system (delta antibody and delta antigen (HDAg)) in HBsAg carriers with severe hepatitis [1, 2]. Further experiments in chimpanzees showed that this HDAg marked transmissible pathogen requires coexistence of HBV infection for its life cycle, proving its defective nature which requires HBsAg for transmission and replication [3]. As the cause of hepatitis D was identified, a virion particle (Figure 1.) composed of outer coat containing HBV envelope proteins (HBsAg) and inner nuclocapsid was described [4]. Internal nuclear like structure is comprised of single stranded, circular RNA molecule of 1700 nucleotides associated with two distinctive forms of hepatitis D antigen (HDAg), small and large subunit [5, 6]. Although HDV in its structure possesses HBsAg, HDV is classified as separate pathogen with own genus called *Deltavirus* [7]. This unusual virus is the smallest infectious pathogen in human virology, with unique replication cycle unknown to animal cells. During replication process a viral RNA is transcribed by hosts RNA polymerases [8], which usually transcribe DNA molecules, and after transcription HDV RNA is cleaved by its own ribozyme [9].

Dependence on the HBsAg presence results in two patterns of HDV infection. HDV can be transmitted simultaneously with HBV (co-infection pattern) or infection may occur at preceding HBV infected individual (super-infection pattern). Due to differences of HDV acquisition clinical course and outcome of HDV infection varies. However, many studies have shown that HDV infection causes more severe liver disease [10] and more rapid progression to cirrhosis [11] than HBV mono-infection alone.

HDV virion

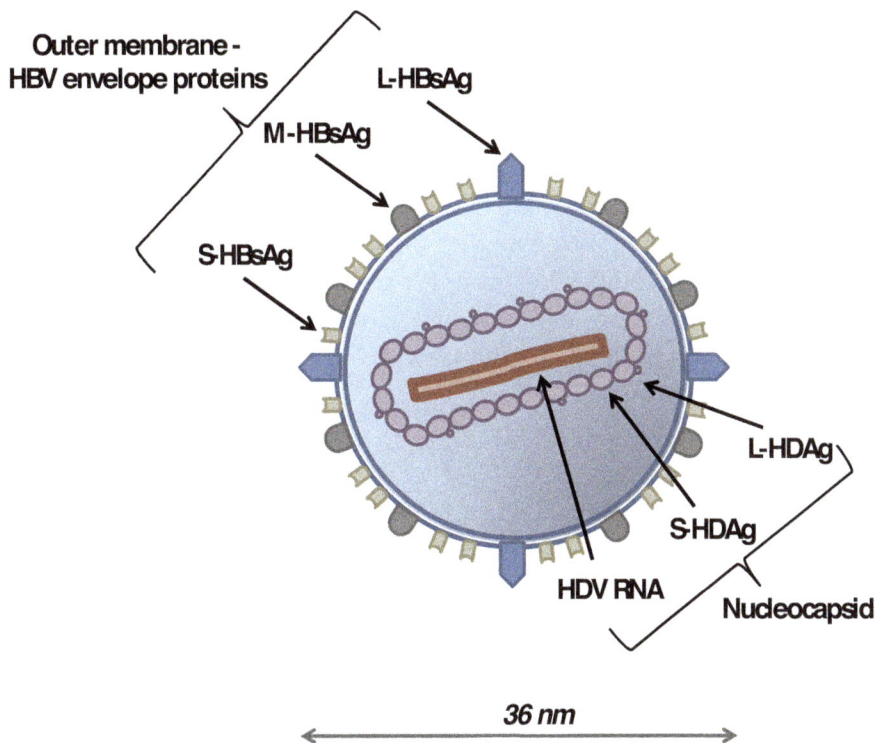

Figure 1. Structure of HDV virion. HDV is composed of outer membrane, HBV envelope proteins within a phospholipid bilayer, and inner nucleocapsid consisting of viral RNA and hepatitis delta antigens. L-HBsAg=large hepatitis B surface antigen. M-HBsAg=medium hepatitis B surface antigen. S-HBsAg=small hepatitis B surface antigen. HDV RNA=hepatitis D virus RNA. L-HDAg=large hepatitis D antigen. S-HDAg=small hepatitis D antigen.

Although many details regarding HDV viral cycle are revealed, therapy of HDV has not progressed. To date, treatment options of HDV infection are limited to interferon regimes with open issues about effectiveness of current approaches. Due to the unsatisfactory results further studies of novel drugs and therapy protocols are required. In this chapter current treatment procedures as well as novel therapeutic strategies to combat chronic HDV infection will be discussed.

2. Epidemiology

It is estimated that 15-20 million of HBsAg positive individuals are infected with HDV, but these numbers are not accurate because of absence of systematic screening in HBV infected individuals [12]. Interestingly, HDV infection is worldwide distributed; however the distribution is not uniform. Areas of HDV high prevalence are: Central Africa, Mediterranean countries, Middle East and South America, while in Western world HDV infection is limited to intravenous drug abusers [13]. Decrease of HDV incidence in industrialized world is caused by improvement of socioeconomic conditions such as implementation of HBV vaccination and systematic screening of blood and blood products. However, reduction in the number of infected individuals in developed countries has stopped, mainly due to the increased immigration from endemic areas [14]. Prevalence of anti-HD among HBsAg positive individuals in Western Europe has been stable during last decade ranging from 8.5 to 11.0 % [15, 16].

So far, eight HDV genotypes have been described. Most frequent is genotype 1 [17], which is prevalent worldwide, while genotypes 2 and 4 are mainly found in the Far East and genotype 3 is limited to Amazonian basin [18]. HDV genotypes 5-8 are found in patients originating from Africa [19]. Different HDV genotypes have impact on variations in clinical course of disease, thus genotypes 1 and 3 cause more severe disease, while genotype 2 is associated with milder form. Also, multiple genotypes of HDV can be found in high risk patients [20].

3. Transmission of HDV

HDV, as its helper HBV, is transmitted parenterally through the exposure to the blood and body fluids. In the developed countries the main route of transmission is by infected syringes among intravenous drug users. Although, there is an evidence for sexual transmission [21], it seems that HDV does not have the same rate of sexual transmission as HBV[22]. Due to the screening of the blood products, there is no more risk of HDV infections for the blood receiving patients. Despite the fact that HDV is parenterally transmitted, inapparent parenteral transmission within household [23] represents major route of transmission in the areas of the high prevalence. Therefore vaccination against HBV of all household members of infected individual is the crucial step in prevention of HDV infections. Vertical transmission from mother to the newborn is rare.

4. Clinical features

As defective virus, HDV replication depends on HbsAg synthesis, therefore HDV can be transmitted only in the presence of accompanied HBV infection. Based on the previous HBsAg status of the infected individual two major patterns of infection are distinguished: simultaneous HBV/HDV co-infection or superinfection by HDV of chronic HBsAg carriers [18].

In the simultaneous infection the fate of HDV depends on the host response to the HBV. When the expression of HBsAg is restrained, the HDV infection may result with abortive response, while abundance of HBsAg enables the full expression of HDV pathogenicity. As a result of this interaction between the two viruses, disease expression may vary. Clinically, HDV/HBV co-infection is usually similar to HBV mono-infection, although acute co-infection can be more severe and can be manifested as acute liver failure [24]. The rate of progression of HDV infection to chronic form is equal to that for acute hepatitis B, less than 5% [19].

Superinfection is defined as HDV infection of a chronically HBV infected individual. Preexisting chronic HBV infection represents perfect environment for replication of defective hepatitis D virus, resulting with abundant HDV expression and suppression of HBV replication. HBV suppression will become permanent, if HDV infection progress to chronic form [20]. Furthermore, superinfection is generally presented as severe acute hepatitis with shorter incubation time and will exceed to chronic HDV infection in high percentage of patients, up to 80% [25]. Clinically, HDV superinfection is manifested as a worsening of present HBV disease or as a new hepatitis in previously undiagnosed HBV infected individual. Along with detection of HDV serum markers, correct diagnosis of superinfection is clarified by negative IgM anti-HBc [21].

5. Symptoms and course

Symptoms of acute hepatits D infection are similar to the other forms of viral hepatitis. Initial phase of acute infection is characterized by nonspecific symptoms such as: fatigue, anorexia, nausea and lethargy accompanied with high increase of serum alanine aminotransferase and aspartate aminotransferase. Sometimes this phase is followed with icteric phase, characterized by jaundice, dark urine, clay-colored stools and elevated levels of serum bilirubin. Acute hepatitis is more severe in superinfection pattern, due to the fact that preceding HBV infection facilitates multiplication of HDV. Furthermore, acute disease can occur as fulminant hepatits, named as acute liver failure (ALF). ALF is a rare form of acute hepatitis; which is more often seen in acute hepatitis caused by HDV than other hepatothropic viruses. Clinically, ALF starts with nonspecific symptoms, such as fatigue and malaise followed by jaundice and hepatic encephalopathy and ultimately leading to coma. ALF is characterized by massive necrosis of hepatocytes, rapid clinical course; ultimately result with death of individual in 2-10 days. Without liver transplantation, ALF has lethal outcome in 80% of cases [26].

Choronic hepatitis D is the rarest form among chronic viral hepatitis, although it is the most severe and most progressive one. Chronic hepatitis D has three times higher risk for cirrhosis development than HBV chronic infection [27]. Clinically it is initially expressed as acute hepatitis in the half of the cases, probably due to initial acute superinfection [28]. However, symptoms of chronic hepatitis D are variable. Chronic hepatitis D can be manifested as fatigue, malaise and anorexia or its clinical course can be without any symptoms [9]. When cirrhosis is developed disease may be stable and asymptomatic for a long period or it can be manifested with complications related to the cirrhotic process. Once developed, a high number of patients with HDV cirrhosis will die of liver failure or hepatocellular carcinoma unless liver transplantation is performed [29].

6. Diagnosis

First step in diagnostic procedures is detection of HDV markers in the blood of HBsAg positive individual, due to the fact that HDV replication is possible only in the presence of HBV.

Actually, guidelines suggest that all HBsAg positive individuals should be screened for HDV infection, as well as members of high-risk group's like intravenous drug users, hemodialysis patients, health care and public safety workers. Also in the case of clinical deterioration of chronic HBV infection, superinfection with HDV should be considered.

Specific markers of HDV infection in serum are: Hepatitis D virus RNA, HDAg and anti-HDV. HDV RNA is detected in serum by molecular hybridization [30] or more sensitive RT-PCR [31], thus serum HDAg and anti-HDV are detected by enzyme-linked immunosorbent assay (ELISA) [32] and radioimmunoassay (RIA). During the diagnostic procedure, along with confirmation of HDV presence, it is necessary to clarify the stage of the infection due to the differences in clinical course and progonosis. Based on the interactions between two viruses, three patterns of HDV infections are distinguished: acute HDV/HBV co-infection, acute HDV infection of HBsAg positive carrier and chronic HDV infection.

Acute HBV/HDV co-infection is characterized with a high titre of IgM anti-HBc, a marker of acute HBV infection which enables to distinguishing confection from acute HDV superinfection. HDAg appears in the early phase of the acute infection and it is only transiently detectable in serum, unless patient is imunodeficient. Then HDAg can be detected for a longer period due to the weak immune system [33]. HDV RNA is also detectable in the early phase of acute infection [34] and represents a sensitive marker for virus replication present in 90% of patients. Nowdays, an active HDV infection is confirmed by detection of HDV RNA in the serum by sensitive real time PCR assays [35]. Although, HDV RNA test can be false negative due to the variability of the genome sequence, so that sero-conversion and detection of IgM anti-HDV is still helpful to establish diagnosis of acute infection.

In chronic HDV infection the high titre of IgG anti-HD antibodies persist even after viral clearance. Also, a large proportion of patients has positive IgM antiHD, a characteristic marker of acute infection. Persistence of anti-HD IgM antibodies indicates progression of disease to the chronic form. HDV RNA is present in the serum of chronically infected patients as HDAg.

Individual's positive for HDV serum markers should be subjected to the liver biopsy to determine histological stage of the liver disease, due to the fact that HDV serum markers or values of liver test do not reflect severity of liver damage [36]. Also, all the HDV positive patients should be tested for HCV and HIV because of the high frequency of co-infection with these parenterally transmitted viruses [37].

7. Treatment

Presence of HBsAg is necessary for the replication of the HDV, hence the therapeutic aim is to eradicate both pathogens. HDV is considered eradicated if HDV-RNA in serum and HDAg in the liver are negative 6 months after therapy [24]. Despite the sustained viral response, there is still a possibility of reactivation of HDV in HBsAg positive individual, due to the limitations of diagnostic procedures to detect a low level of HDV copies (1000 copies/ml). Experimentally in animal model, the posibillity to transfer HDV infection with serum diluted up to 10^{-11} was demonstrated [38]. Although HDV is considered eradicated when serum HDV RNA and HDAg in the liver are persistently undetectable, only eradication of HBsAg represents a complete cure and it is ultimate goal of HDV treatment. Eradication of virus results in normalization of ALT levels and stopping of liver fibrosis process, while developed anti HD antibodies will prevent re-infections [24].

So far only approved therapy for Hepatits D is standard interferon-α (IFN- α). Long-term administration of high-dose standard IFN- α, 5 million units daily or 9 million units three times per week for 12 months, results in normalization of alanine aminotransferase serum values, clearance of serum HDV RNA, and histological improvement in 50 percent of patients with chronic hepatitis D [39]. High-dose IFN therapy improves the long-term clinical outcome and survival rate of the patients, even if they have advanced disease and active cirrhosis before therapy induction [40]. There are still arguments going on with regard to duration of interferon treatment. Interferon therapy administered through 12 months has better results comparing to 6 months therapy [39], although prolongation of IFN therapy to 24 months does not result with increasing response to the treatment [41]. Unfortunately, large number of patients will appear relapse usually 2-6 months after termination of treatment [39]. Thus interferon therapy is insufficient for the majority of patients with chronic HDV, characterized with incomplete sustained viral response and common biochemical and virological relapses after cessation of treatment [42, 43]. Interferon treatment is often accompanied with numerous side effects, which requires a continuous supervision of the patients during treatment. Most common side effects are influenza like symptoms such as fatigue and weight loss [44]. Severe psychiatric disorders can appear as a result of prolonged high dose interferon therapy [42, 45], which disables interferon application to the certain number of patients. Another compulsory reason for cessation of interferon therapy is decompensation of liver disease, due to the fact that high number of patients has advanced disease and cirrhosis [46, 47].

Lately, pegylated form of interferon-α (Peg-IFN-α) is introduced in therapy of HDV. It is characterized by longer half-life, which allows longer intervals between drug administrations. Treatment with Peg-IFN-α showed better response in naive patients and in previous nonres-ponders compared to standard IFN-α treatment [48, 49]. Patients not achieving SVR with standard interferon therapy, may eradicate serum HDV RNA after a 6-month treatment with Peg-IFN-α [50]. For the lowering of HDV RNA beyond detectable level, it is demonstrated that even standard doses of Peg-IFN- α are more successful than high doses of standard IFN- α, although in that case seroconversion of HBsAg is not taken into consideration [51]. However, the rate of clearance of HBsAg is greater with Peg-IFN-α, but overall clearance and serocon-version of HBsAg is low, only in 3-5% of cases [52]. Generally, it is difficult to assess the effectiveness of IFN-α therapy due to differences in study strategies that examined the effect of the treatment. Studies usually differ in forms of drugs, doses, duration of the treatment and patient follow-up period, making comparison of results a difficult task (Table 1.). Considering these differences in the previous studies, overall sustained viral response varies from 17 to 43 % [53]. Currently the largest hepatitis delta multicenter study is HIDIT I trial, which is carried out by the German Network of Competence for Viral Hepatitis (Hep-Net) in collaboration with centers from Turkey and Greece. In total of 90 patients with hepatitis D, the effect of Peg-IFN-

α-2a in combination with adeofovir versus either drug alone was examined. Overall, 28% of the patients had sustained viral response after treatment with Peg-IFN-α-2a for 48 weeks, with no difference in efficacy between combined therapy compared with Peg-IFN-α-2a monotherapy [54]. From the results of current studies it is evident that treatment with Peg-IFN-α-2a has limited efficacy as a therpy of hepatitis delta, thus further investigations of potential tretment options are needed.

Study and year	Patients (n)	Therapy	Duration (weeks)	Results
Yurdaydin, 2008. [74]	39	1st group (n=14), Lamivudine (100mg/day) plus IFN-α-2a (9 MU/3x week) vs. 2nd group (n=8), IFN-α-2a vs. 3rd group (n=17), Lamivudine	48	BR: 1st(64%), 2nd(63%), 3rd(18%) EOTR: 1st(50%), 2nd(50%), 3rd(12%) SVR: 1st(36%), 2nd(50%), 3rd(12%) Combination treatment was not superior to IFN therapy.
Gheorghe, 2011. [75]	49	Peg-IFN-α-2b (1.5µg/kg/week)	48	BR: 50% EOTR: 33.3% SVR: 25%
Ormeci, 2011. [76]	18	Peg-IFN-α-2b (1.5µg/kg/week)	96 weeks (n=11) and 48 weeks (n=7)	No significant difference between two groups in terms of HDV-RNA suppression and ALT normalisation.
Wedemeyer, 2011. [77]	90	1st group (n=31) Peg-IFN-α-2a (180 µg/week) plus Adeofovir (10 mg/ daily) vs. 2nd group (n=29) Peg-IFN-α-2a vs. 3rd group(n=30) Adeofovir	48	BR: 1st(32%), 2nd(28%), 3rd(7%) EOTR: 1st(23%), 2nd(24%), 3rd(0%) SVR: 1st(26%), 2nd(31%), 3rd(0%)
Karaca, 2012. [78]	32	Peg-IFN-α-2a (180 µg) or Peg-IFN-α-2b (1.5 µg/kg) per week	96	EOTR: 50% SVR: 47%
Kabaçam, 2012. [79]	13	Entecavir (1 mg/day)	48	Ineffective in chronic hepatitis delta.
Samiullah, 2012. [80]	238	Peg-IFN-α-2b (1.5 µg/kg/week)	48	BR: 51.3% EOTR: 29.8% SVR: 29.4%

BR: Biochemical response is determined by a normalization of ALT at the end of the treatment.

EOTR: The end of treatment response is defined by a HDV-RNA negative status.

SVR: A sustained virological response is defined by undetectable serum HDV-RNA at six months after the end of treatment.

Table 1. Recent studies for treatment of chronic delta hepatitis

Last 30 years many antiviral drugs are tested in the therapy of hepatitis D, but with limited succsess. Particulary it was tested efficiency of nucleoside and nucleotide analogues (NUCs) such as: lamivudine, adeofovir, famciclovir and entecavir; due to the fact that NUCs have some therapeutic efficancy against HBV. The effect of tenofovir was observed in a group of patients with concomitant presence of HCV, HBV and HDV infection. It seems that the prior long term treatment with lamivudine and tenofovir before introduction of IFN therapy might help fastering decline of HDV RNA copies in such patients. However, seroconversion of HBsAg was not observed. Patients who suffer from multiple infections with HCV, HBV and HDV present another group difficult to treat. Unfortunately, the consequence is a progressive liver fibrosis. It is shown that neither IFN monotherapy or combination therapy with NUCs and IFN are effective. Those patients are less sensitive to IFN therapy [55]. Babiker et al. report the case of successful depletion of serum HDV RNA in a patient with acute HDV superinfection due to 65 weeks treatment with tenofovir and lamivudine. But, after the cessation of the treatment HDV RNA levels began to increase [56]. Another combination therapy is the therapy with entecavir and PEG IFNα-2a. In this case also, quantitative HBsAg was used as the treatment response guidance for dual infection with HBV and HDV. The seroconversion of HBsAg and undetectable HDV RNA levels were achieved after 35 months of such therapy. In this patient, the stage of liver fibrosis has also improved significantly. The consolidation therapy during next 12 months after the seroconversion was continued and the patient remained seronegative during 12 months after cessation of the therapy [57].

Possible new drug candidates for the therapy are the ones affecting the interaction between HD virion and HBsAg, as well as posttranslational modifications of HDV proteins, such as prenylation. Also, it seems IFN- λ could be possible alternative for IFN-α because in the treatment of chronic hepatitis C, IFN- λ proved to cause less side effects [53].

8. Liver transplantation in HDV patients

HDV infection is characterized with more severe disease than HBV monoinfection. Studies showed two times higher relative risk of cirrhosis and threefold risk increase of hepatocellular carcinoma in patients coinfected with HBV and HDV compared with HBV monoinfection [27, 58]. Consequently, liver transplantation (LT) represents only therapeutic option for the patients with end-stage liver disease, as well as for hepatocellular carcinoma and fulminant hepatitis due to the coinfection or superinfection with HDV and HBV.

Prevention of allograft reinfection is the main requirement for the long term survival. Major risk factor predicitng HBV-HDV recurrence after LT is a high level of HBV DNA (>10^5 copies/ml) at transplant, fortunately that is unusal feature of HDV disease course [59]. Therefore, patients coinfected with HBV and HDV generally do not require pretransplant antiviral B therapy. In case when pretransplant antiviral treatment is needed, entecavir or teneofovir are preferred rather than lamivudine, while IFN therapy is not recommended during the pre-transplant period. Other predictors of a low risk of HBV-HDV recurrence are low levels of HBV replication markers, HDV coinfection and fulminant hepatitis [60]. Coinfection with human immunodeficiency virus and recurrence of HCC represent a risk factors for HBV recurrence [61, 62].

The patient's prognosis and overall outcome after LT is on satisfactory level with current posttransplant therapy. Golden standard for prevention of recurrent disease is combination of hyperimmune serum against HBV(HBIg) and potent nucleoside analogue. Therapeutic strategy of low dose intramuscular HBIg in combination with lamivudine is the most cost-effective profilaxis [63], with the rates of the recurrence level as low as 4% at 4 years [64]. Therefore, the outcome of LT due to HDV related liver disease is similar to or better than in other indications of LT [65, 66].

Due to LT, HDV RNA becomes negative within the first days after transplantation, followed by a decline of HbsAg with almost identical pattern. However, HDVAg can be detected in the hepatocytes of the graft for several months after treatment [54]. This HDV latency in the graft represents a potential source of HDV recurrence, because of possible HBV superinfection and reexpression of HBsAg. Thus, transplanted patients should be monitored for HbsAG and HBV DNA every 3 months and for HDV RNA every 6 months.

9. Perspectives for a vaccine development against HDV

Since the details in pathophysiologic respose to HDV infection still aren't enlightened, there are difficulties in finding the effective vaccine against it. In the case of HDV infection, the antigen is nucleoprotein and the imunization means the activation of T cells (CD4+ and CD8+) which would destroy infected cells and prevent replication of the virus. Preclinical studies have been done on woodchuks. In this model of chronically infected woodchuks with woodchuck hepatitis virus (WHV), it is possible to achieve the superinfection with HDV. So far, T cell vaccine prevented the coinfection with WHV- HDV, but it failed to prevent the superinfection of chronic carriers of WHV. Further studies have to be done to resolve the problem of preventing the superinfection by stimulating T cells. This would mean that chronic carriers would have to be vaccinated frequently to activate a large number of T cells before the patient is exposed to HDV. [67]

10. Novel therapeutic strategies for future treatment

So far, the treatment outcome of hepatitis delta is not satisfactory. Thus, new therapy aproaches are necessary (Figure 2.). Interferon-α targets the HbsAg, whose depletion is crucial for succesful treatment of hepatitis delta. The major difficulty with such therapy are numerous adverse effects, since IFN-α receptors are also present in other tissues than hepatic. Additional problem is the necessity of long term application of IFN-α to achieve therapeutic response. Better candidate could be IFN- λ, since its receptors are present only on epithelial cells [68]. It has been shown that pegylated IFN- λ used as monotherapy, or in combination with ribavirin, has significant antiviral activity against hepatitis C virus. Also, as expected, it causes less undesirable side effects. [69] Further studies must be done to evaluate the effectivness of IFN-λ in treatment od chronic hepatitis delta.

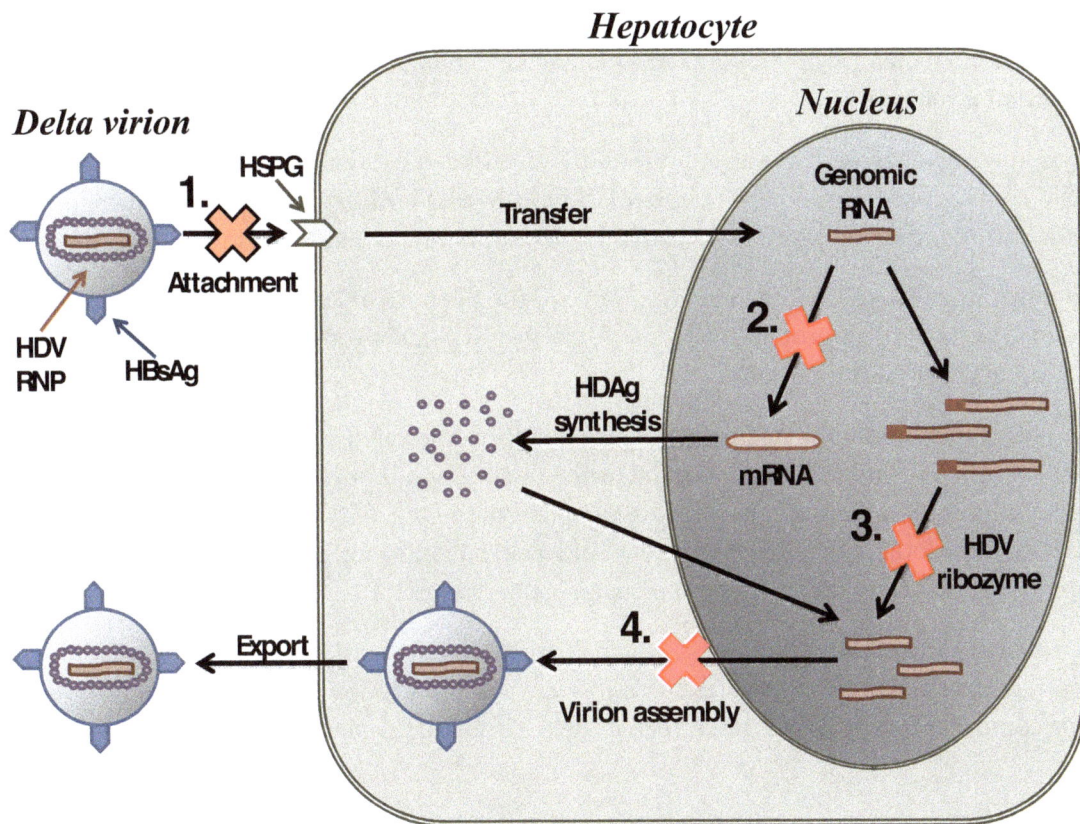

HDV RNP= hepatitis D virus ribonucleoprotein. HBsAg= hepatitis B surface antigen. HSPG=highly sulphated proteoglycans. HDAg=hepatitis D antigen.

Figure 2. Potential drug targets in HDV treatment. 1. Neutralizing of negativly charged HSPG may prevent HDV and HBV attachment to hepatocyte membrane. 2. Gene therapy targets genes which encode HDAg 3. Inhibition of HDV ribozymes would prevent virus replication, 4. Interferring with posttranslational modifications of HDVAg enables virion assembly.

Other strategy for therapy development is to interfere with posttranslational modifications of HDVAg. Such modifications are prenylation, acetylation, metylation and phosphorylation of HDVAg. Prenylation inhibitors proved effective in cell culture model and are currently in clinical studies. [54] Drugs interferring with other types of HDV posttranslational modifications haven't been developed yet. [70]

Since HDV genome is too small to code all the necessary particles for it's own replication, it almost entirely depends on the host's replication mechanisms. For example, it deceives host's RNA polymerases so they copy HDV genome. HDV replication is known as rolling replication mechanism, meaning that HDV circular genome is elongated into multimeric linear transcripts and than cleaved into multiple genome size monomers by it's own RNA. This type of RNA is known as ribozyme, which is actually HDV RNA with enzymatic activity.

Small interfering RNAs (siRNAs) are up to 25 nucleotides long double stranded RNAs which silence particular gene by binding to mRNA. After binding to target mRNA,siRNA causes it's degradation. In therapy of HDV infection, silencing gene which codes LHD-Ag would disable HD virion replication [16].

Ribozymes can also serve as target for therapy. It has been shown that amoxicillin, apramycin and ristomycin in complex with copper (II) bind to HDV ribozymes and inhibit them. [71] Further studies are necessary to investigate the therapeutic potential of such treatment.

Not only large HDAg (LHDAg) is important for the lifecycle of hepatitis delta virus, but also the small delta antigen protein (SHDAg). Therefore, it can also be the target for new drugs in development for HDV treatment.

It has been shown that the negatively charged highly sulphated proteoglycanes (HSPG) play a role in both HBV and HDV attachement to hepatocyte membrane. Those weak forces between opposite charged subjects enable virus attachment to the cell. [72] This kind of target could be good for developing the drug which would prevent binding of both HBV and HDV to hepatocyte surface by neutralizing the negative charge of HSPG.

Gene therapy would target HDVAg, which is proved to have crucial role in lifecycle of HDV. Design of specific molecule which binds to gene which encodes delta antigen is in progess. Some computational analyses have been done to simulate the silencing of target gene. [73]

11. Conclusions

HDV is an unusal, defective hepatotropic virus which causes severe acute hepatitis and most progressive chronic viral hepatitis. Despite the efforts in eradication of HDV, as its obligatory helper HBV, prevalence of HDV in developed countries remains stable and represents a relevant public health concern. Current conventional therapy of hepatitis delta is characterized with poor overall response, thus further investigations of novel treatment options are needed. Continuous research of virology and pathogenesis is necessary to provide fundamentals for development of novel approaches in treatment of HDV.

Acknowledgements

The support of the J. J. Strossmayer University of Osijek research grant (to MS) and Ministry of science, education and sport research grant (to AV) are gratefully acknowledged.

Author details

Hrvoje Roguljic[1], Sonja Sarcevic[2], Robert Smolic[1,2], Nikola Raguz Lucic[2], Aleksandar Vcev[1,3] and Martina Smolic[1,2*]

*Address all correspondence to: martina.smolic@mefos.hr

1 Department of Mineral Research, Faculty of Medicine, J. J. Strossmayer University of Osijek, Croatia

2 Department of Pharmacology, Faculty of Medicine, J. J. Strossmayer University of Osijek, Croatia

3 Department of Medicine, Faculty of Medicine, J. J. Strossmayer University of Osijek, Croatia

Authors declare no conflict of interest

References

[1] Rizzetto M, Canese MG, Aricò S, Crivelli O, Trepo C, Bonino F, et al. Immunofluorescence detection of new antigen-antibody system (delta/anti-delta) associated to hepatitis B virus in liver and in serum of HBsAg carriers. Gut. 1977;18(12):997-1003.

[2] Rizzetto M, Shih JW, Gocke DJ, Purcell RH, Verme G, Gerin JL. Incidence and significance of antibodies to delta antigen in hepatitis B virus infection. Lancet. 1979;2(8150):986-90.

[3] Rizzetto M, Canese MG, Gerin JL, London WT, Sly DL, Purcell RH. Transmission of the hepatitis B virus-associated delta antigen to chimpanzees. J Infect Dis. 1980;141(5):590-602.

[4] Rizzetto M, Hoyer B, Canese MG, Shih JW, Purcell RH, Gerin JL. delta Agent: association of delta antigen with hepatitis B surface antigen and RNA in serum of delta-infected chimpanzees. Proc Natl Acad Sci U S A. 1980;77(10):6124-8.

[5] Gudima S, Chang J, Moraleda G, Azvolinsky A, Taylor J. Parameters of human hepatitis delta virus genome replication: the quantity, quality, and intracellular distribution of viral proteins and RNA. J Virol. 2002;76(8):3709-19.

[6] Ryu WS, Netter HJ, Bayer M, Taylor J. Ribonucleoprotein complexes of hepatitis delta virus. J Virol. 1993;67(6):3281-7.

[7] Alvarado-Mora MV, Locarnini S, Rizzetto M, Pinho JR. An update on HDV: virology, pathogenesis and treatment. Antivir Ther. 2013;18(3 Pt B):541-8.

[8]   Lai MM. RNA replication without RNA-dependent RNA polymerase: surprises from hepatitis delta virus. J Virol. 2005;79(13):7951-8.

[9]   Taylor JM. Structure and replication of hepatitis delta virus RNA. Curr Top Microbiol Immunol. 2006;307:1-23.

[10] Govindarajan S, Chin KP, Redeker AG, Peters RL. Fulminant B viral hepatitis: role of delta agent. Gastroenterology. 1984;86(6):1417-20.

[11] Fattovich G, Boscaro S, Noventa F, Pornaro E, Stenico D, Alberti A, et al. Influence of hepatitis delta virus infection on progression to cirrhosis in chronic hepatitis type B. J Infect Dis. 1987;155(5):931-5.

[12] Hadziyannis SJ. Review: hepatitis delta. J Gastroenterol Hepatol. 1997;12(4):289-98.

[13] Rizzetto M, Ponzetto A, Forzani I. Hepatitis delta virus as a global health problem. Vaccine. 1990;8 Suppl:S10-4; discussion S21-3.

[14] Wedemeyer H, Heidrich B, Manns MP. Hepatitis D virus infection--not a vanishing disease in Europe! Hepatology. 2007;45(5):1331-2; author reply 2-3.

[15] Heidrich B, Deterding K, Tillmann HL, Raupach R, Manns MP, Wedemeyer H. Virological and clinical characteristics of delta hepatitis in Central Europe. J Viral Hepat. 2009;16(12):883-94.

[16] Ciancio A, Rizzetto M. Chronic hepatitis D at a standstill: where do we go from here? Nat Rev Gastroenterol Hepatol. 2014;11(1):68-71.

[17] Shakil AO, Hadziyannis S, Hoofnagle JH, Di Bisceglie AM, Gerin JL, Casey JL. Geographic distribution and genetic variability of hepatitis delta virus genotype I. Virology. 1997;234(1):160-7.

[18] Ito T, Tahara SM, Lai MMC. The 3'-untranslated region of hepatitis C virus RNA enhances translation from an internal ribosomal entry site. Journal of Virology. 1998;72(11):8789-96.

[19] Radjef N, Gordien E, Ivaniushina V, Gault E, Anaïs P, Drugan T, et al. Molecular phylogenetic analyses indicate a wide and ancient radiation of African hepatitis delta virus, suggesting a deltavirus genus of at least seven major clades. J Virol. 2004;78(5): 2537-44.

[20] Su CW, Huang YH, Huo TI, Shih HH, Sheen IJ, Chen SW, et al. Genotypes and viremia of hepatitis B and D viruses are associated with outcomes of chronic hepatitis D patients. Gastroenterology. 2006;130(6):1625-35.

[21] Wu JC, Chen CM, Sheen IJ, Lee SD, Tzeng HM, Choo KB. Evidence of transmission of hepatitis D virus to spouses from sequence analysis of the viral genome. Hepatology. 1995;22(6):1656-60.

[22] Weisfuse IB, Hadler SC, Fields HA, Alter MJ, O'Malley PM, Judson FN, et al. Delta hepatitis in homosexual men in the United States. Hepatology. 1989;9(6):872-4.

[23] Niro GA, Casey JL, Gravinese E, Garrubba M, Conoscitore P, Sagnelli E, et al. Intrafamilial transmission of hepatitis delta virus: molecular evidence. J Hepatol. 1999;30(4): 564-9.

[24] Pascarella S, Negro F. Hepatitis D virus: an update. Liver Int. 2011;31(1):7-21.

[25] Smedile A, Farci P, Verme G, Caredda F, Cargnel A, Caporaso N, et al. Influence of delta infection on severity of hepatitis B. Lancet. 1982;2(8305):945-7.

[26] Lee WM. Acute liver failure. N Engl J Med. 1993;329(25):1862-72.

[27] Fattovich G, Giustina G, Christensen E, Pantalena M, Zagni I, Realdi G, et al. Influence of hepatitis delta virus infection on morbidity and mortality in compensated cirrhosis type B. The European Concerted Action on Viral Hepatitis (Eurohep). Gut. 2000;46(3):420-6.

[28] Farci P, Niro GA. Clinical features of hepatitis D. Semin Liver Dis. 2012;32(3):228-36.

[29] Rosina F, Conoscitore P, Cuppone R, Rocca G, Giuliani A, Cozzolongo R, et al. Changing pattern of chronic hepatitis D in Southern Europe. Gastroenterology. 1999;117(1):161-6.

[30] Zignego AL, Dubois F, Samuel D, Georgopoulou U, Reynes M, Gentilini P, et al. Serum hepatitis delta virus RNA in patients with delta hepatitis and in liver graft recipients. J Hepatol. 1990;11(1):102-10.

[31] Wu JC, Chen TZ, Huang YS, Yen FS, Ting LT, Sheng WY, et al. Natural history of hepatitis D viral superinfection: significance of viremia detected by polymerase chain reaction. Gastroenterology. 1995;108(3):796-802.

[32] Shattock AG, Morgan BM. Sensitive enzyme immunoassay for the detection of delta antigen and anti-delta, using serum as the delta antigen source. J Med Virol. 1984;13(1):73-82.

[33] Grippon P, Ribiere O, Cadranel JF, Pelletier S, Pillot B, Emerit J, et al. Long-term delta antigenaemia without appearance of delta antibody in two immunodeficient patients. Lancet. 1987;1(8540):1031.

[34] Buti M, Esteban R, Roggendorf M, Fernandez J, Jardi R, Rashofer R, et al. Hepatitis D virus RNA in acute delta infection: serological profile and correlation with other markers of hepatitis D virus infection. Hepatology. 1988;8(5):1125-9.

[35] Mederacke I, Bremer B, Heidrich B, Kirschner J, Deterding K, Bock T, et al. Establishment of a novel quantitative hepatitis D virus (HDV) RNA assay using the Cobas TaqMan platform to study HDV RNA kinetics. J Clin Microbiol. 2010;48(6):2022-9.

[36]   Zachou K, Yurdaydin C, Drebber U, Dalekos GN, Erhardt A, Cakaloglu Y, et al. Quantitative HBsAg and HDV-RNA levels in chronic delta hepatitis. Liver Int. 2010;30(3):430-7.

[37]   Boyd A, Lacombe K, Miailhes P, Gozlan J, Bonnard P, Molina JM, et al. Longitudinal evaluation of viral interactions in treated HIV-hepatitis B co-infected patients with additional hepatitis C and D virus. J Viral Hepat. 2010;17(1):65-76.

[38]   Ponzetto A, Hoyer BH, Popper H, Engle R, Purcell RH, Gerin JL. Titration of the infectivity of hepatitis D virus in chimpanzees. J Infect Dis. 1987;155(1):72-8.

[39]   Farci P, Mandas A, Coiana A, Lai ME, Desmet V, Van Eyken P, et al. Treatment of chronic hepatitis D with interferon alfa-2a. N Engl J Med. 1994;330(2):88-94.

[40]   Farci P, Roskams T, Chessa L, Peddis G, Mazzoleni AP, Scioscia R, et al. Long-term benefit of interferon alpha therapy of chronic hepatitis D: regression of advanced hepatic fibrosis. Gastroenterology. 2004;126(7):1740-9.

[41]   Yurdaydin C, Bozkaya H, Karaaslan H, Onder FO, Erkan OE, Yalçin K, et al. A pilot study of 2 years of interferon treatment in patients with chronic delta hepatitis. J Viral Hepat. 2007;14(11):812-6.

[42]   Gaudin JL, Faure P, Godinot H, Gerard F, Trepo C. The French experience of treatment of chronic type D hepatitis with a 12-month course of interferon alpha-2B. Results of a randomized controlled trial. Liver. 1995;15(1):45-52.

[43]   Madejón A, Cotonat T, Bartolomé J, Castillo I, Carreño V. Treatment of chronic hepatitis D virus infection with low and high doses of interferon-alpha 2a: utility of polymerase chain reaction in monitoring antiviral response. Hepatology. 1994;19(6): 1331-6.

[44]   Romeo R, Del Ninno E, Rumi M, Russo A, Sangiovanni A, de Franchis R, et al. A 28-year study of the course of hepatitis Delta infection: a risk factor for cirrhosis and hepatocellular carcinoma. Gastroenterology. 2009;136(5):1629-38.

[45]   Lau JY, King R, Tibbs CJ, Catterall AP, Smith HM, Portmann BC, et al. Loss of HBsAg with interferon-alpha therapy in chronic hepatitis D virus infection. J Med Virol. 1993;39(4):292-6.

[46]   Rizzetto M. Hepatitis D: thirty years after. J Hepatol. 2009;50(5):1043-50.

[47]   Niro GA, Rosina F, Rizzetto M. Treatment of hepatitis D. J Viral Hepat. 2005;12(1): 2-9.

[48]   Castelnau C, Le Gal F, Ripault MP, Gordien E, Martinot-Peignoux M, Boyer N, et al. Efficacy of peginterferon alpha-2b in chronic hepatitis delta: relevance of quantitative RT-PCR for follow-up. Hepatology. 2006;44(3):728-35.

[49] Erhardt A, Gerlich W, Starke C, Wend U, Donner A, Sagir A, et al. Treatment of chronic hepatitis delta with pegylated interferon-alpha2b. Liver Int. 2006;26(7): 805-10.

[50] Ferenci P, Formann E, Romeo R. Successful treatment of chronic hepatitis D with a short course of peginterferon alfa-2a. Am J Gastroenterol. 2005;100(7):1626-7.

[51] Alavian SM, Tabatabaei SV, Behnava B, Rizzetto M. Standard and pegylated interferon therapy of HDV infection: A systematic review and meta- analysis. J Res Med Sci. 2012;17(10):967-74.

[52] Li WC, Wang MR, Kong LB, Ren WG, Zhang YG, Nan YM. Peginterferon alpha-based therapy for chronic hepatitis B focusing on HBsAg clearance or seroconversion: a meta-analysis of controlled clinical trials. BMC Infect Dis. 2011;11:165.

[53] Rizzetto M. Current management of delta hepatitis. Liver Int. 2013;33 Suppl 1:195-7.

[54] Mederacke I, Filmann N, Yurdaydin C, Bremer B, Puls F, Zacher BJ, et al. Rapid early HDV RNA decline in the peripheral blood but prolonged intrahepatic hepatitis delta antigen persistence after liver transplantation. J Hepatol. 2012;56(1):115-22.

[55] Riaz M, Idrees M, Kanwal H, Kabir F. An overview of triple infection with hepatitis B, C and D viruses. Virol J. 2011;8:368.

[56] Babiker ZO, Hogan C, Ustianowski A, Wilkins E. Does interferon-sparing tenofovir disoproxil fumarate-based therapy have a role in the management of severe acute hepatitis delta superinfection? J Med Microbiol. 2012;61(Pt 12):1780-3.

[57] Chen GY, Su TH, Kao JH. Successful treatment of chronic hepatitis B and D with pegylated-interferon plus entecavir. J Formos Med Assoc. 2013.

[58] Fattovich G, Bortolotti F, Donato F. Natural history of chronic hepatitis B: special emphasis on disease progression and prognostic factors. J Hepatol. 2008;48(2):335-52.

[59] Samuel D, Muller R, Alexander G, Fassati L, Ducot B, Benhamou JP, et al. Liver transplantation in European patients with the hepatitis B surface antigen. N Engl J Med. 1993;329(25):1842-7.

[60] Degertekin B, Han SH, Keeffe EB, Schiff ER, Luketic VA, Brown RS, et al. Impact of virologic breakthrough and HBIG regimen on hepatitis B recurrence after liver transplantation. Am J Transplant. 2010;10(8):1823-33.

[61] Faria LC, Gigou M, Roque-Afonso AM, Sebagh M, Roche B, Fallot G, et al. Hepatocellular carcinoma is associated with an increased risk of hepatitis B virus recurrence after liver transplantation. Gastroenterology. 2008;134(7):1890-9; quiz 2155.

[62] Coffin CS, Stock PG, Dove LM, Berg CL, Nissen NN, Curry MP, et al. Virologic and clinical outcomes of hepatitis B virus infection in HIV-HBV coinfected transplant recipients. Am J Transplant. 2010;10(5):1268-75.

[63] Roche B, Samuel D. Liver transplantation in delta virus infection. Semin Liver Dis. 2012;32(3):245-55.

[64] Gane EJ, Angus PW, Strasser S, Crawford DH, Ring J, Jeffrey GP, et al. Lamivudine plus low-dose hepatitis B immunoglobulin to prevent recurrent hepatitis B following liver transplantation. Gastroenterology. 2007;132(3):931-7.

[65] Steinmüller T, Seehofer D, Rayes N, Müller AR, Settmacher U, Jonas S, et al. Increasing applicability of liver transplantation for patients with hepatitis B-related liver disease. Hepatology. 2002;35(6):1528-35.

[66] Kim WR, Poterucha JJ, Kremers WK, Ishitani MB, Dickson ER. Outcome of liver transplantation for hepatitis B in the United States. Liver Transpl. 2004;10(8):968-74.

[67] Roggendorf M. Perspectives for a vaccine against hepatitis delta virus. Semin Liver Dis. 2012;32(3):256-61.

[68] Donnelly RP, Dickensheets H, O'Brien TR. Interferon-lambda and therapy for chronic hepatitis C virus infection. Trends Immunol. 2011;32(9):443-50.

[69] Muir AJ, Shiffman ML, Zaman A, Yoffe B, de la Torre A, Flamm S, et al. Phase 1b study of pegylated interferon lambda 1 with or without ribavirin in patients with chronic genotype 1 hepatitis C virus infection. Hepatology. 2010;52(3):822-32.

[70] Hughes SA, Wedemeyer H, Harrison PM. Hepatitis delta virus. Lancet. 2011;378(9785):73-85.

[71] Stokowa-Sołtys K, Gaggelli N, Nagaj J, Szczepanik W, Ciesiołka J, Wrzesiński J, et al. High affinity of copper(II) towards amoxicillin, apramycin and ristomycin. Effect of these complexes on the catalytic activity of HDV ribozyme. J Inorg Biochem. 2013;124:26-34.

[72] Lamas Longarela O, Schmidt TT, Schöneweis K, Romeo R, Wedemeyer H, Urban S, et al. Proteoglycans act as cellular hepatitis delta virus attachment receptors. PLoS One. 2013;8(3):e58340.

[73] Singh S, Gupta SK, Nischal A, Khattri S, Nath R, Pant KK, et al. Identification and characterization of novel small-molecule inhibitors against hepatitis delta virus replication by using docking strategies. Hepat Mon. 2011;11(10):803-9.

[74] Yurdaydin C, Bozkaya H, Onder FO, Sentürk H, Karaaslan H, Akdoğan M, et al. Treatment of chronic delta hepatitis with lamivudine vs lamivudine + interferon vs interferon. J Viral Hepat. 2008;15(4):314-21.

[75] Gheorghe L, Iacob S, Simionov I, Vadan R, Constantinescu I, Caruntu F, et al. Weight-based dosing regimen of peg-interferon α-2b for chronic hepatitis delta: a multicenter Romanian trial. J Gastrointestin Liver Dis. 2011;20(4):377-82.

[76] Ormeci N, Bölükbaş F, Erden E, Coban S, Ekiz F, Erdem H, et al. Pegylated interferon alfa-2B for chronic delta hepatitis: 12 versus 24 months. Hepatogastroenterology. 2011;58(110-111):1648-53.

[77] Wedemeyer H, Yurdaydìn C, Dalekos GN, Erhardt A, Çakaloğlu Y, Değertekin H, et al. Peginterferon plus adefovir versus either drug alone for hepatitis delta. N Engl J Med. 2011;364(4):322-31.

[78] Karaca C, Soyer OM, Baran B, Ormeci AC, Gokturk S, Aydin E, et al. Efficacy of pegylated interferon-α treatment for 24 months in chronic delta hepatitis and predictors of response. Antivir Ther. 2013;18(4):561-6.

[79] Kabaçam G, Onder FO, Yakut M, Seven G, Karatayli SC, Karatayli E, et al. Entecavir treatment of chronic hepatitis D. Clin Infect Dis. 2012;55(5):645-50.

[80] Samiullah S, Bikharam D, Nasreen. Treatment of chronic hepatitis delta virus with peg-interferon and factors that predict sustained viral response. World J Gastroenterol. 2012;18(40):5793-8.

8

Targeting Bacterial Persistence to Develop Therapeutics Against Infectious Disease

Elizabeth Hong-Geller and Sofiya N. Micheva-Viteva

Additional information is available at the end of the chapter

1. Introduction

The application of the prototype antibiotics penicillin and streptomycin to bacterial infection in the 1940's marked a historic milestone in medicine and heralded a new era of antimicrobial therapy as the modern standard for infectious disease management. Yet, even in those early days of discovery, scientist Joseph Bigger noted an unexplained phenomenon. Although penicillin treatment of *Staphylococcus aureus* infection killed the great majority of the bacterial population, a small subset of cells (~1 in 10^5) continued to persist and remained recalcitrant to antibiotic-mediated killing.[1] When re-grown in the absence of antibiotic, the bacterial community once again became sensitive to antibiotic-mediated killing and resembled the original culture (~1 in 10^5 persisters), providing conclusive proof that these organisms were not drug-resistant strains that had evolved via genetic mutations (in which case all bacteria in the final population would be drug-resistant). (Fig. 1) Instead, persister cells are phenotypic variants that are genetically identical to the susceptible bacterial population, but have modified their physiology to survive environmental stress. These bacteria exhibit antibiotic tolerance that is non-heritable and reversible upon removal of the antibiotic, a completely different phenomenon than the more well-studied antibiotic resistance mechanisms mediated by genetic mutation. Persistence is akin to a community "insurance policy" in which surviving persister cells hedge against unlikely but catastrophic events, while still maintaining near optimal growth at the population level.[2, 3]

In this review, we will discuss the known molecular mechanisms that underlie bacterial persistence, the impact of persistence on infectious disease, and the different strategies that are being developed to target persisters in disease. The human toll of pathogen infection has been compounded by the rampant use of antibiotics in the last half-century, leading to the rapid evolution of drug-resistant strains to practically every approved antibiotic. There is a

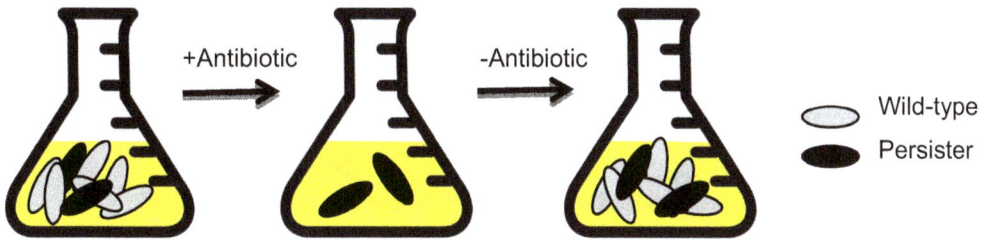

Figure 1. Bacterial persisters are recalcitrant to antiiotic killing. After removal of antibiotic, bacterial community expands to contain both wild-type and persister sub-groups, indicating that the persisters are phenotypic variants instead of containing genetic mutations.

great public health need to identify novel strategies for development of therapeutics to treat pathogen infection. Development of novel therapies that either kill persisters directly or stimulate their reversion to logarithmic growth may effectively reduce disease relapse and shorten the treatment period.[4] It may be the case that a combination therapy comprised of conventional antibiotics that kill replicating pathogens and new drugs that target the metabolically-inactive persisters can also reduce the rate of emergence of antibiotic resistance.

2. Impact of bacterial persistence on infectious disease

Without question, bacterial persistence greatly contributes to the burden of infectious disease, where persisters survive antibiotic treatment to re-infect patients in a frustrating cycle of chronic infection. Many antibiotics have been shown to be only active against dividing bacteria. [5] Persisters are thought to be dormant cells that greatly slow down essential cellular functions that antibiotics generally target, including trancription, translation, cell wall synthesis, and DNA replication. Persisters are found at relatively higher levels in stationary phase compared to logarithmic cultures, consistent with a dormant state. The persistence state has been found in many different bacterial species, including *E. coli*, *Mycobacterium tuberculosis*, and *Pseudomonas aeruginosa*, underscoring the evolution of persistence as a survival strategy in different stressful environments.[6]

There is also increasing evidence that persisters mediate drug tolerance in biofilm formation associated with chronic diseases, including endocarditis, gingivitis, and osteomyelitis.[7] Biofilms form a protective environment for persisters, shielding them from the host immune system.[8] (Fig. 2) Biofilms can form readily on in-dwelling devices, such as catheters and prostheses, or on physiological surfaces, such as *P. aeruginosa* infection of the lung in cystic fibrosis patients. The dormancy of persisters and the different pathways that lead to their formation contribute to the unique challenge in treatment of chronic infections, especially in immunocompromised patients where biofilms can form deep in the soft tissues. In addition, the presence of different subpopulations of persistent pathogens with varying antiobiotic susceptibilities further complicates treatment with optimizing drug efficiencies.

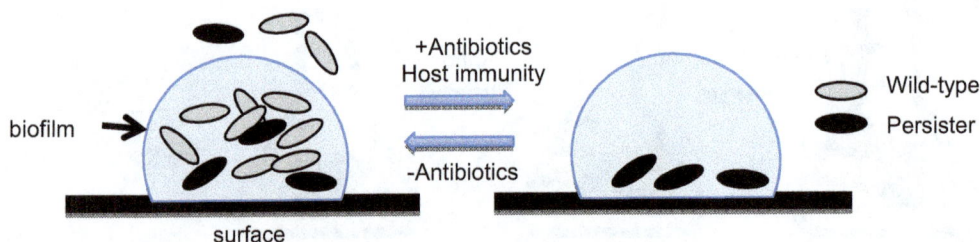

Figure 2. Biofilm formation with persisters. Biofilms can contain both wild-type replicating and persister cells. Addition of antibiotics and host immunity can kill both wild-type and persister cells in the biofilm and extracellular milieu. The biofilm matrix can protect persisters from killing and can lead to re-population of pathogen in the biofilm after antibiotics are removed.

3. Molecular mechanisms of bacterial persistence

Despite observance of the persister phenotype since the 1940's, the genetic regulatory pathways that switch bacteria into the persister phenotype remain poorly understood. Further research on bacterial persistence rapidly declined with the availability of potent antibiotics. Furthermore, there were technical difficulties in obtaining sufficient numbers of persister cells for analysis and a lack of sophisticated and sensitive methods to study rare biological events at single cell resolution. With the recent emergence of antibiotic-resistant bacterial strains, interest in the mechanisms of bacterial persistence has slowly resurged, amid rapid advances in microfluidics and advanced imaging that can be applied to single cell analysis. [9, 10] A list of genes and pathways linked to persistence is listed in Table 1.

In the 1980's, a genetic screen was performed to select for *E. coli* mutants that exhibited increased persistence in response to ampicillin exposure.[11] *hipA* (high persistence) was the first gene identified that modulated the frequency of persister formation, with the gain-of-function allele *hipA7* inducing ~1% persisters in culture, an ~1000 fold increase in persisters compared to a wild-type strain. HipA is a component of a toxin-antitoxin (TA) module that plays a role in inhibition of protein and nucleic acid synthesis in response to stress. HipA functions as a kinase that phosphorylates the essential translation factor Elongation Factor Tu (EF-Tu) to inhibit translation.[12]

The increased level of persister cells has led to the use of *hipA* mutants in multiple studies on bacterial persistence, including integration of microfluidics and single cell microscopy[13] and microarray analysis.[14] These types of studies can enable quantitative analysis of single cell behavior and gene expression dynamics to measure cell-to-cell heterogeneity in a clonal cell population. For example, growth patterns of fluorescently-labeled *E. coli hipA* mutants in the channels of a microfluidic device suggested that slow-growing persister cells were already present in the bacterial culture prior to antibiotic exposure, suggesting that the persistent state may partially stem from stochastic mechanisms.[13] This study led to the identification of two different persister types. Type I persisters are non-growing cells that enter at stationary phase, a dormant state that protects them from the lethal action of several antibiotics known to affect mainly actively growing cells. Type II persisters do not require a starvation signal to enter the persister state and are continuously generated during exponential growth in a fashion that seems to depend on the population size. Although Type I and II persisters exist in wild-type populations of *E. coli*, their differentiation has only been achieved using time lapse single cell microscopy. Bacterial cells were also shown to still express proteins for a short period of time prior to entering into full dormancy, indicating a gradual downregulation of essential cellular processes during switching to the persistence state.[15]

While HipA contributes to persistence in *E. coli*, the absence or poor conservation of *hipA* in other bacteria that have exhibited persistence suggested the existence of other persistence mechanisms. Several other genetic screens have led to identification of additional metabolic genes that function in cell dormancy, including GlpD[16], an enzyme that functions in glycerol-3-phosphate metabolism, PhoU[17], a negative regulator that inhibits energy metabolism and nutrient transport, the global regulators DksA and DnaKJ[18], and the HipA-like toxin proteins RelE and MazF.[19 - 21] Transient ectopic overexpression of chaperone DnaJ and PmrC were also shown to increase the number of persisters by up to 1000-fold.[19]

There is also increasing evidence that bacterial communication via chemical signaling may play a role in establishing persistence. Recently, indole signaling has been implicated in triggering persistence, leading to enhancement of persister formation in *E. coli* by ~10-fold in response to multiple antibiotics.[22] This indole signaling is dependent on activation of the OxyR and phage-shock pathways and enables the bacterial community to alter its frequency of persistence as a survival mechanism. Another mediator of bacterial cell-cell communications, the quorum-sensing peptide CSP pheromone was also implicated in the formation of stress-induced multidrug-tolerant persisters in the oral pathogen *Streptococcus mutans*, the leading etiological agent of dental biofilm.[23] In addition, gaseous ammonia released by stationary phase bacterial cultures was found to modify the antibiotic resistance spectrum of bacterial neighbors.[24] Ammonia release increases the level of intracellular polyamines, which modulates membrane permeability to different antibiotics.

These results suggest that persisters may form through independent parallel mechanisms and do not follow a single linear regulatory pathway. The underlying commonality is that each of these mechanisms leads to a small subset of quiescent or slowly-dividing cells within an otherwise rapidly dividing population. The fact that the great majority of candidate persister genes have been identified in *E. coli* leaves open the question of whether persistence mechanisms are universal or species-specific. For example, *P. aeruginosa* infection in cystic fibrosis patients is thought to be exacerbated by persister cells in biofilm formation and subsequent recalcitrance to antibiotic treatment.[25] However, the majority the *E. coli* persister gene candidates do not have confirmed homologs in *P. aeruginosa*. An independent screen of a transposon insertion library from *P. aeruginosa* identified a separate list of genes, including a putative DNA helicase and type IV pilus response regulator, as putative persister genes.[26] Another study developed computational algorithms based on systems biology data such as transcriptomics profiles and functional interactions networks to predict novel *M. tuberculosis* genes required for long-term persistence in mouse lungs.[27] In this study, 18 novel genes were experimentally validated to play a role in persistence. To date, clear understanding of the molecular mechanisms that regulate persister formation has yet to emerge.

Key gene/pathway	Mechanism	Ref
Toxin/antitoxin		
HipA/B	Kinase that phosphorylates EF-Tu	[11-12]
RelE	Ribosome-dependent endonuclease	[20]
RelA	(p)ppGpp synthetase	[35-36]
TisB	Antimicrobial peptide that opens membrane channel	[38-40]
MazF	Endonuclease	[21]
Other genes		
GlpD	Glycerol-3-phosphate metabolism	[16]
PhoU	Negative regulator of energy metabolism	[17]
DksA	Transcriptional regulator of rRNA	[18]
DnaKJ	Chaperone	[18]
PmrC	Transfer of phosphoethanolamine to lipidA	[19]
DinG	DNA helicase in *P. aeruginosa*	[26]
PilH	Type IV pilus response regulator in *P. aeruginosa*	[26]
Other molecules		
Indole	Activation of OxyR and phage-shock pathways	[22]
CSP	Quorom-sensing peptide	[23]
Ammonia gas	Increase in intracellular polyamines	[24]

Table 1. Selected molecular pathways that lead to bacterial persistence

4. Toxin/Anti-toxin (TA) modules

One common gene family that has been linked to bacterial persistence is the TA loci, which function in adaptation to rapidly changing environmental conditions in many bacteria and Archaea.[28] TA modules are present in the genome of diverse bacteria, with more than 50 modules in *Mycobacterium tuberculosis*, a pathogen that enters dormancy as part of its disease lifecycle. Type II TA modules typically encode for a pair of co-transcribed stress-inducible proteins, a stable toxin that inhibits cell growth, and a more labile anti-toxin that regulates the activity of its cognate toxin. (Fig. 3) The toxin and anti-toxin form a tight complex and repress their own expression. Depletion of the anti-toxin leads to release of its cognate toxin, which interferes with an essential cellular target, such as mRNA, DNA gyrase, or DNA helicase, to induce cell cycle arrest or inhibit metabolic functions. There are three types of antitoxins: type I TA antitoxins encode small antisense RNAs that repress toxin gene translation, type II loci encode protein antitoxins, and type III loci express small RNA antitoxins.[29 - 31] It should be noted that the term 'toxin' can be considered a misnomer, since the toxin genes do not kill the bacteria, but rather repress cell growth.

Since the initial mapping of the *hipA* toxin to a TA locus, several other studies have linked TA function to bacterial persistence. *E. coli* becomes dormant if toxin levels exceed a specific threshold, with the amount determining the length of time bacteria remains in dormancy.[32] Persister cells increased their TA expression levels, and deletion of ten TA loci that encoded for mRNA endonucleases in *E. coli* led to a marked reduction in frequency of persister formation.[33] Furthermore, overexpression of the toxin can induce a persistence state from which cells can be resuscitated by expression of anti-toxin gene transcription.[34] This evidence supports a model in which TA loci play a key role in switching on the persistence state in response to environmental stressors.

Other TA loci, in addition to *hipA/B*, have been implicated in mediating persistence. For example, the toxin RelA has been shown to be required for the long-term survival and persistence of *M. tuberculosis* in mice.[35] Interestingly, RelA encodes for (p)ppGpp synthetase, which functions in the synthesis of (p)ppGpp, or guanosine tetra-and pentaphosphate, a signaling molecule that has been shown to be indicative of the persistent state.[36] (p)ppGpp is a central mediator of the stringent response, which modulates cell expression to survive stress and nutrient limitations.[37] Persisters exhibit relatively higher levels of (p)ppGpp, which is consistent with the slowed growth rate and metabolically inactive state in persisters. Damage of DNA induces the SOS response and expression of the TisB toxin, an endogenous antimicrobial peptide that causes persister formation by opening an ion channel.[38 - 40] This decreases the proton motive force and ATP levels, leading to target shutdown and a dormant, drug-tolerant state.

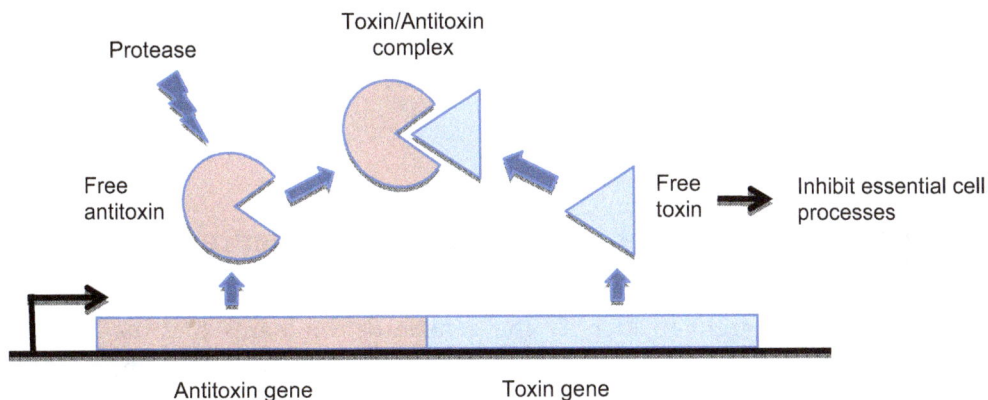

Figure 3. Co-expression and regulation of the TA loci. The anti-toxin regulates toxin activity by forming a tight complex with the toxin. The antitoxin is generally produced at a higher rate than the toxin and is degraded by cellular proteases.

Since both toxin and anti-toxin transcripts are co-expressed from a single promoter, the imbalance between the two transcripts is primarily caused by accumulation of specific proteases, such as the Lon protease in *E. coli*, that target the anti-toxin for degradation. Deletion of *lon*, but not other protease-encoding genes, led to a decrease in persistence, indicating that Lon plays in specific role in induction of persistence.[33] Lon was also identified in a screen of a *P. aeruginosa* PAO1 luciferase fusion library as a differentially-regulated gene upon exposure to a sub-inhibitory concentration of gentamicin and was shown to be essential for biofilm formation.[41]

5. Isolation of bulk and single cell persisters

Persisters are a difficult cell population to manipulate, due to their transient nature, low frequency, and mechanistic heterogeneity. A variety of methods have been utilized for persister enrichment and have leveraged *hipA* mutant *E. coli* strains as the starting material to maximize persister numbers. Persister cells have been isolated based on sedimentation of surviving cells following antibiotic treatment.[3, 14] Transcriptomics profiling from the persister population indicated that genes involved in energy production were downregulated, consistent with a dormant phenotype. However, since each antibiotic and microbe exhibits unique killing and survival kinetics, respectively, treatment to isolate persisters is highly dependent on the individual system. Prolonged exposure to antibiotic agents may also activate stress response mechansims, which have been recently linked to induction of persistence. Another isolation method utilized an *E. coli* strain expressing a green fluorescent protein (GFP) reporter fused to a ribosomal RNA promoter *rrnBP1*.[42] Since persisters display low metabolic activty, sorting of dimly green cells by FACS will concentrate persisters that exhibit little of no transcription from the *rrnBP1* promoter. Finally, persisters have also been isolated by using a combination of alkaline and enzymatic lysis that targets the cell membrane and kills normally growing cells.[43] This strategy took 25 min compared to >3 hrs for previous methods and hence is less likely to induce a stable stress response. Furthermore, persisters isolated with this protocol did not exhibit activation of the SOS response, indicating that stress response was not activated.

6. Therapeutic strategies that target bacterial persistence

Initially, investigators sought to identify the genetic determinants that mediate persister formation as potential targets to prevent or reverse persistence. Given the number of disparate genes that appear to be involved in persistence, such an approach may prove to be difficult. Nevertheless, identification of bacterial proteins that are essential even in persisters can provide novel targets for drug development. Since persisters exist in a slowed metabolic state, it is likely that changes in environmental parameters can shift pathogen metabolism from persistence to a replicating state. In the last several years, compounds have been identified that have exhibited promise in the switching of persisters into growing cells susceptible to antibiotic killing or in the direct killing of persisters. (Table 2) These strategies can be integrated with current antibiotics regimens to develop novel viable therapies for treatment of infectious disease.

6.1. Metabolite stimulation of aminoglycoside-mediated bacterial killing

A promising strategy for the eradication of persistent bacteria is the combination of an antibiotic that kills actively replicating bacteria with a metabolite that may enhance the susceptibility of the persistent bacteria to antibiotics. An elegant example of this strategy was the addition of metabolites to stimulate cellular metabolism and switch *E. coli* and *S. aureus* persisters back to the wild-type state to be susceptible to aminoglycosides.[44] Multiple carbon sources that maximize coverage of glycolysis, the pentose-phosphate pathway and the Entner-Doudoroff pathway were tested for their ability to potentiate aminoglycosides against *E. coli* persisters. Metabolites that enter upper glycolysis, including glucose, mannitol, and fructose, and one that enters lower glycolysis, pyruvate, led to a reduction in persister viability in response to the aminoglycoside gentamicin, by three orders of magnitude. Other metabolites that enter the latter two pathways (e.g. arabinose and ribose) did not have a significant effect on persister death. This potentiation was found to be specific to aminoglycosides, and did not occur in persisters exposed to quinolone or β-lactam antibiotics, which target DNA and the cell wall, respectively. The metabolic stimuli were found to generate a proton-motive force (PMF), which facilitates aminoglycoside uptake and subsequent bacterial killing. Treatment of persisters with an inhibitor of PMF, the ionophore CCCP, abolished aminoglycoside potentiation by the metabolite/gentamicin treatment. These results indicate that persisters, although dormant, are nevertheless primed for metabolic uptake and energy metabolism.

In both an *E. coli* biofilm model and a chronic biofilm-associated infection in mice, a combination of mannitol and gentamicin reduced biofilm viability by several orders of magnitude compared to antibiotic alone. In the infected mice, the dual treatment inhibited bacterial spread to the kidneys, compared to no treatment or antibiotic alone, demonstrating the feasibility for potential clinical use. Metabolite-enabled killing of persisters was also shown to be effective in the Gram-positive pathogen *Staphylococcus aureus*, although with fructose as the most effective metabolite, due to the differential expression of metabolite transporters in *S. aureus*. Thus, delivery of PMF-stimulating metabolites may be a novel strategy to complement current aminoglycoside treatments to generate more effective antibacterial therapies.

6.2. Hyperactivation of ClpP protease kills persisters

Modulation of target protein function that is lethal for microbes is a novel approach for persister cell elimination. In a recent paper, activation of the ClpP protease by the antibiotic acyldepsipeptide 4 (ADEP4) was shown to kill persister cells by degrading over 400 cellular proteins.[45] ADEP exhibits anti-bacterial activity against Gram-positive bacteria *in vitro* and in several rodent models of bacterial infection.[46] ClpP is a proteolytic subunit that normally pairs with different ATPase regulatory subunits to degrade misfolded proteins in the bacterial cytoplasm. Binding of ADEP to ClpP maintains the catalytic chamber of ClpP in an open configuration to enable promiscuous cleavage of proteins and decouple protein degradation from dependence on ATP hydrolysis. Null mutants of *clpP* were resistant to ADEP4, but were found to be highly resistant to killing by multiple antibiotics. This uncontrolled proteolysis ultimately resulted in bacterial autolysis and cell death. Treatment with ADEP4 exhibited a decrease in cell count of *S. aureus* stationary cells by 4 $\log_{10}$ in two days. Conventional antibiotics, including rifampicin, linezolid, and ciprofloxacin, were inactive against stationary phase *S. aureus*. However, treatment with a combination of ADEP4 and a conventional antibiotic led to eradication of *S. aureus* persisters in growing and stationary cultures. Furthermore, this combination treatment cleared a chronic biofilm infection in a mouse model that was previously untreatable with just conventional antibiotics.[45] These studies demonstrate that persisters are not invulnerable to killing and that ADEP4 is an effective antibiotic against persisters in a deep-seated biofilm infection. Conventional antibiotics were likely not effective against persisters due to pathogen tolerance rather than the inability to diffuse within the biofilm.

Compound	Mechanism	Ref
Metabolites (e.g. mannitol, fructose)	Metabolite stimulation to generate a proton-motive force for aminoglycoside-mediated killing	[44]
ADEP4	Activation of the Clp protease to promiscuously cleave target proteins in persisters	[45]
HT61	Drug compound depolarizes and breaks down bacterial cell wall	[47]
C10	Drug compound killed persisters in combination with antibiotics	[48]
Pyrazinamide	Byproduct pyrazinoic acid activates multiple essential cellular processes	[53]
Diarlyquinolines (TMC207)	Inhibitor of ATP synthase to block energy metabolism in TB	[55]
Imidazopyridines Benzimidazoles Thiopenes	Drug compounds that reduced ATP content in both replicating and persistent Mycobacteria	[58]
Muropeptides	Activation of PrkC to stimulate translation	[60]
Rpf (Resuscitation promotion factor)	Degradation of peptidoglycan as mediators to induce cell growth	[61]

Table 2. Strategies to defeat bacterial persistence

6.3. Drug screening against metabolically-inactive bacteria

Small molecule library screens have been performed to identify compounds that specifically target persisters. A quinolone-derived library was screened against non-multiplying *S. aureus* using a long-term stationary phase culture.[47] One compound in particular, termed HT61, exhibited 6 logs killing compared to 1 log for commercially-available antibiotics, such as amoxicillin and linezolid, in *S. aureus* persisters and clinical methillicin-resistant *S. aureus* strains. HT61 acts via depolarization of the bacterial cell membrane and subsequent break-down of the cell wall. HT61 also displayed significant bactericidal effects against other Gram positive pathogens, including *Streptococcus pyogenes* and *Streptococcus agalactiae*, but was less potent for actively-replicating *S. aureus* and not effective against Gram negative bacteria such as *E. coli* and *Klebsiella aerogenes*. In a mouse skin bacterial colonization model, HT61 effectively killed surface *S. aureus* and did not induce adverse effects in a minipig skin model. Importantly, HT61-resistant *S. aureus* were not detected even after 50 passages of exposure, suggesting that compounds that target persisters may bypass development of antibiotic resistance in normally replicating bacteria.

Another screen was performed to identify compounds from a library composed of 6800 chemicals, based on scaffolds and physicochemical properties, that can effectively kill persist-ers.[48] Compounds were downselected based on enhanced killing of *E. coli* K-12 in combi-nation with both ampicillin and norfloxacin, two antibiotics with different mechanisms of action. In particular, one compound denoted C10, 3-[4-(4-methoxyphenyl)piperazin-1-yl]piperidin-4-yl biphenyl-4-carboxylate, exhibited a marked decrease in *E. coli* and *Pseudomonas aeroginosa* persistence frequency in combination with fluoroquinolone antibiotics, but did not affect normal antibiotic-sensitive cells. While persisters were killed when treated with a combination of C10 and norfloxacin, they also exhibited fast re-growth in the presence of C10 alone, suggesting that C10 may induce reversion of dormant persisters into replicating antibiotic-sensitive cells. It will be necessary to identify the binding target of C10 to more fully understand the mechanism of action on bacterial persistence.

6.4. Combination therapy to treat tuberculosis

Combination treatments that target both replicating and persistent bacteria will likely prove to be an effective strategy to combat chronic infections. A good example of this approach is the multiple drug treatment of tuberculosis (TB), a global disease mediated by *Mycobacterium tuberculosis*, that causes ~2 million deaths per year. Dormant TB can survive within a host for decades, thus requiring long-term treatment. Treatment of active *M. tuberculosis* by a front-line cocktail of four drugs, isozianid, rifampicin, pyrazinamide, and ethambutol, can be effective in controlling the disease in the first several months. Isoniazid is effective against rapidly growing bacilli in lesions, whereas rifampicin and pyrazinamide are thought to be more effective in killing persistent bacilli.[49] These persistent bacilli localize in macrophages within tissue cavities. Upon exposure in a low O_2 (hypoxic) and nutrient environment, they enter a low-metabolic, dormant state by downregulation of protein and nucleic acid synthesis and formation of a thick cell wall. TB persister cells escape both host immune detection and killing by isoniazid, which can lead to disease relapse upon exit out of the dormant state in the host.

Interestingly, the mechanism of action of the front-line drug pyrazinamide, known for >50 yrs, has only recently been deciphered. Pyrazinamide is activated by a mycobacterial amidase to yield the bioactive compound pyrazinoic acid, which has been linked to multiple essential cellular processes, including ribosome function[50], fatty acid synthase II[51], and respiratory activity.[52] Trapping of pyrazinoic acid in the cell leads to a rise in acidity, which kills the pathogen.[53] Other existing antibiotics, such as moxifloxacin and gatifloxacin, have also been shown to enhance rates of *M. tuberculosis* persister death when combined with conventional drug treatments.[54]

Although in a latent state, *M. tuberculosis* still performs respiratory energy conversion to maintain requisite metabolic functions, providing a potential target for novel drug development. Dormant mycobacteria were found to express a functional ATP synthase to generate energy that drives basal cellular reactions. A newly-discovered inhibitor of ATP synthase, diarylquinoline TMC207, was recently identified as a potent anti-mycobacterial compound against replicating *M. tuberculosis*.[55] Significantly, nanomolar concentrations of TMC207 were able to kill dormant pathogen by blocking ATP synthase activity at a higher efficacy than observed for replicating mycobacteria, despite ATP synthase being transcriptionally downregulated in latent *M. tuberculosis*.[56] TMC207 also exhibited potent sterilization in an infected lung mouse model, comparable to the triple drug combination of rifampicin, isozianid, and pyrazinamide. The high efficacy of TMC207 may stem from killing of both actively-growing and dormant pathogen. These results suggest that basal ATP synthase activity is essential for the survival of dormant *M. tuberculosis,* and ATP homeostasis may represent a viable target for development of persister-directed drugs. TMC207 is presently in Phase II clinical trials for TB treatment. Furthermore, medicinal chemistry optimization efforts led to generation of novel diarylquinoline chemotypes that targeted Gram-positive pathogens, including *S. aureus* in replicating planktonic and metabolically resting biofilm states, potentially broadening the antibacterial spectrum of diarylquinoline-based antibiotics.[57]

To further identify novel inhibitors against dormant mycobacteria, a hypoxic model system was established to screen >600,000 compounds for those that lowered ATP content in a non-replicating *M. bovis* BCG recombinant strain.[58] The screen yielded 140 non-cytotoxic compounds, including imidazopyridines, benzimidazoles, and thiopenes, which modulated respiratory function against both replicating and non-replicating mycobacteria. Reduction of cellular ATP levels was shown to correlate with cell death in bacteria treated with the three compound clusters. Thus, these clusters may form the basis of antibiotic compound development against mycobacteria.

6.5. Bacterial factors that trigger exit from dormancy

Sporulation is another form of persistence in which both pathogen and environmental microbes enter a metabolically-inactive state and become resistant spores under unfavorable conditions. For example, in nutrient-poor environments, *Bacillus* and *Clostridium* species undergo tightly regulated transcriptional and morphological changes to form a dormant but robust spore that is resistant to extreme stress conditions, such as high temperatures, desiccation, and toxicity. In the laboratory, *Bacillus subtilis* spores have been shown to germinate and exit the spore state in response to treatment with various nutrients, such as amino acids.[59] Binding of these nutrients to receptors on the inner membrane of the spore leads to rehydration of the cell interior and breakdown of the peptidoglycan spore layer. *B. subtilis* has also been shown to exit dormancy in response to peptidoglycan-derived muropeptides, consisting of a disaccharide-tripeptide with a meso-diaminopimelic acid (m-DAP) residue in the third position.[60] Peptidoglycan from growing cells, but not stationary cells, have been shown to more effectively induce germination, suggesting that these muropeptides may function as signaling molecules that can stimulate dormant cells. In response to muropeptide binding to its extracellular domain, the serine/threonine kinase PrkC has been shown to phosphorylate elongation factor G (EF-G), which modulates ribosomal activity and initiation of translation to induce microbial exit from dormancy.[60]

Other protein factors expressed by microbes have been reported to stimulate growth of dormant cells. The environmental microbe, *Micrococcus luteus*, secretes a resuscitation-promoting factor (Rpf), which can stimulate exit from dormancy when added to *M. luteus* cultures.[61] *M. luteus* Rpf has been shown to hydrolyze peptidoglycan at picomolar concentrations and stimulate aged cultures of *M. tuberculosis*, thus exhibiting cross-species activity. [62, 63] *M. tuberculosis* expresses five endogenous Rpfs that function in reactivation of chronic tuberculosis in animal models.[64] Although the exact function of Rpfs remains unclear, it has been suggested that Rpf-mediated proteolysis of peptidoglycan can generate muropeptides for PrkC-like kinases to activate protein translation.[65]

7. Conclusion

The rise in antimicrobial drug resistance, alongside the failure of conventional research efforts to discover new antibiotics, will eventually lead to a public health crisis that can drastically curtail our ability to combat infectious disease. Bacterial persistence is an underexplored mechanism by which to develop novel treatments to complement or extend the current repertoire of antibiotics.[66 - 68] Although persisters do not cause overt disease, they act as a pool from which bacteria can emerge from dormancy to cause recurrent infection. Mechanisms of persister formation appear to be highly redundant across different bacterial species, which contributes to the difficulty in identification of universal mechanisms to target and eradicate persistence. To date, the more successful strategies in the lab have been to target cell functions, such as basal energy metabolism and cell wall integrity, that are also essential for persister cell maintenance.[69] Of particular note, addition of metabolites such as mannitol or fructose was shown to potentiate aminoglycoside-mediated killing by generating a proton motive force to stimulate aminoglycoside uptake.[44] Several medicinal chemistry strategies to screen for small molecules effective against persisters have also identified lead targets for potential optimization and rational drug design.

By developing treatments against both persisters and replicating pathogens, it may be possible to shorten antibiotic regimens, especially for deep-seated diseases such as tuberculosis, and reduce relapse rates in patients. Another advantage to combination therapies is potential extension of the useful life of current antibiotics to kill pathogen at a faster rate, and thus slow down the further emergence of antibiotic resistance. Additional strategies to optimize pulse-dosing regimens using multiple antibiotics that include anti-persister drugs may be able to sterilize particularly recalcitrant chronic infections. These types of therapies may be designed for the individual patient as part of an increasingly personalized approach to medicine. Aside from the clinical relevance of bacterial persisters, non-genetic heterogeneity has been found to play important roles in other systems, including susceptibility of cancer cells to treatment[70], host response to viral infection[71], and bacterial responses to other stresses.[72] Thus, understanding the mechanisms of cell-to-cell variability will provide insights into the general adaptation of life to variable environments.

Acknowledgements

The writing of this review was supported by a Defense Threat Reduction Agency (DTRA) grant to EH-G to study molecular mechanisms of bacterial persistence and develop therapeutics stratagies to defeat persistence.

Author details

Elizabeth Hong-Geller* and Sofiya N. Micheva-Viteva

*Address all correspondence to: ehong@lanl.gov

Los Alamos National Laboratory, Bioscience Division, Los Alamos, NM, USA

References

[1] Bigger J. Treatment of staphylococcal infections with penicillin by intermittent sterilisation. Lancet 1944;244 497-500.

[2] Levin B, Rozen D. Non-inherited antibiotic resistance. Nat Rev Microbiol 2006;4 556-62.

[3] Lewis K. Persister cells. Annual review of microbiology 2010;64 357-72.

[4] Coates A, Hu Y. Targeting non-multiplying organisms as a way to develop novel antimicrobials. Trends Pharmacol Sci 2008;29 143-50.

[5] Gilbert P, Collier P, Brown M. Influence of growth rate on susceptibility to antimicrobial agents: biofilm, cell cycle, dormancy, and stringent response. Antimicrob Agents Chemo 1990;34 1865-8.

[6] Dhar N, McKinney J. Microbial phenotypic heterogeneity and antibiotic tolerance. Cur Opin Microbiol 2007;10 30-8.

[7] Hall-Stoodley I, Costerton J, Stoodley P. Bacterial biofilms: from the natural environment to infectious disease. Nature Rev Microbiol 2004;2 95-108.

[8] Mah T. Biofilm-specific antibiotic resistance. Future Microbiol 2012;7 1061-72.

[9] Bennett M, Hasty J. Microfluidic devices for measuring gene network dynamics in single cells. Nat Rev Genet 2009;10 628-38.

[10] Young J, Locke J, Altinok A, Rosenfeild N, Bacarian T, Swain P, Mjolsness E, Elowitz M. Measuring single-cell gene expression dynamics in bacteria using fluorescence time-lapse microscopy. Nat Protoc 2012;7 80-8.

[11] Moyed HS, Bertrand KP. hipA, a newly recognized gene of *Escherichia coli* K-12 that affects frequency of persistence after inhibition of murein synthesis. J Bacteriol 1983;155 768-75.

[12] Schumacher M, Piro R, Xu W, Hansen S, Lewis K, Brennan R. Molecular mechanisms of HipA-mediated multidrug tolerance and its neutralization by HipB. Science 2009;323 396-401.

[13] Balaban N, Merrin J, Chait R, Kowalik L, Leibler S. Bacterial persistence as a phenotypic switch. Science 2004;305 1622-162.

[14] Keren I, Shah D, Spoering A, Kaldalu N, Lewis K. Specialized persister cells and the mechanism of multidrug tolerance in *E. coli*. J Bacteriol 2004;186 8172-80.

[15] Gefen O, Gabay C, Mumcuoglu M, Engel G, Balaban N. Single-cell protein induction dynamics reveals a period of vulnerability to antibiotics in persister bacteria. Proc Natl Acad Sci 2008;105 6145-9.

[16] Spoering A, Vulic M, Lewis K. GlpD and PlsB participate in persister cell formation in *E. coli*. J Bacteriol 2006;188 5136-44.

[17] Li Y, Zhang Y. PhoU is a persistence switch involved in persister formation and tolerance to multiple antibiotics and stresses in *E. coli*. Antimicrob Agents Chemother 2007;51 2092-9.

[18] Hansen S, Lewis K, Vulic M. Role of global regulators and nucleotide metabolism in antibiotic tolerance in *E. coli*. Antimicrob Agents Chemo 2008;52 2718-26.

[19] Vasquez-Laslop N, Lee H, Neyfakh A. Increased persistence in *E. coli* caused by controlled expression of toxins or other unrelated proteins. J Bacteriol 2006;188 3494-7.

[20] Griffin M, Davis J, Strobel S. Bacterial toxin RelE: a highly efficient ribonuclease with exquisite specificity using atypical catalytic residues. Biochem 2013;52 8633-42.

[21]   Aizenman E, Engelberg-Kulka H, Glaser G. An *E. coli* chromosomal "addiction module" regulated by guanosine 3',5'-bispyrophosphate: a model for programmed bacterial cell death. Proc Natl Acad Sci 1996;93 6059-63.

[22]   Vega N, Allison K, Khalil A, Collins J. Signaling-mediated bacterial persister formation. Nat Chem Biol 2012;8 431-3.

[23]   Leung V, Levesque C. A stress-inducible quorum-sensing peptide mediates the formation of persister cells with noninherited multidrug tolerance. J Bacteriol 2012;194 2265-74.

[24]   Bernier S, Letoffe S, Delepierre M, Ghigo J. Biogenic ammonia modifies antibiotic resistance at a distance in physically separated bacteria. Mol Microbiol 2011;81 705-16.

[25]   Spoering A, Lewis K. Biofilms and planktonic cells of *Pseudomonas aeruginosa* have similar resistance to killing by antimicrobials. J Bacteriol 2001;183 6746-51.

[26]   De Groote V, Verstraeten N, Fauvart M, Kint C, Verbeeck A, Beullens S, Cornelis P, Michiels J. Novel persistence genes in *Pseudomonas aeruginosa* identified by high-throughput screening. FEMS Microbiol Lett 2009;297 73-9.

[27]   Dutta N, Bandyopadhyay N, Veeramani B, Lamichhane G, Karakousis P, Bader J. Systems-biology-based identification of *Mycobacterium tuberculosis* persistence genes in mouse lungs. mBio 2014;5 e01066-13.

[28]   Gerdes K, Maisonneuve E. Bacterial persistence and toxin-antitoxin loci. Annu Rev Microbiol 2012;66 103-23.

[29]   Fozo E, Hemm M, Storz G. Small toxic proteins and the antisense RNAs that repress them. Microbiol Mol Biol Rev 2008;72 579-89.

[30]   Gerdes K, Christensen S, Lebner-Olesen A. Prokaryotic toxin-antitoxin stress response loci. Nat Rev Microbiol 2005;3 371-82.

[31]   Fineran P, Blower T, Folds I, Humphreys D, Lilley K, Salmond G. The phage abortive infection system, ToxIN, functions as a protein-RNA toxin-antitoxin pair. Proc Natl Acad Sci 2009;106 894-9.

[32]   Rotem E, Loinger A, Ronin I, Levin-Reisman I, Gabay C, Shoresh N, Biham O, Balaban N. Regulation of phenotypic variability by a threshold-based mechanism underlies bacterial persistence. Proc Natl Acad Sci 2010;107 12541-6.

[33]   Maisonneuve E, Shakespeare L, Jorgensen M, Gerdes K. Bacterial persistence by RNA endonucleases. Proc Natl Acad Sci 2011;108 13206-11.

[34]   Pedersen K, Christensen SK, Gerdes K. Rapid induction and reversal of a bacteriostatic condition by controlled expression of toxins and antitoxins. Mol Microbiol 2002;45 501-10.

[35]   Dahl J, Kraus C, Boshoff H, Doan B, Foley K, Avarbock D, Kaplan G, Mizrahi V, Rubin H, Barry C. The role of RelMtb-mediated adaptation to stationary phase in long-

term persistence of *Mycobacterium tuberculosis* in mice. Proc Natl Acad Sci 2003;100 10026-31.

[36] Korch S, Henderson T, Hill T. Characterization of the hipA7 allele of *E. coli* and evidence that high persistence is governed by (p)ppGpp synthesis. Mol Microbiol 2003;50 1199-213.

[37] Baracchini F, Bremer H. Stringent and growth control of rRNA synthesis in *E. coli* are both mediated by ppGpp. J Biol Chem 1988;263 2597-602.

[38] Dorr T, Vulic M, Lewis K. Ciprofloxacin causes persister formation by inducing the TisB toxin in *Escherichia coli*. PLoS Biol 2010;8 e1000317.

[39] Unoson C, Wager E. A small SOS-induced toxin is targeted against the inner membrane in *Escherichia coli*. Mol Microbiol 2008;70 258-70.

[40] Gurnev P, Ortenberg R, Dorr T, Lewis K, Bezrukov S. Persister-promoting bacterial toxin TisB produces anion-selective pores in planar lipid bilayers. FEBS Lett 2012;586 2529-34.

[41] Marr A, Overhage H, Bains M, Hancock R. The Lon protease of *Pseudomonas aeruginosa* is induced by aminoglycosides and is involved in biofilm formation and motility. Microbiol 2007;153 474-82.

[42] Shah D, Zhang Z, Khodursky A, Kaldalu N, Kurg K, Lewis K. Persisters: a distinct physiological state of *E. coli*. BMC Microbiol 2006;6 53.

[43] Canas-Duarte S, Restrepo S, Pedraza J. Novel protocol for persister cells isolation. PLoS One 2014;9 e88660.

[44] Allison KR, Brynildsen MP, Collins JJ. Metabolite-enabled eradication of bacterial persisters by aminoglycosides. Nature 2011;473 216-20.

[45] Conlon B, Nakayasu E, Fleck L, LaFleur M, Isabella V, Coleman K, Leonard S, Smith R, Adkins J, Lewis K. Activated ClpP kills persisters and eradicates a chronic biofilm infection. Nature 2013;503 365-70.

[46] Brotz-Oesterhelt H, Beyer D, Kroll H, Endermann R, Ladel C, Schroeder W, Hinzen B, Raddatz S, Paulsen H, Henninger K, Bandow J, Sahl H, Labischinski H. Dysregulation of bacterial proteolytic machinery by a new class of antibiotics. Nat Med 2005;11 1082-7.

[47] Hu Y, Shamaei-Tousi A, Liu Y, Coates A. A new approach for the discovery of antibiotics by targeting non-multiplying bacteria: a novel topical antibiotic for staphylococcal infections. PLos One 2010;5 e11818.

[48] Kim J, Heo P, Yang T, Lee K, Cho D, Kim B, Suh J, Lim H, Shin D, Kim S, Kweon D. Selective killing of bacterial persisters by a single chemical compound without affecting normal antibiotic-sensitive cells. Antimicrob Agents Chemo 2011;55 5380-3.

[49] Mitchison D. Pyrazinamide-on the antituberculosis drug frontline. Nat Med 1996;6 635-6.

[50] Shi W, Zhang X, Jiang X, Yuan H, Lee J, Barry C, Wang H, Zhang W, Zhang Y. Pyrazinamide inhibits trans-translation in *Mycobacterium tuberculosis*. Science 2011;333 1630-2.

[51] Sayahi H, Zimhony O, Jacobs W, Shekhtman A, Welch J. Pyrazinamide, but not pyrazinoic acid, is a competitive inhibitor of NADPH binding to *Mycobacterium tuberculosis* fatty acid synthase I. Bioorg Med Chem Lett 2011;21 4804-7.

[52] Lu P, Haagsma A, Pham H, Maaskant J, Mol S, Lili H, Bald D. Pyrazinoic acid decreases the proton motive force, respiratory ATP synthesis activity, and cellular ATP levels. Antimicrob Agents Chemo 2011;55 5354-7.

[53] Zhang Y, Mitchison D. The curious characteristics of pyrazinamide: a review. Int J Tuber Lung Dis 2003;7 6-21.

[54] Hu Y, Coates A, Mitchison D. Sterilizing activities of fluoroquinolones against rifampicin-tolerant populations of *Mycobacterium tuberculosis*. Antimicrob Agents Chemo 2003;47 653-7.

[55] Andries K, Verhasselt P, Guillemont J, Gohlmann H, Neefs J, Winkler H, Van Gestel J, Timmerman P, Zhu M, Lee E, Williams P, de Chaffoy D, Huitric E, Hoffner S, Cambau E, Truffot-Pernot C, Lounis N, Jarlier V. A diarylquinoline drug active on the ATP synthase of *Mycobacterium tuberculosis*. Science 2005;307 223-7.

[56] Koul A, Vranckx L, Dendouga N, Balemans W, Van den Wyngaert I, Vergauwen K, Gohlmann H, Willebrords R, Poncelet A, Guillemont J, Bald D, Andries K. Diarylquinolines are bactericidal for dormant mycobacteria as a result of disturbed ATP homeostasis. J Biol Chem 2008;283 25273-80.

[57] Balemans W, Vranckx L, Lounis N, Pop A, Guillemont J, Vergauwen K, Mol S, Gilissen R, Motte M, Lancois D, De Bolle M, Bonroy K, H L, Andries K, Bald D, Koul A. Novel antibiotics targeting respiratory ATP synthesis in Gram-positive pathogenic bacteria. Antimicrob Agents Chemo 2012;56 4131-9.

[58] Mak P, Rao S, Tan M, Lin X, Chyba J, Tay J, Ng S, Tan B, Cherian J, Duraiswamy J, Bifani P, Lim V, Lee B, Ma N, Beer D, Thayalan P, Kuhen K, Chatterjee A, Supek F, Glynne R, Zheng J, Boshoff H, Barry C, Dick T, Pethe K, Camacho L. A high-throughput screen to identify inhibitors of ATP homeostasis in non-replicating *Mycobacterium tuberculosis*. ACS Chem Biol 2012;7 1190-7.

[59] Setlow P. Spore germination. Curr Opin Microbiol 2003;6 550-6.

[60] Shah I, Laaberki M, Popham D, Dworkin J. A eukaryotic-like Ser/Thr kinase signals bacteria to exit dormancy in response to peptidoglycan fragments. Cell 2008;135 486-96.

[61] Mukamolova G, Kaprelyants A, Young D, Young M, Kell D. A bacterial cytokine. Proc Natl Acad Sci 1998;95 8916-21.

[62] Mukamolova G, Murzin A, Salina E, Demina G, Kell D, Kaprelyants A, Young M. Muralytic activity of *Micrococcus luteus* Rpf and its relationship to physiological activity in promoting bacterial growth and resuscitation. Mol Microbiol 2006;59 84-98.

[63] Shieeva M, Bagramyan K, Telkov M, Mukamolova G, Young M, Kell D, Kaprelyants A. Formation and resuscitation of "non-culturable" cells of *Rhodococcus rhodochrous* and *Mycobacterium tuberculosis* in prolonged stationary phase. Microbiol 2002;148 1581-91.

[64] Russell-Goldman E, Xu J, Wang X, Chan J, Tufariello J. *Mycobacterium tuberculosis* Rpf double-knockout strain exhibits profound defects in reactivation from chronic tuberculosis and innate immunity phenotypes. Microbiol 2008;148 1581-91.

[65] Kana B, Mizrahi V. Resuscitation-promoting factors as lytic enzymes for bacterial growth and signaling. FEMS Immunol Med Microbiol 2010;58 39-50.

[66] Bald D, Koul A. Advances and strategies in discovery of new antibacterials for combating metabolically resting bacteria. Drug Disc Today 2013;18 250-5.

[67] Smith P, Romesberg F. Combating bacteria and drug resistance by inhibiting mechanisms of persistence and adaptation. Nat Chem Biol 2007;3 549-56.

[68] Allison K, Brynildsen M, Collins J. Heterologous bacterial persisters and engineering approaches to eliminate them. Cur Opin Microbiol 2011;14 593-8.

[69] Hurdle J, O'Neill A, Chopra I, Lee R. Targeting bacterial membrane function: an underexploited mechanism for treating persistence infections. Nat Rev Microbiol 2011;9 62-75.

[70] Kessler D, Austin R, Levine H. Resistance to chemotherapy: patient variability and cellular heterogeneity. Cancer Res 2014;74 4663-70.

[71] Snidjer B, Sacher R, Ramo P, Damm E, Liberali P, Pelkmans L. Population context determines cell-to-cell variability in endocytosis and virus infection. Nature 2009;461 520-3.

[72] Booth I. Stress and the single cell: intrapopulation diverisity is a mechanism to ensure survivial upon exposure to stress. Int J Food Microbiol 2002;78 19-30.

9

Challenges of Patient Selection for Phase I Oncology Trials

Mark Voskoboynik and Hendrik-Tobias Arkenau

Additional information is available at the end of the chapter

1. Introduction

The modern era of oncology has seen an enormous increase in the number of therapeutic agents being tested on cancer patients with a broad variety of mechanisms of action, indications and rationale for their use. For an oncology drug to gain approval by the relevant government drug authority such as the United States Food and Drugs Administration (FDA) or the European Medicines Agency (EMA) it must demonstrate adequate safety and efficacy as well as have a favourable risk-benefit profile. As a result, all new oncology drugs must go through a process of investigation, usually beginning with pre-clinical laboratory and animal testing all the way through to the required clinical trials. The average time taken for a new drug to progress through clinical testing until the time it is approved is approximately 7.6 years [1]. The costs of drug development are large, estimated at up to $1 billion per approved drug and ever-increasing, placing an increasing burden on health care services [2, 3]. This has tremendous impacts on the cost of health-care provision with novel anticancer drugs often coming with a large price tag of more than $10,000 per month of treatment [4, 5]. Offsetting these costs are the tremendous improvements in patient outcomes that have been made in recent times with targeted therapies such as imatinib, trastuzumab and crizotinib to name just a few [6-8]. Patient selection for early phase oncology trials is of utmost importance because of the cascading effects it has on subsequent drug development and a drug's ultimate success as a safe, beneficial and cost-effective treatment.

2. Oncology clinical trials — Background

New drugs are developed in a sequential and rationale manner from the moment of their discovery in the pre-clinical phase through the various phases of clinical trials hopefully leading to their ultimate approval and availability for patients.

2.1. Clinical trial phases

Drugs are developed through several phases of clinical trials with each phase designed to answer specific questions and meet various endpoints (Figure 1). Each clinical trial phase can take a variable period of time to complete depending on the treatment setting, particular indication, trial drug and overall patient accrual rates. Each trial phase has specific challenges although a detailed discussion with regards to phase II and III trials is beyond the scope of this chapter.

Phase I trials, including first-in-human (FIH) trials, focus on a small group of patients to attempt to define the safety and tolerability of a particular treatment as well as the optimal dose, usually called the maximum tolerated dose (MTD).

Phase II trials use the information garnered from the Phase I trial, particularly in terms of appropriate dosing and sometimes with regards to patient selection, and a particular treatment is investigated on a larger number of patients, often with more specific disease characteristics than in Phase I patients. Increasingly so, phase II trials have multiple arms and the focus of these trials is on demonstrating a signal for treatment efficacy and consolidating the early safety data yielded from the phase I trial.

If a strong signal for the effectiveness of the trial treatment is obtained from the phase II trial, an even larger phase III trial is then conducted. Phase III trials are designed to establish the efficacy, or lack thereof, a trial treatment. As a result, a larger patient population is required and the trial treatment is compared with an established standard-of-care treatment or placebo if there is no standard treatment available to the particular patient group. Usually, it is the data and results from this study that will be relied upon to gain drug approval.

2.2. Phase I clinical trials

The primary aim of a phase I oncology clinical trial is to identify the maximum-tolerated dose (MTD) of a particular drug, defined as the dose level where greater than one-third of patients treated experience a dose-limiting toxicity (DLT). This allows the identification of the optimal and safe drug dose to take forward for further drug development – this is called the recommended phase II dose (RP2D). For cytotoxic drugs, the RP2D is usually the highest dose that can be delivered without exposing patients to unacceptable levels of toxicity. For targeted drugs, the dose of the drug that causes a treatment response and clinical activity may be very different to the MTD [9]. An important component of phase I trials is to provide patients with a safe treatment at doses that are as close to therapeutic as possible. There are often multiple secondary endpoints in phase I trials including the tolerability, response to treatment, pharmacokinetics of the study drug(s) and pharmacodynamics.

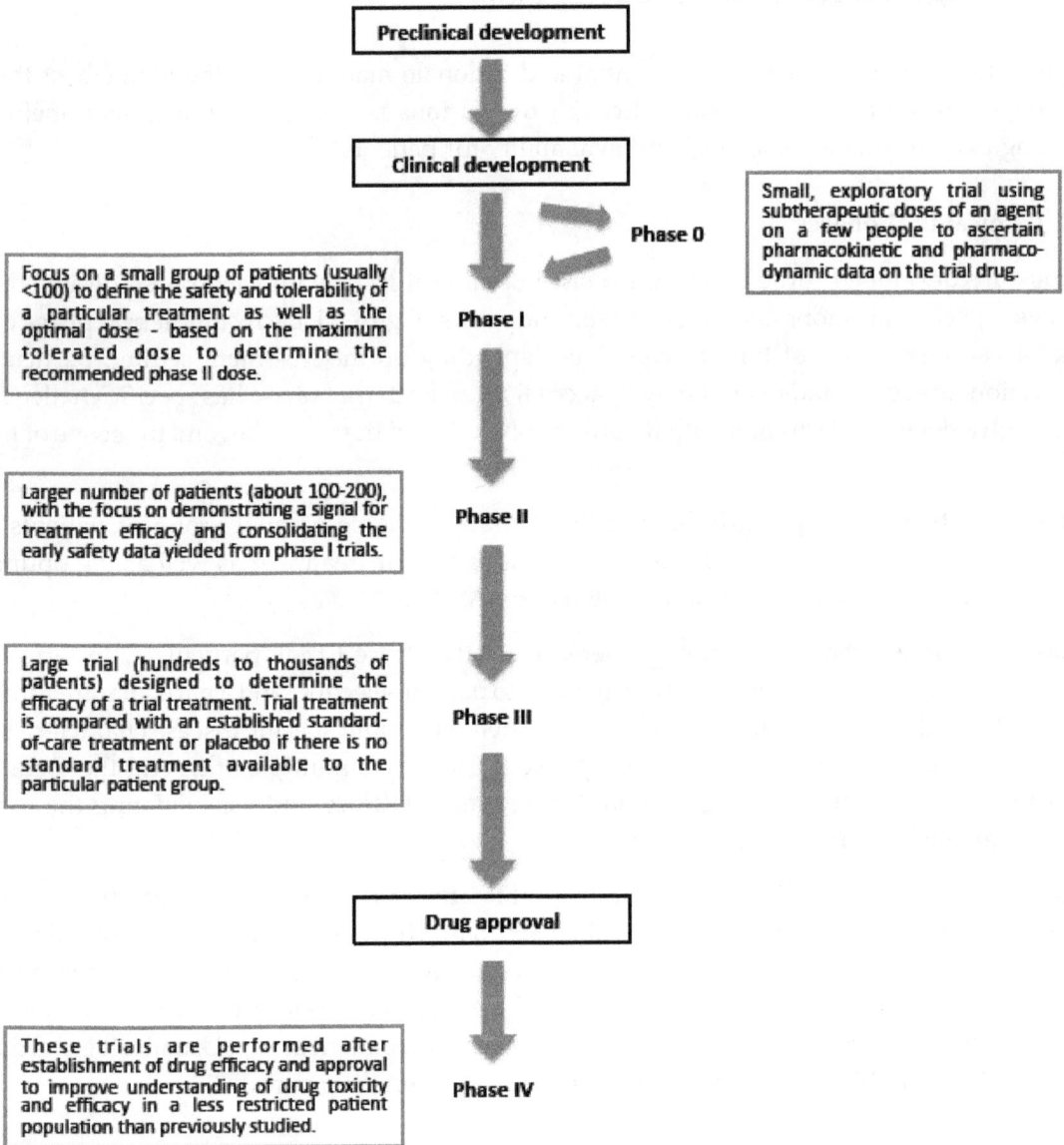

Preclinical development

Clinical development

Phase 0 — Small, exploratory trial using subtherapeutic doses of an agent on a few people to ascertain pharmacokinetic and pharmacodynamic data on the trial drug.

Phase I — Focus on a small group of patients (usually <100) to define the safety and tolerability of a particular treatment as well as the optimal dose - based on the maximum tolerated dose to determine the recommended phase II dose.

Phase II — Larger number of patients (about 100-200), with the focus on demonstrating a signal for treatment efficacy and consolidating the early safety data yielded from phase I trials.

Phase III — Large trial (hundreds to thousands of patients) designed to determine the efficacy of a trial treatment. Trial treatment is compared with an established standard-of-care treatment or placebo if there is no standard treatment available to the particular patient group.

Drug approval

Phase IV — These trials are performed after establishment of drug efficacy and approval to improve understanding of drug toxicity and efficacy in a less restricted patient population than previously studied.

Figure 1. The standard pathway for oncology drug development, including the various clinical trial phases.

The aims of phase I oncology trials clearly impact significantly upon trial design. The intention of phase I trial design is to minimise the number of patients exposed to either sub-therapeutic drug doses or severe treatment-related toxicity. With phase I trial design there is a basic tension between escalating drug doses too quickly, exposing more patients to toxicity, and escalating too slowly, exposing patients to doses of treatment that are sub-therapeutic and ineffective [10]. The design of phase I trials is therefore critical in order to minimise the risk of a negative outcome for each individual patient and at the same time controlling the number of patients required for trial enrolment in order to accomplish the aims of the trial.

The traditional design incorporating the '3 + 3' method of dose escalation is still the most widely used. This involves treating 3 patients at a time at each dose-level. The dose level should be increased for each subsequent group of 3 patients until at least 1 dose limiting toxicity (DLT) occurs in a group of 3 patients. If only 1 of 3 patients have a DLT, a further 3 patients are treated at the same dose level. If 2 or more DLTs occur per dose level, the dose escalation is stopped and occasionally a further 3 patients are treated at the dose level below. The highest dose level (where ≤1 out of 6 patients had a DLT) below the maximally administered dose had a DLT is considered the MTD and the RP2D. Dose levels are traditionally defined using a Fibonacci dose escalation whereby dose is increased by increments of 100%,67%, 50%, 40% followed by 33% for all subsequent levels.

Novel designs include accelerated titration designs, continual reassessment method and adaptive trial designs [11]. Accelerated titration phase I trial designs attempt to make phase I trials more efficient and more accurate when determining the RP2D. A group of proposed accelerated titration designs were developed by Simon and colleagues in 1997 [12]. The key features of these designs are rapid dose escalation, intra-patient dose escalation and the ability to analyse trials using a dose-toxicity model [11]. The most popular of these designs, 'design 4', starts with an initial accelerated phase that doubles the dose at each dose level, comprising of single patients. When the first DLT is experienced, the cohort for that particular dose level is expanded to include 3 patients and subsequent to this, standard phase I dose escalation and design is employed. This design also allows intra-patient dose escalation if a particular patient has no toxicity at their current dose. By use of a simulated phase I trial, as presented by Simon and colleagues in this paper, there was a significant reduction in the number of patients that were treated at sub-therapeutic doses, without a significant increase in the proportion of patients exposed to significant treatment toxicity. Other adaptive trial design methods exist, including the continual reassessment method (CRM) introduced by O'Quigley and colleagues in 1990 [13].

The potential benefits of novel designs are that fewer patients are treated with sub-therapeutic or nontherapeutic doses however they do not seem to have the reduced the number of patients that are enrolled onto trials. By adapting these novel trial designs, the most appropriate recruitment structure can be used for the particular drug under investigation.

3. Patient selection for clinical trials

3.1. Estimation of prognosis in oncology

Selecting the appropriate patient for early phase clinical trials is a fundamental component of any clinical trial design. A key component, in particular for phase I trials, but probably true for all phases of drug development, is the assessment of an individual patients prognosis. Many patients being considered for enrolment onto a phase I oncology trial have had progressive metastatic disease through all standard lines of treatment and often have a limited life expectancy. Standard trial eligibility criteria have been designed largely with the intention of minimising the number of patients enrolled onto these studies that have a poor prognosis and a greater potential for toxicity.

Estimating prognosis is inherently challenging for a clinician and estimates are often made based on intuition and experience rather than in a scientific or an evidence-based manner. Physicians' often make inaccurate estimates of a patient's prognosis, usually by being optimistic and overestimating survival. Various studies have shown that overestimation of the prognosis of terminal patients can be up to 5 times longer than their actual survival, exemplifying just how difficult making these estimates are [14-16].

Routine trial eligibility criteria include good performance status, adequate organ function (including haematological, kidney and liver etc.), and typically an anticipated life expectancy of greater than 12 weeks. Performance status is most commonly assessed using the Eastern Cooperative Oncology Group (ECOG) performance status score that is a score graded 0-5 [17]. It is a validated assessment of a patients ability to perform routine activities of daily living. A performance status (PS) of 0 indicates that the patient is fully active, ambulant and able to carry all activities without restriction whereas a PS of 5 is applied to a patient that is deceased. Most trials would permit a patient with a PS of between 0 and 1 or 2 (partially restricted in physical activity (PS = 1) and unable to carry out work activities but remain ambulatory and self-caring (PS = 2)). Another commonly used assessment score for performance status is the Karnofsky Performance Status (KPS) score which has more specific gradations between 0% (dead) and 100% (asymptomatic without complaints) in 10% increments [18, 19].

It is well documented that patients with a poorer performance status have an inferior prognosis overall when using either the KPS or ECOG PS [20-23]. It has been shown that an ECOG PS of 3 indicates a prognosis of less than 3 months and a PS of 4 of less than 1 month.

A number of other factors can be used to predict the prognosis of oncology patients. For example, the primary malignancy impacts greatly on the prediction of patient survival. For instance, patients diagnosed with metastatic carcinoid tumours often survive for a number of years compared to patients with metastatic pancreatic cancer who have a median overall survival of less than 12 months even with the best treatment currently available [24, 25]. Various laboratory data has also been associated with a poor prognosis such as hypoalbuminaemia, raised inflammatory markers (including leukocytosis, raised C-reactive peptide (CRP), lymphopenia and certain metabolic abnormalities such as hypercalcaemia [26, 27].

A number of tumour-specific prognostic scores have been developed to help stratify patients into various treatments based on their risk. A good illustrative example of this is the Memorial Sloan-Kettering Cancer Center (MSKCC) risk criteria for metastatic clear cell renal cell carcinoma. These criteria, published by Motzer and colleagues in 1999, were developed with five pre-treatment features that were associated with a shorter patient survival [28]. The five prognostic factors were low performance status (KPS <80%), high serum lactate dehydrogenase (>1.5 times upper limit of normal), low haemoglobin (< lower limit of normal), high corrected serum calcium (>10 mg/dL) and absence of prior nephrectomy. Patients with three or more risk factors were considered to be in a 'poor risk' category with a median survival time of 4 months compared to the 'favorable-risk category containing patients with zero risk factors and a median survival of 20 months.

A large number of molecular tests have been shown to have prognostic value in various malignancies. Examples of molecular results that confer a poorer prognosis in advanced cancers include BRAF mutations in colorectal cancer and melanoma, human epidermal growth factor receptor 2 (HER2) positivity in breast cancer and phosphatidylinositol-3,4,5-triphosphate 3-phosphatatse (PTEN) deficiency in prostate cancer to name a few [29-32]. Interestingly, recent developments in targeted therapies have led to the use of newer agents directed against some of these molecular or genetic abnormalities, in some cases resulting in significant improvements in prognosis and overcoming the negative prognostic implications of the result in the first place.

In addition to various clinical, molecular and genetic factors, circulating tumour cells (CTCs) can be used and have been shown to be prognostics in a variety of malignancies. CTCs are shed from solid tumours in to the circulation. Recent improvements in technology has led to a variety of laboratory methods that are able to effectively detect and isolate these CTCs which are usually very rarely found in the circulation. The CellSearch System® (Janssen Diagnostics, Inc) is the most frequently used and is the only FDA cleared device for measuring CTCs as an aid for clinicians treating patients with prostate, breast and colon cancers. A series of key studies conducted approximately 10 years ago showed that patients with higher levels of CTCs in the circulation had a poorer prognosis. For example, patients with castrate refractory prostate cancer and a CTC count lower than 5 / 7.5mL had a median overall survival of 21.7 months compared to patients with a CTC count greater than 5 that had a survival of 11.5 months [33]. Similar results were seen in patients with breast and colon cancer whereby a particular cut-point of CTC counts could be used to clearly differentiate patients with a favourable prognosis from those patients with an unfavourable prognosis [34, 35]. Although there are currently limitations with the technology and its implementation into routine clinical practice, this field is developing rapidly and will likely play a part in patient selection in the future.

Overall, the prediction of a patient's individual prognosis is challenging, complex and involves a variety of factors related to their clinical situation, the characteristics of the cancer, the molecular biology of the cancer as well as other factors including circulating tumour cells (Figure 2).

3.2. Phase I patient selection criteria

A number of prognostic scores have been published in recent times with the aim of improving patient selection for phase I clinical trials [36-40]. Probably the most important of these scores and the only one that has been prospectively validated is the Royal Marsden Hospital (RMH) score (see Table 1).

Arkenau and colleagues initially performed a retrospective analysis of 212 patients that were enrolled onto phase I trials and reviewed their demographic data as well as a number of clinical and analytic variables [38]. Using a multivariate analysis model, three independent variables

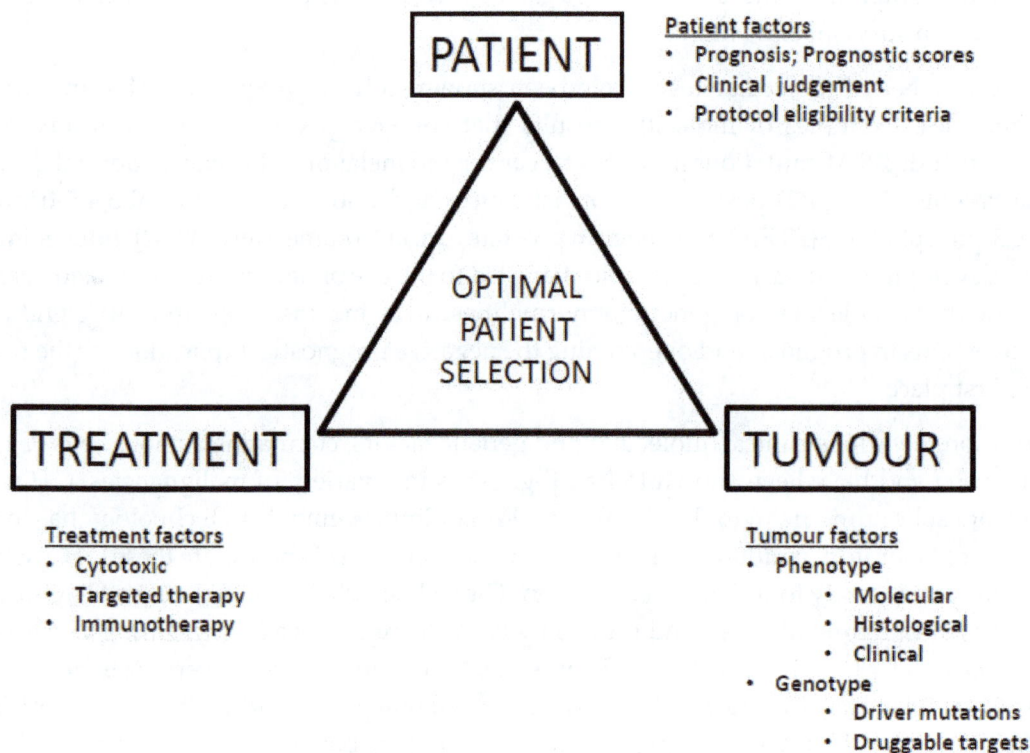

Figure 2. Factors impacting on optimal patient selection for phase I clinical trials in oncology.

were determined to be associated with a poor overall survival – an elevated lactate dehydrogenase [LDH] (above the upper limit of normal [ULN]), low albumin (< 35 g/L), and more than two sites of metastases. Using these variables, a score was developed that could separate these patients broadly into two groups, those patients with a good prognosis (RMH score 0 to 1) and those with a poor prognosis (RMH score 2 to 3). This retrospective analysis subsequently led to the prospective validation of this score in a separate publication by the same group. In this validation study, 78 prospective patients that were treated within one of 19 phase I trials were evaluated [36]. 95% of patients had an ECOG performance score of 0 to 1 and were mostly treated with new biologic agents (68%) with a minority (32%) receiving cytotoxic-based treatment. The patients had a broad range of malignancies with over 80% having gastrointestinal, breast, gynecologic, sarcoma or urologic cancers. All patients were required to have evidence of disease progression before study entry. Five patients had a partial response to their treatment (7.5%) and fourteen (17.9%) achieved stable disease at three months as per the Response Evaluation Criteria in Solid Tumours (RECIST). The median overall survival for the entire study population was 27.1 weeks with an OS of 33.0 weeks for patients with a score of 0 to 1, compared to an OS of 15.7 weeks with a score of 2 to 3 (P=0.036). These findings represent the first prospectively validated prognostic score that might assist in the optimal selection of patients for entry into phase I trials.

The RMH prognostic score was further validated at the MD Anderson Cancer Center in their Phase I trials patients [41]. They retrospectively reviewed 229 consecutive patients with lung, pancreatic and head and neck tumours that were treated on 57 phase I trials. They applied the RMH score to these patients and found that the patients with a good RMH prognostic score had a longer median survival than those with a poor prognostic score (33.9 weeks vs 21.1 weeks, P<0.0001). The authors of this study therefore showed that the RMH prognostic score can be accurately applied to patients treated at a separate institution across a range of malignancies treated in a range of trials.

Stavraka and colleagues used a multivariate approach to attempt to identify variables that predicted survival in patients referred to the phase I oncology unit at their institution to devise the Hammersmith Score (HS) [37]. Analyses were carried out on 118 patients with 52 patients (44%) treated in one of 7 phase I trials. Of these patients that actually entered a study, only 1 (2%) had a partial response and 15 (28%) had stable disease. The median OS in patients that entered a study was 22 weeks compared to 11 weeks in those patients that did not enter a study. The multivariate analysis identified four independent negative predictive factors for OS – albumin <35 g/dL (P=0.01), LDH >450 IU/dL (P<0.001), sodium <135 mmol/dL (P=0.06) and ECOG PS≥2 (P=0.04). Based on three of these variables, excluding ECOG PS, a scoring system was devised to stratify patients into either low-risk (HS score 0 to 1) or high-risk groups (HS score 2-3). Patients in the low risk group had a median OS of 31.2 weeks compared to a median OS of 8.9 weeks in the high-risk group (P<0.001).

Chau and colleagues from the Princess Margaret Hospital in Toronto, Canada, assessed 17 potential clinical characteristics in 233 patients enrolled in phase I trials to create their own risk score – the Princess Margaret Hospital Index (PMHI) [39]. In their cohort of patients, the median overall survival was 320 days, significantly longer than the 27 weeks reported by Arkenau for the Royal Marsden group. In the multivariate analysis they found that high LDH (p=0.001), > 2 metastatic sites (p=0.004) and ECOG PS > 0 (p=0.05) were significantly associated with OS. They found that 3 variables were associated with 90-day mortality – albumin <35g/L (p=0.008), > 2 metastatic sites (p=0.02) and ECOG >1 (p=0.001). A single point was assigned to each of these variables and patients with a PMHI score of 0-1 had lower 90-day mortality rate compared to patients with a score of 2-3 (7% and 37% respectively).

A large, European, multicenter study was designed to generate and validate a prognostic model for 90-day mortality which is a common eligibility criterion in phase I oncology trials [42]. Data from 2,232 patients enrolled in phase I trials across 14 oncology units was evaluated. The median overall survival was 38.6 weeks with a 90-day mortality rate of 16.5%. Two prognostic models were derived using a variety of variables including ECOG performance status, albumin, LDH, alkaline phosphatase, number of metastatic sites, lymphocytes, white cell count and time per treatment index (TPTi). TPTi is a log ratio of the time interval between diagnosis of advanced / metastatic and phase I trial entry over the number of lines of systemic treatment. The most predictive combination of variables includes albumin, LDH with ECOG PS or number of metastatic sites – similar to the RMH score. When compared to the RMH score using receiving operator characteristic (ROC) curves, there were no statistically significant differences seen. When the two models derived in this study (models A and B) were applied to patients with PS 0 to 1, patients with higher scores identified patients with OS of less than 11 weeks. When the RMH score was used to define the poorest risk group, their median OS was 14.6 weeks. The prognostic score (derived from model B – 'European score B') was assessed for its performance on a group of 200 patients that were eligible for phase I trials (PS 0-1) and it reduced the 90-mortality by half and the total number of patients recruited by 20%. This score performed almost identically to the RMH score when applied to the same population of patients.

Along a similar but distinct line, prediction models have been devised to try to identify patients at particularly high risk of drug toxicity. In one additional attempt to improve prediction of a patients risk for serious drug-related toxicity (SDRT), a nomogram was developed by Hyman and colleagues [43]. The data from 3,104 patients treated in 127 trials sponsored by the National Cancer Institute Cancer Therapeutics Evaluation Program (CTEP) between 2000 and 2010 was used for the derivation of a nomogram that could potentially estimate a patient's risk for developing serious toxicity. Data was from a large, prospectively maintained database. Trials that were evaluating cytotoxic or molecularly targeted agents were included. Standard phase I eligibility criteria were used to select appropriate patients. SDRT was defined as a grade ≥ 3 non-haematologic or grade ≥ 4 haematologic toxicity attributed to study treatment which is similar to the definition of a dose-limiting toxicity used by the majority of phase I trials. 728 patients (23.5%) experienced a SDRT and a total of 13 (0.4%) patients died as a result of drug related toxicity. Several factors were found to be reliable (p<0.10) predictors of serious drug-related toxicities in cycle one of trial treatment. Using a variety of statistical methods, a nomogram was built incorporating ECOG PS, WBC, creatinine clearance, albumin, aspartate transaminase (AST), number of study drugs and agent type (biologic or nonbiologic). This nomogram was independently validated using an independent data set of 234 patients. The authors concluded that by using their nomogram, improvements can be made in patient selection for phase I trials, in particular by prospectively identifying patients at high risk for drug toxicity.

There are a number of older retrospective series published and in a systematic review, Ploquin and colleagues summarised the published literature regarding prognostic models for life expectancy of patients enrolled in phase I trials up till the end of 2009 [44]. Nine publications were identified with all of them being retrospective analyses, except for the RMH score by Arkenau and colleagues in 2009 as described previously [36, 45-51]. Most of these studies fairly consistently identified that patients at greatest risk of death included those with a poorer performance status and greatest tumour volume (for example: increased number of metastatic sites, raised LDH). A consistent limitation of these studies, with one notable exception, is the use of retrospective data almost all were from single centre series which limits the generalizability of these studies.

One of the standard inclusion criteria in clinical trials is a life expectancy of greater than 12 weeks so it would be interesting to see how these scores might apply for this particular inclusion criterion. The RMH score shows that patients in the good prognosis group have a survival of 33 weeks, exceeding this particular criteria but even the median survival of the poor prognosis group exceeds the 12-week threshold (15.7 weeks). The patients in the high-risk group as defined by the HS, albeit retrospectively, had a survival shorter than 12 weeks (8.9 weeks) so potentially patients that fall into this category can be excluded from phase I trials.

With a number of scores now published it is unclear which of these is superior in predicting patient survival and this would require a separate prospective trial to clarify this question. As it currently stands, the RMH score is the only score that has been prospectively validated and therefore has the strongest evidence supporting its use. This is reflected in its more widespread use however further research is required to validate its utility in sites outside the Royal Marsden Hospital and indeed across other countries and across a broad cross-section of patient populations.

Score	Prospective validation	Parameters	Overall Survival (weeks)	P-value	HR
Royal Marsden Hospital Score [36] Arkenau 2008	Yes	LDH (>ULN) = 1 Albumin (<35 g/L) = 1 > 2 sites of metastases = 1	Score 0-1: 33.0 Score 2-3: 15.7	0.036	1.4
Hammersmith Score [37] Stavraka 2014	No	LDH >450 IU/dL = 1 Albumin <35 g/dL = 1 Sodium <135 mmol/dL = 1	Score 0-1: 31.2 Score 2-3: 8.9	<0.001	
Princess Margaret Hospital Index [39] Chau 2011	No	High LDH >2 metastatic sites ECOG PS > 0			
European Model B [42] Olmos 2012	No	Albumin <35 g/dL = 1 LDH (>ULN) = 1 ≥ 3 sites of metastases = 1 Low TPTi (<24 weeks/treatment) = 1 Increased ALP (>ULN) = 1 Low lymphocyte count (<18%) = 1 High WBC (>10,500/uL)	Score 0: 141 Score 1: 61 Score 2: 54 Score 3: 37 Score 4: 29 Score 5: 21 Score 6: 11 Score 7: 10	0.036 (log-rank)	- 2.00 2.54 3.24 4.57 6.20 14.1 14.1

Abbreviations: LDH = lactate dehydrogenase; PS = performance status; TPTi = time per treatment index, a log ratio of the time interval between diagnosis of advanced / metastatic and phase I trial entry over the number of lines of systemic treatment; ULN = upper limit of normal; WBC = white blood cell count

Table 1. Key publications of prognostic scores for phase I oncology trial patients.

4. Challenges

4.1. Impact of novel agents — Targeted therapies

Conducting phase I oncology trials has a number of inherent challenges. Traditionally, patients enrolled into these trials have exhausted all prior standard available therapies and by virtue of them having an incurable malignancy and very limited future treatment options, have a shortened life expectancy. There has therefore existed a paradoxical situation whereby the ideal patient has an advanced and often heavily pre-treated cancer but requires a prognosis that is suitable for the exposure of a novel investigational drug. The landscape in this field has shifted over recent years with phase I trials increasingly investigating targeted, biological agents as opposed to cytotoxic agents. The result of this change is that patients are being enrolled into phase I trials earlier in their disease course, including in the first line setting. The implications of these changes in practice will in some ways make the task of predicting a patient's prognosis slightly more straightforward as they are earlier in their disease course. On the other hand, predicting the prognosis of treatment-naïve patients might be more unpredictable as the natural history of their cancer has not been allowed enough time to be established.

Further complicating the situation is the advent of targeted agents that have rapid and significant responses. Examples of this include crizotinib in ALK-rearranged metastatic lung adenocarcinoma, vemurafenib in metastatic melanoma harbouring BRAF V600 mutations, EGFR inhibitors such as gefitinib and erlotinib in EGFR mutated lung cancer and idelalisib, a PI3K-delta inhibitor, for indolent lymphomas [7, 52-54]. These new agents increasingly have biomarkers that strongly predict for a response to treatment that can be quite rapid. The presence of these predictive biomarkers might mean that patient selection could potentially be relaxed because of the higher likelihood of a response. An illustrative example of this is the use of EGFR inhibitors in non-small-cell lung cancer. In the initial, large phase III trial of erlotinib, an EGFR inhibitor, compared to placebo in previously treated metastatic non-small-cell lung cancer, an unselected group of patients were treated [55]. The objective response rate in the erlotinib group was only 8.9% although it did result in an improved overall survival in this group of patients. This was an important trial but it certainly did not represent a large step forward for this group of patients. At the same time as these EGFR inhibitors were being developed, it was becoming apparent that the presence of an EGFR mutation, either a base-pair deletion at exon 19 or a point mutation at exon 21 (L858R) predicted for a good response to these targeted agents [56]. Mok and colleagues subsequently published a trial comparing another EGFR inhibitor, gefitinib, to chemotherapy in patients with metastatic adenocarcinoma [54]. In this trial, patients found to be harbouring an EGFR mutation had a 71% response rate to gefitinib, far higher than the 8.9% response rate seen in an unselected group of patients.

The advent of these targeted agents and their improved response rates and often improved safety profiles means that the traditional paradigm of patient selection will need be adapted and should evolve with this change in therapeutic agents. A potential consequence of more clearly defining the patient selection criteria for phase I trials is that the criteria could become too selective. If patients that are entered onto phase I trials are 'super-selected' for the best prognostic population, the toxicity that would be seen might not be entirely reflective of the general population. This might mean that the resulting maximum tolerated dose (MTD) and therefore the recommended phase II dose (RP2D) of the trial drugs would be too high and would potentially create more drug toxicity in the phase II and phase III patients. As we have expressed previously, the cascading effects of an increased rate of drug toxicity due to overly aggressive calculation of MTD could impact on drug development and trial costs and could ultimately have a bearing on the success or failure of that drug [57].

4.2. Impact of novel agents — Immunotherapies

Another major advance in the treatment of advanced malignancies has been the development of so-called 'immune-checkpoint inhibitors'. Modern immunotherapy agents include CTLA-4 inhibitors such as ipilimumab and tremelimumab which block the CTLA-4 molecule which is important for down-regulating T-cell activation, thereby enhancing immune activation. Inhibition of the programmed cell death 1 (PD-1) receptor and its primary ligand (PD-L1) with an ever growing number of drugs such as nivolumab, lambrolizumab and pembrolizumab improves the anti-tumour T-cell immune response in a more specific mode of action than CTLA-4 inhibitors. This class of compounds have provided significant improvements in patient outcomes with gains being made in tumour responses and most importantly in patient survival in a broad range of malignancies such as melanoma, renal cell carcinoma and lung cancer amongst others [58-60].

These immunotherapies, in particular the PD-1 and PD-L1 inhibitors, seem to be largely well tolerated, particularly when compared to chemotherapy, and can induce deep tumour responses that are durable [61]. From the initial trials of these agents there appear to be a significant minority of patients that have very prolonged durations of response, far greater than would otherwise be expected with 'traditional' treatments or previous standards of care. For example, patients with metastatic melanoma that were treated with Ipilimumab, a CTLA-4 inhibitor, of the approximately 10% of patients that achieved a response to treatment, many of these continued to have a response more than 12-24 months (median 19.3 months) after treatment was commenced. This is in sharp contradistinction to the patients treated in the 'standard' therapy arm with chemotherapy (dacarbazine) where the median duration of response was 8.1 months [62]. It is not entirely clear how the above patient selection such as the RMH and PMH scores would perform for this class of agents and whether they are applicable. Further research is required to determine the applicability of the phase I prognostic scores to patients enrolled onto trials using these immunotherapies.

5. Future of trial design

With the enormous number of novel therapeutic agents being developed and studied in phase I trials, the future for oncology patients seems bright. With the new immunotherapies, including combination therapies, the concept of curing patients with advanced malignancies has even been considered [61]. Adapting trial eligibility criteria and optimising patient selection is vital for the future of a safe and cost-effective drug development process. It is clear that determining the appropriateness of a particular patient for a particular phase I trial is more complex than applying a variety of scores or nomograms. When studying treatments that are personalised for a particular tumour or biomarker or even a mutation it is also important to individualise patient selection. The tendency and temptation is have an easily generalisable patient selection criteria because of its simplicity and reproducibility. The reality is that the behaviour of malignancies differ not only between organ of origin (for example prostate cancer compared to pancreatic cancer) but also within the same cancer type based on its phenotype (for example oestrogen receptor positive breast cancer compared with oestrogen / progesterone / HER-2 negative breast cancer) or genotype (for example BRAF mutated compared to BRAF wild type melanoma).

Given the complexity of patient selection described above, patients should be rationally selected with consideration given to tumour characteristics, patient factors as well as the investigational agents being assessed. Importantly, a degree of flexibility is essential when designing phase I trials for unselected populations to allow for the often extensive inter-patient and inter-tumour variability. The best way forward for optimizing patient selection is to rapidly adapt, in an evidence-based way, to the ever-evolving drug classes being developed as well as the ongoing financial pressures of drug development and not least of all patient expectations and the need for ongoing patient safety.

Author details

Mark Voskoboynik[1,2] and Hendrik-Tobias Arkenau[1,3]

*Address all correspondence to: tobias.arkenau@hcahealthcare.co.uk

1 Sarah Cannon Research Institute UK, London, UK

2 Department of Medical Oncology, Guy's Hospital, London, UK

3 University College London, London, UK

References

[1] Kaitin KI, DiMasi JA. Pharmaceutical innovation in the 21st century: new drug approvals in the first decade, 2000-2009. Clinical pharmacology and therapeutics. 2011;89(2):183-8. Epub 2010/12/31.

[2] Kantarjian HM, Fojo T, Mathisen M, Zwelling LA. Cancer drugs in the United States: Justum Pretium--the just price. J Clin Oncol. 2013;31(28):3600-4. Epub 2013/05/08.

[3] Goozner M. The $800 million pill: The truth behind the cost of new drugs: Univ of California Press; 2004.

[4] Smith TJ, Hillner BE. Bending the cost curve in cancer care. N Engl J Med. 2011;364(21):2060-5. Epub 2011/05/27.

[5] Fojo T, Grady C. How much is life worth: cetuximab, non-small cell lung cancer, and the $440 billion question. J Natl Cancer Inst. 2009;101(15):1044-8. Epub 2009/07/01.

[6] Demetri GD, von Mehren M, Blanke CD, Van den Abbeele AD, Eisenberg B, Roberts PJ, et al. Efficacy and safety of imatinib mesylate in advanced gastrointestinal stromal tumors. N Engl J Med. 2002;347(7):472-80. Epub 2002/08/16.

[7] Shaw AT, Kim DW, Nakagawa K, Seto T, Crino L, Ahn MJ, et al. Crizotinib versus chemotherapy in advanced ALK-positive lung cancer. N Engl J Med. 2013;368(25): 2385-94. Epub 2013/06/04.

[8] Piccart-Gebhart MJ, Procter M, Leyland-Jones B, Goldhirsch A, Untch M, Smith I, et al. Trastuzumab after adjuvant chemotherapy in HER2-positive breast cancer. N Engl J Med. 2005;353(16):1659-72. Epub 2005/10/21.

[9] Postel-Vinay S, Arkenau HT, Olmos D, Ang J, Barriuso J, Ashley S, et al. Clinical benefit in Phase-I trials of novel molecularly targeted agents: does dose matter? Br J Cancer. 2009;100(9):1373-8. Epub 2009/04/30.

[10] LoRusso PM, Boerner SA, Seymour L. An overview of the optimal planning, design, and conduct of phase I studies of new therapeutics. Clin Cancer Res. 2010;16(6): 1710-8. Epub 2010/03/11.

[11] Ivy SP, Siu LL, Garrett-Mayer E, Rubinstein L. Approaches to phase 1 clinical trial design focused on safety, efficiency, and selected patient populations: a report from the clinical trial design task force of the national cancer institute investigational drug steering committee. Clin Cancer Res. 2010;16(6):1726-36. Epub 2010/03/11.

[12] Simon R, Freidlin B, Rubinstein L, Arbuck SG, Collins J, Christian MC. Accelerated titration designs for phase I clinical trials in oncology. J Natl Cancer Inst. 1997;89(15): 1138-47. Epub 1997/08/06.

[13] O'Quigley J, Pepe M, Fisher L. Continual reassessment method: a practical design for phase 1 clinical trials in cancer. Biometrics. 1990;46(1):33-48. Epub 1990/03/01.

[14] Christakis NA, Lamont EB. Extent and determinants of error in doctors' prognoses in terminally ill patients: prospective cohort study. BMJ. 2000;320(7233):469-72. Epub 2000/03/04.

[15] Vigano A, Dorgan M, Bruera E, Suarez-Almazor ME. The relative accuracy of the clinical estimation of the duration of life for patients with end of life cancer. Cancer. 1999;86(1):170-6. Epub 1999/07/03.

[16] Glare P, Virik K, Jones M, Hudson M, Eychmuller S, Simes J, et al. A systematic review of physicians' survival predictions in terminally ill cancer patients. BMJ.
2003;327(7408):195-8. Epub 2003/07/26.

[17] Oken MM, Creech RH, Tormey DC, Horton J, Davis TE, McFadden ET, et al. Toxicity
and response criteria of the Eastern Cooperative Oncology Group. American journal
of clinical oncology. 1982;5(6):649-55. Epub 1982/12/01.

[18] Karnofsky D, Burchenal J. The clinical evaluation of chemotherapeutic agents in cancer. In: Evaluation of chemotherapeutic agents.. New York Columbia University
Press; 1949.

[19] Schag CC, Heinrich RL, Ganz PA. Karnofsky performance status revisited: reliability,
validity, and guidelines. J Clin Oncol. 1984;2(3):187-93. Epub 1984/03/01.

[20] Yates JW, Chalmer B, McKegney FP. Evaluation of patients with advanced cancer using the Karnofsky performance status. Cancer. 1980;45(8):2220-4. Epub 1980/04/15.

[21] Mor V, Laliberte L, Morris JN, Wiemann M. The Karnofsky Performance Status Scale.
An examination of its reliability and validity in a research setting. Cancer. 1984;53(9):
2002-7. Epub 1984/05/01.

[22] Reuben DB, Mor V, Hiris J. Clinical symptoms and length of survival in patients with
terminal cancer. Archives of internal medicine. 1988;148(7):1586-91. Epub 1988/07/01.

[23] Miller RJ. Predicting survival in the advanced cancer patient. Henry Ford Hospital
medical journal. 1991;39(2):81-4. Epub 1991/01/01.

[24] Conroy T, Desseigne F, Ychou M, Bouche O, Guimbaud R, Becouarn Y, et al. FOL-
FIRINOX versus gemcitabine for metastatic pancreatic cancer. N Engl J Med.
2011;364(19):1817-25. Epub 2011/05/13.

[25] Zuetenhorst JM, Taal BG. Metastatic carcinoid tumors: a clinical review. The oncolo-
gist. 2005;10(2):123-31. Epub 2005/02/15.

[26] Ralston SH, Gallacher SJ, Patel U, Campbell J, Boyle IT. Cancer-associated hypercal-
cemia: morbidity and mortality. Clinical experience in 126 treated patients. Annals of
internal medicine. 1990;112(7):499-504. Epub 1990/04/01.

[27] Al Murri AM, Bartlett JM, Canney PA, Doughty JC, Wilson C, McMillan DC. Evaluation of an inflammation-based prognostic score (GPS) in patients with metastatic
breast cancer. Br J Cancer. 2006;94(2):227-30. Epub 2006/01/13.

[28] Motzer RJ, Mazumdar M, Bacik J, Berg W, Amsterdam A, Ferrara J. Survival and
prognostic stratification of 670 patients with advanced renal cell carcinoma. J Clin
Oncol. 1999;17(8):2530-40. Epub 1999/11/24.

[29] Richman SD, Seymour MT, Chambers P, Elliott F, Daly CL, Meade AM, et al. KRAS
and BRAF mutations in advanced colorectal cancer are associated with poor progno-

sis but do not preclude benefit from oxaliplatin or irinotecan: results from the MRC FOCUS trial. J Clin Oncol. 2009;27(35):5931-7. Epub 2009/11/04.

[30] Long GV, Menzies AM, Nagrial AM, Haydu LE, Hamilton AL, Mann GJ, et al. Prognostic and clinicopathologic associations of oncogenic BRAF in metastatic melanoma. J Clin Oncol. 2011;29(10):1239-46. Epub 2011/02/24.

[31] Slamon DJ, Clark GM, Wong SG, Levin WJ, Ullrich A, McGuire WL. Human breast cancer: correlation of relapse and survival with amplification of the HER-2/neu oncogene. Science. 1987;235(4785):177-82. Epub 1987/01/09.

[32] McMenamin ME, Soung P, Perera S, Kaplan I, Loda M, Sellers WR. Loss of PTEN expression in paraffin-embedded primary prostate cancer correlates with high Gleason score and advanced stage. Cancer Res. 1999;59(17):4291-6. Epub 1999/09/15.

[33] de Bono JS, Scher HI, Montgomery RB, Parker C, Miller MC, Tissing H, et al. Circulating tumor cells predict survival benefit from treatment in metastatic castration-resistant prostate cancer. Clin Cancer Res. 2008;14(19):6302-9. Epub 2008/10/03.

[34] Cristofanilli M, Hayes DF, Budd GT, Ellis MJ, Stopeck A, Reuben JM, et al. Circulating tumor cells: a novel prognostic factor for newly diagnosed metastatic breast cancer. J Clin Oncol. 2005;23(7):1420-30. Epub 2005/03/01.

[35] Cohen SJ, Punt CJ, Iannotti N, Saidman BH, Sabbath KD, Gabrail NY, et al. Relationship of circulating tumor cells to tumor response, progression-free survival, and overall survival in patients with metastatic colorectal cancer. J Clin Oncol. 2008;26(19):3213-21. Epub 2008/07/02.

[36] Arkenau HT, Barriuso J, Olmos D, Ang JE, de Bono J, Judson I, et al. Prospective validation of a prognostic score to improve patient selection for oncology phase I trials. J Clin Oncol. 2009;27(16):2692-6. Epub 2009/04/01.

[37] Stavraka C, Pinato DJ, Turnbull SJ, Flynn MJ, Forster MD, O'Cathail SM, et al. Developing an objective marker to optimize patient selection and predict survival benefit in early-phase cancer trials. Cancer. 2014;120(2):262-70. Epub 2014/01/09.

[38] Arkenau HT, Olmos D, Ang JE, de Bono J, Judson I, Kaye S. Clinical outcome and prognostic factors for patients treated within the context of a phase I study: the Royal Marsden Hospital experience. Br J Cancer. 2008;98(6):1029-33. Epub 2008/03/20.

[39] Chau NG, Florescu A, Chan KK, Wang L, Chen EX, Bedard P, et al. Early mortality and overall survival in oncology phase I trial participants: can we improve patient selection? BMC cancer. 2011;11:426. Epub 2011/10/07.

[40] Fussenich LM, Desar IM, Peters ME, Teerenstra S, van der Graaf WT, Timmer-Bonte JN, et al. A new, simple and objective prognostic score for phase I cancer patients. Eur J Cancer. 2011;47(8):1152-60. Epub 2011/03/01.

[41] Garrido-Laguna I, Janku F, Vaklavas C, Falchook GS, Fu S, Hong DS, et al. Validation of the Royal Marsden Hospital prognostic score in patients treated in the Phase I

Clinical Trials Program at the MD Anderson Cancer Center. Cancer. 2012;118(5): 1422-8. Epub 2011/08/09.

[42]   Olmos D, A'Hern R P, Marsoni S, Morales R, Gomez-Roca C, Verweij J, et al. Patient selection for oncology phase I trials: a multi-institutional study of prognostic factors. J Clin Oncol. 2012;30(9):996-1004. Epub 2012/02/23.

[43]   Hyman DM, Eaton AA, Gounder MM, Smith GL, Pamer EG, Hensley ML, et al. Nomogram to predict cycle-one serious drug-related toxicity in phase I oncology trials. J Clin Oncol. 2014;32(6):519-26. Epub 2014/01/15.

[44]   Ploquin A, Olmos D, Ferte C, Cassier PA, Kramar A, Duhamel A, et al. Life-expectancy of patients enrolled in phase 1 clinical trials: a systematic review of published prognostic models. Critical reviews in oncology/hematology. 2012;83(2):242-8. Epub 2012/01/10.

[45]   Janisch L, Mick R, Schilsky RL, Vogelzang NJ, O'Brien S, Kut M, et al. Prognostic factors for survival in patients treated in phase I clinical trials. Cancer. 1994;74(7): 1965-73. Epub 1994/10/01.

[46]   Yamamoto N, Tamura T, Fukuoka M, Saijo N. Survival and prognostic factors in lung cancer patients treated in phase I trials: Japanese experience. Int J Oncol. 1999;15(4):737-41. Epub 1999/09/24.

[47]   Bachelot T, Ray-Coquard I, Catimel G, Ardiet C, Guastalla JP, Dumortier A, et al. Multivariable analysis of prognostic factors for toxicity and survival for patients enrolled in phase I clinical trials. Ann Oncol. 2000;11(2):151-6. Epub 2000/04/13.

[48]   Han C, Braybrooke JP, Deplanque G, Taylor M, Mackintosh D, Kaur K, et al. Comparison of prognostic factors in patients in phase I trials of cytotoxic drugs vs new noncytotoxic agents. Br J Cancer. 2003;89(7):1166-71. Epub 2003/10/02.

[49]   Penel N, Vanseymortier M, Bonneterre ME, Clisant S, Dansin E, Vendel Y, et al. Prognostic factors among cancer patients with good performance status screened for phase I trials. Investigational new drugs. 2008;26(1):53-8. Epub 2007/09/25.

[50]   Wheler J, Tsimberidou AM, Hong D, Naing A, Jackson T, Liu S, et al. Survival of patients in a Phase 1 Clinic: the M. D. Anderson Cancer Center experience. Cancer. 2009;115(5):1091-9. Epub 2009/01/24.

[51]   Penel N, Delord JP, Bonneterre ME, Bachelot T, Ray-Coquard I, Blay JY, et al. Development and validation of a model that predicts early death among cancer patients participating in phase I clinical trials investigating cytotoxics. Investigational new drugs. 2010;28(1):76-82. Epub 2009/02/12.

[52]   Gopal AK, Kahl BS, de Vos S, Wagner-Johnston ND, Schuster SJ, Jurczak WJ, et al. PI3Kdelta inhibition by idelalisib in patients with relapsed indolent lymphoma. N Engl J Med. 2014;370(11):1008-18. Epub 2014/01/24.

[53] McArthur GA, Chapman PB, Robert C, Larkin J, Haanen JB, Dummer R, et al. Safety and efficacy of vemurafenib in BRAF(V600E) and BRAF(V600K) mutation-positive melanoma (BRIM-3): extended follow-up of a phase 3, randomised, open-label study. The lancet oncology. 2014;15(3):323-32. Epub 2014/02/11.

[54] Mok TS, Wu YL, Thongprasert S, Yang CH, Chu DT, Saijo N, et al. Gefitinib or carboplatin-paclitaxel in pulmonary adenocarcinoma. N Engl J Med. 2009;361(10):947-57. Epub 2009/08/21.

[55] Shepherd FA, Rodrigues Pereira J, Ciuleanu T, Tan EH, Hirsh V, Thongprasert S, et al. Erlotinib in previously treated non-small-cell lung cancer. N Engl J Med. 2005;353(2):123-32. Epub 2005/07/15.

[56] Inoue A, Suzuki T, Fukuhara T, Maemondo M, Kimura Y, Morikawa N, et al. Prospective phase II study of gefitinib for chemotherapy-naive patients with advanced non-small-cell lung cancer with epidermal growth factor receptor gene mutations. J Clin Oncol. 2006;24(21):3340-6. Epub 2006/06/21.

[57] Voskoboynik M, Arkenau HT. Improving patient selection for phase I oncology trials. J Clin Oncol. 2014;32(28):3198-9. Epub 2014/07/30.

[58] Hamid O, Robert C, Daud A, Hodi FS, Hwu WJ, Kefford R, et al. Safety and tumor responses with lambrolizumab (anti-PD-1) in melanoma. N Engl J Med. 2013;369(2):134-44. Epub 2013/06/04.

[59] Hodi FS, O'Day SJ, McDermott DF, Weber RW, Sosman JA, Haanen JB, et al. Improved survival with ipilimumab in patients with metastatic melanoma. N Engl J Med. 2010;363(8):711-23. Epub 2010/06/08.

[60] Bailey A, McDermott DF. Immune checkpoint inhibitors as novel targets for renal cell carcinoma therapeutics. Cancer J. 2013;19(4):348-52. Epub 2013/07/23.

[61] Eggermont AM, Kroemer G, Zitvogel L. Immunotherapy and the concept of a clinical cure. Eur J Cancer. 2013;49(14):2965-7. Epub 2013/07/31.

[62] Robert C, Thomas L, Bondarenko I, O'Day S, M DJ, Garbe C, et al. Ipilimumab plus dacarbazine for previously untreated metastatic melanoma. N Engl J Med. 2011;364(26):2517-26. Epub 2011/06/07.

10

Advanced Human *In vitro* Models for the Discovery and Development of Lung Cancer Therapies

Samuel Constant, Song Huang,
Ludovic Wisniewski and Christophe Mas

Additional information is available at the end of the chapter

1. Introduction

Lung cancer is the leading cause of cancer deaths in both men and women, with more than 1 million deaths worldwide each year [1]. Unfortunately, this difficult therapeutic area has shown the highest failure rate in clinical trials over the last 30 years [2] and hitherto, there is no effective treatment for patients with lung cancer. The reasons for this drug attrition are multiple, but one major explanation is considered to be the lack of relevant preclinical models to appropriately validate potential drug targets and rank novel therapeutic agents before engaging in clinical trials [3].

Genetically engineered mice, ectopic and orthotopic xenotransplantation of tumors into immunodeficient mice are common models used as surrogate of patients to evaluate drug candidates before clinical testing. Although animal models can recapitulate important facets of human responses, their limitations as preclinical cancer models have now been widely documented [4-7]. Fundamental differences in transcriptional regulation [8], telomerase activity [9], neoplastic transformation mechanisms [10], cytokines production [11] as well as matrix metalloproteinases biology [12] are but a few features which compromise the design of efficient cancer therapies. Even the patient derived xenograft model (PDX), which better recapitulate the phenotypic features of the human tumor, displays a number of inherent limitations [13]. In this system, the tumorgraft established from primary tumor fragments has to be maintained through serial transplantations into mice, which will lead to the loss of the human stroma environment after 2-3 passages [14]. Clearly, such a replacement of the original tumor microenvironment by murine host components has significant consequences on growth features as well as response to therapies. Indeed, a number of oncogenic mouse ligands fail to cross-activate their related human receptors [15, 16] while stromal mediators have been identified as a critical source triggering tumour cells resistance to treatment [17, 18]. These observations highlight the importance of considering tumor-extracellular matrix interactions in the design of *in vitro* cancer models. Modern tumor biology has moved away from the traditionalist view conveyed for years by 2D cultures saturated with growth factors by revealing that the many varieties of cells that compose a tumor don't just grow on their own but constantly integrate and react to signals coming from the extracellular matrix components. Solid tumors are now regarded as complex organs able to instruct the surrounding tissue to promote their own growth and progression, but also dependent on both molecular and mechanical signals coming from the adjacent healthy environment [19, 20]. Therefore, experimental models recapitulating true human cancer biology are mandatory for the validation of therapeutic agents in order to keep away from the risk of studying no more than adaptive cancer biology in a wrong environment that will eventually result in translation failure.

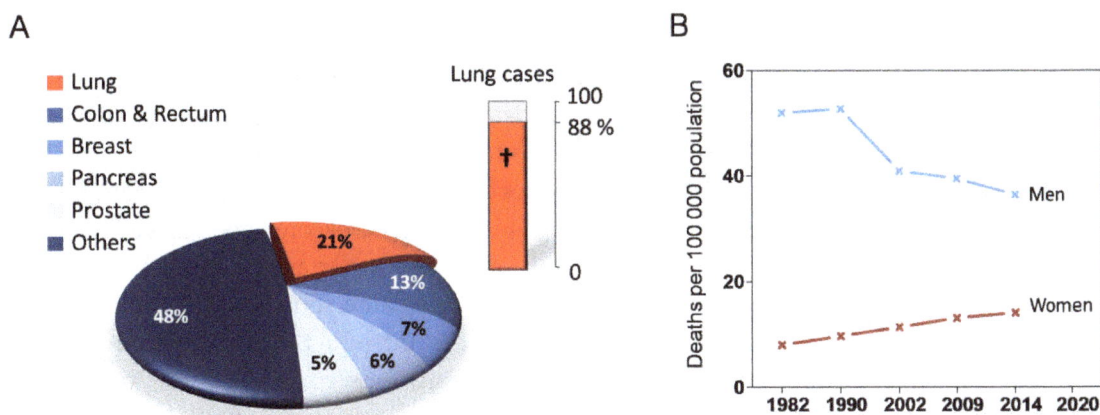

Figure 1. (A) Cancer deaths anticipated in 2014. Estimated leading cancer sites mortality in European Union for the year 2014 expressed as percent of total cancer deaths. Column diagram highlights the mortality rate within the population specifically affected by lung cancer. (B) Age-standardized (world population) EU male (blue) and female (red) lung cancer death rates per 100,000 from 1982 to 2014. The graph shows the unfavourable trend for female lung cancer with a regular increase in case numbers over the last 30 years. Source: Malvezzi et al, Annals of oncology, 2014; 25(8): 1650-6. and Bosetti et al, Annals of oncology, 19: 631–640, 2008.

In this article we report the significant efforts ongoing within academia and industry to developing *in vitro* novel complex human tumor models that should improve the identification and selection of efficient lung cancer therapies. We first focus on the human lung cancer cell lines currently available, their contribution to lung cancer biology and their use in research. Then, we will move from cell monolayers to three-dimensional (3D) cultures, exploring at first the function of natural and synthetic extracellular matrix before to document some recent advances in the field, including spheroids, bioscaffolds, decellularized lung matrix models and precision-cut lung tumor slices. Finally, we will present the bioengineering of a new generation of lung cancer models: OncoCilAir™. These 100% human models, which combine *in vitro* both tumor nodules surrounded by a functional airway epithelium and stroma, open new ways to test simultaneously drug efficacy, side toxicity and tumor recurrence in a single, integrated and accessible 3D model.

2. Lung cancer, current treatments and perspectives

Lung cancer (LC) is one of the major health concerns in the western world. LC is the most frequently diagnosed cancer in men and women and represents the most common cause of cancer-related deaths, both in the United States and in Europe, with a significant rate of 27% and 21% of total cancer deaths, respectively [21] (Fig.1A). The LC epidemic has been clearly linked to tobacco smoking [22], and while mortality rate in men has regularly fallen over the last decades (53 lung cancer deaths for every 100,000 European males in the late 1980s to 41.1/100,000 in 2009) thanks to strong measures for smoking control and prevention in middle-aged men, female LC rates are predicted to rise 8% in 2015 [1] (Fig.1B). There are two main types of lung cancer: non-small lung cancer (NSCLC) which account for about 85% of all lung cancers and small cell lung cancer (SCLC, 15%). SCLC is the most aggressive form of LC, with fast growing cells leading to large tumors. Histologically, NSCLC includes 3 subgroups: adenocarcinoma, squamous cell and large cell carcinoma [23]. As in many other forms of cancer, LC does not display too many symptoms, develops slowly over a period of several years, and only manifests itself in advanced stages (III or IV), where five-year survival rates are less than 10% because of high degree of metastasis. The overall median survival in stage IV is only about 8-10 months [24]. Platinum and taxane based chemotherapies (cisplatin, paclitaxel) has remained for years the treatments of choice, but more recently LC patients have been selected based on their tumor mutation profile. In most cases, oncogene driver mutations are exclusives (EGFR, ALK/EML4, KRAS, PTEN, etc...) and importantly, they divided patient populations into molecular subsets that do not show the same sensitivity to different treatments [25]. This patient stratification has enabled the introduction of targeted therapies directed against specific signaling pathways whose tumors are dependent on. Indeed, humanized recombinant antibodies directed against the vascular endothelial growth factor (VEGF) (bevacizumab) or small molecule inhibitors of EGFR-TK (erlotinib, gefitinib and afatinib), ALK and MET (crizotinib, ceritinib) have recently been used as a promising new line of therapies to treat lung cancer. Unfortunately, this drug portfolio extends survival only by a few months (Table 1) since most of the patients develop resistance to treatments, leading invariably to the recurrence of the disease [26-32]. Huge efforts are now undertaken to understand and circumvent drug resistance mechanisms. First observations have pointed out two main mechanisms for drug resistance acquisition: the selection of another pre-existing oncogene mutation or the activation of a bypass track, i.e. the deregulation of an alternative growth signaling pathway to maintain cell proliferation and tumor progression [33]. In *EGFR*-mutant lung cancer treated with the EGFR-TK inhibitors erlotinib and gefitinib, resistance is generally mediated by the T790M EGFR second-site mutation (~50% of the cases) [34] or phosphatidylinositol 3-kinase PI3K–AKT pathway activation via focal amplification of MET as second signaling pathway (~5%) [35]. For *ALK*-mutant lung cancer treated with crizotinib, mechanisms of resistance include the gatekeeper mutation L1196M (~30% of the cases) and KIT and EGFR signaling pathways activation as bypass track (~45%) [36]. Overall, these findings argue for the use of combined therapies in a manageable way. But recent data based on the analysis of tumor specimens at the time of acquired resistance suggest a much more complex landscape. In fact, multiple mechanisms, as diverse as epigenetic changes [37], epithelial to mesenchyme transition (EMT) or conversion from a LC histological type to another (EGFR-dependent NSCLC to SCLC), are induced under the selective pressure of targeted therapies [38, 39]. These observations imply the arrival of a personalized medicine, where a careful profiling of patient tumor's mutation status (germline and somatic) and epigenetic signature will be mandatory all along the therapy to identify and adapt the correct treatment strategy. However, such scheduled combinatorial regimen would require the development of multiple-generation inhibitors to overcome specific subsets of resistance mutations and induce durable remissions. But the ability to escape multiple types of treatment could well be a hallmark of cancer cells. With this in mind, alternative strategies are worth considering. Instead of constraining tumor cells signalling through exogenous therapies making them overreact, a different approach might be to restrict tumor progression through its own microenvironment. The original 1975's experiment of teratocarcinoma injection into blastocysts from Mintz and Illmensee was the first example of tumor repression by the microenvironment [40]. Today, tumor reprogramming through stroma instruction is emerging as a new treatment paradigm [41-43]. From this perspective, advanced human three-dimensional (3D) cell culture approaches modelling tumor-stroma communication could be key to accelerate the development of new lung cancer therapeutics.

Generic	Trade Name	Indication	Type	Class	Target	PFS	Ref
▶ Afatinib	Gilotrif	NSCLC	small molecule	antineoplastic antiangiogenesis	EGFR HER2-4	3.3-13.6	[32]
▶ Crizotinib	Xalkori	NSCLC	small molecule	antineoplastic	ALK MET, ROS1	9.7	[29]
▶ Ceritinib	Zykadia	NSCLC	small molecule	antineoplastic	ALK IGF1R	7	[31]
▶ Erlotinib	Tarceva	NSCLC	small molecule	antineoplastic antiangiogenesis	EGFR	12-14	[26;27]
▶ Gefitinib	Iressa	NSCLC	small molecule	antineoplastic antiangiogenesis	EGFR	7.7-12.9	[26]
▶ Bevacizumab	Avastin	NSCLC	rHMAb	antiangiogenesis	VEGF	6.2	[28]

Table 1. Targeted therapies approved by the Food and Drug Administration in the treatment of lung cancer. The median time to progression on targeted therapy (Progression Free Survival - PFS) is given in months. rHMAb: recombinant human monoclonal antibody. Source: National Cancer Institute database, 2014.

3. Lung cancer cell lines

Cell lines derived from human tumors provide an unlimited, self-replicating source of malignant cells that can be studied by investigators throughout the world. Therefore, even if cell lines represent only a highly selected fraction of the original tumor, their ease of access has resulted in the production of a very large body of literature. Indeed, it is acknowledged that most of our understanding of the molecular mechanisms involved in LC comes from studies done on mouse or human cell lines [44].

3.1. Lung cancer cell lines collection

To date, more than 250 LC cell lines have been established, mainly from Western population. Currently, the American Type Culture Collection (ATCC, Manassas, VA) catalog lists 121 human lung tumor cell lines. Among this panel, SCLC is less represented, first due to the lower frequency of the disease, and second because SCLC tumors are rarely surgically resected. Indeed, only small tissue samples from biopsy examinations, malignant aspirates, and rare malignant effusions are available for research use. Moreover, the fact that SCLC tumor cells lack the ability to adhere to culture dishes and required to be grown *in vitro* as floating cell aggregates or spheroids has precluded for a long time their expansion as cell lines. SCLC was first successfully cultured in Japan in 1971 [45].

Regarding NSCLC, primary and metastatic tumor materials are more easily accessible, even through routine bronchoscopy [38, 39]. However, although cells from metastatic tumors, especially from malignant effusions, are relatively easy to culture, cell cultures from primary solid tumor are not obvious to establish, with success rates ranging from 2.6 to 5% [46, 47]. Various protocols are in use, but on the whole, tumor tissues minced in small pieces are either directly cultured as fragments in a matrix (e.g. Matrigel®) or subjected to enzymatic dissociation (collagenase/hyaluronidase) and then suspended in culture medium. Clearly, positive results are higher when starting from material corresponding to advanced stages as MHC III and IV [46]. The culture medium composition is also critical and the development of serum-free chemically defined media (e.g. ACL4) has significantly improved success rates [48].

The resulting current LC cell lines depository represent therefore a unique resource that can be extremely valuable in term of genetic manipulation, high-throughput screening and development of more complex co-culture models.

3.2. Lung cancer cell lines as *in vitro* model

LC cell lines have been used for decades in functional studies with the aim to identify new oncogene drivers or tumor suppressors. Thus, LC cell lines compared to normal human bronchial epithelial cells were instrumental to generate list of differentially expressed genes that could account for tumorigenicity and represent therefore new therapeutic targets. As an example, this strategy lead to the detection of *ERBB3*, a gene associated with the EGF signaling pathway, among the genes over-expressed in LC cell lines [49]. Interestingly, this result was validated later on by another study that identified the activation of ERBB3 signaling as a mechanism of resistance to gefitinib [35]. Since these initial findings, ERBB3 has been recognized as a key node of LC progression and several humanized anti-ErbB3 antibodies are currently in pre-clinical development [50].

However, cell lines limitations have emerged as our knowledge about the disease increased. As an example, several studies have shown that differences in genetic background are important in defining cancer biology as well as in drug sensitivity [51]. Thus, a potential shortcoming of the current LC collection may reside in its under-representation of some populations, like the East Asian population, possibly introducing bias in research and drug discovery. Indeed, epidemiologic surveys have revealed that in the US, 10% of patients with NSCLC have tumour associated with EGFR mutations, while this number increases to 35% in

East Asia, suggesting different selection mechanisms or sensitivity for lung cancer subtypes among different ethnic groups.

Accordingly, the recent classification of lung cancers into genetic subsets based on mutations in driver oncogenes (*see previous section*) prompted the community to accurately characterize the LC cell lines collection at the genomic and genetic levels. In this perspective, the Sanger Cancer Institute has initiated the genetic characterization of a panel of cancer cell lines (The Cancer Genome Project, http://cancer.sanger.ac.uk/cancergenome/projects/cell_lines/). Using current high throughput techniques this program provides information on mutations, copy number variations, single nucleotide polymorphisms (SNPs) and microsatellite instability of 136 cell lines representative of the different type of lung cancers (adenocarcinoma, small cell carcinoma, etc...) with the aim to define a genetic profile predictive of drug sensitivity. Such a signature should contribute to stratify patient population and to identify efficient targeted therapies.

Another emerging use of LC cell line is related to the identification of resistance mechanisms. As documented in section 2, so far all the approaches used in the treatment of lung cancer have resulted in the acquisition of resistance by the patients. One successful approach to discovering resistance mechanisms has been to culture sensitive cell lines with increasing concentrations of the drug until resistance emerges. The resistant cell line can subsequently be analysed to identify the resistance mechanisms, leading to the identification of resistance biomarkers and new strategies to overcome resistance [36].

Undoubtedly, cell lines have proven to be useful in elucidating important aspect of lung cancer biology. However, thanks to modern deep-sequencing technologies, we now know that lung tumors are composed of population of cells with distinct molecular and phenotypic properties [52] and consequently, that cell lines do not fully recapitulate human tumor biology. Clearly, the scientific community has taken into account these limitations, as shown by the growing interest for the establishment of complex *in vitro* cell models intended to bridge the gap between animal models and human studies.

4. Biocompatible matrices for 3D cell culture

In this section, we will try to briefly resume different ways and techniques used to culture the cells in 3D. Maintaining a 3D structure is critical to reproduce the tumour-stroma environment, communication between tumour cells, and the interaction with other surrounding cell types such as epithelial cells or fibroblasts [19]. Advances in materials chemistry and processing technologies, as well as developmental biology have led to the design of 3D cell culture matrices and bioscaffolds that better represent the geometry, chemistry, and signaling environment of natural extracellular matrix.

To obtain 3D cell cultures, cells are generally seeded onto/into biocompatible scaffolds or matrices. The 3D differentiation of cells depends on various parameters but it is generally accepted that best results are obtained when the natural environment is closely imitated [53]. Natural extracellular matrices are mainly composed of fibrous network made of collagen, elastic fibers, water and other materials like glycosaminoglycans, proteoglycans and glycoproteins [54]. To mimic the natural extracellular environment of the cells important parameters have to be taken into account [55]:

1. The matrix composition (collagen, fibrin, alginate, etc.)

2. The structure (pore size, pore distribution, pore geometry, etc.)

3. The manufacturing method (electrospinning, 3D printing, inverted colloidal crystal, spontaneous polymerization, etc.)

4. The biocompatibility

As the fate of a cell is largely determined by its environment, the elaboration of the right extracellular context is critical to promote the correct differentiation of a cell population.

For example, it is well known that epithelial cells have to be cultured at the air-liquid interface to differentiate. This could be easily obtained by seeding cells onto micro porous supports or scaffolds allowing nutrients to come from the back. The apical side of the cells remains generally exposed to the air [56]. This basic principle of air-liquid interface cultivation can be transposed to most of epithelial cells such as airway, vaginal, buccal, intestinal, etc. However, this approach is no more suitable when the cells are not from epithelial origin [57, 58].

It is typically the case for fibroblasts that are not able to survive when directly exposed to the air. To culture fibroblasts in 3D, a different type of environment is required. Cells can be embedded into a biocompatible matrix based on various components [53]. Among the most used we find collagen and fibrin. Collagen is the major component of connective tissues, it is naturally produced by fibroblasts and can be easily isolated from many type of tissues such as dermis, bone, tendon, etc...

Whereas collagen is easily obtained, applications for human therapies and 3D cell culture remain limited because of contamination risks between animals and humans (e.g. Creutzfeldt-Jakob). Moreover, the gel polymerization can be difficult to control thus reducing the field of applicability. Another drawback is the variation between batches to batches. These weaknesses have led to the development of new generations of synthetic matrices and scaffolds where polymerization as well as intrinsic properties of materials (elasticity, porosity, permeability, hydration, etc.) can be more easily controlled. The matrices used today for 3D cell culture can be divided into 3 groups:

a. Natural compounds: collagen, gelatin, hyaluronate, glycosaminoglycan, chitosan, alginate, silk, fibrin, dextran, matrigel®, etc...

b. Synthetic compounds: polyglycolic acid (PGA), polylactic acid (PLA), polylactic-co-glycolic acid (PLGA), polycarpolactone (PCL), polyethylene glycol (PEG), polyvinyl alcohol (PVA), polypropylene fumarate (PPF), polyacrylic acid (PAA), etc...

c. Mixed compounds, made of natural compounds synthetically modified. These included peptide-coupled alginates, chitosan, hyluranan, tyrosine-derived polymers, etc...

Each material has its own strengths and weaknesses and therefore it is fundamental to select matrix components in function of the needs. In the context of lung tumor cell model, it is pertinent to determine the final end-point studied. For example, if cells invasion has to be studied, it is necessary to use matrix components where cells are able to adhere, migrate and proliferate [59]. Moreover, some cells have the ability to digest and transform the scaffold and elaborate a new environment adapted to their needs. In that case it will be valuable to select a natural matrix component like collagen or fibrin. If the goal of the experiment is to obtain a 3D scaffold for human therapy, the best choice will be the use of synthetic matrices where all components can be defined and controlled [60]. If the sensitivity of a cancer cell to a drug has to be studied, a relevant choice could be the use of cell spheroids embedded into a non degradable matrix component, like alginate [61]. In that case, cells are immobilized and their drug susceptibility can be determined using a simple viability test. Alginate scaffold has been optimized for 3D tumor modeling using H460, A549 and H1650 NSCLC cell lines [62]. In this study the anticancer effects of various chemotherapeutic agents were studied and compared with conventional 2D cell culture models. Results have shown that cells grown in 3D demonstrated a more realistic drug response with higher resistance to chemotherapy [62].

Clearly, there is a tremendous flexibility to reconstitute a scaffold and the choice of synthesis should be guided by the type of cells, the application and the desired physical properties [53]. In addition, new perspectives are offered by bioprinting technologies. The possibility to organize extracellular matrix into precise geometries should help engineering 3D complex tumor tissues for *in vitro* assays [63].

5. Tumor spheroid models for lung cancer research

Numerous anchorage-independent assays have been developed for drug discovery. The most popular is the spheroid model because it allows both 3D self-organization of tumor cells and drug screening in high-throughput format. Many normal and malignant cell types can be grown as sphere-shaped cell colonies, so called spheroids. Cells that don't form spheroids spontaneously can be induced to do so by co-culturing with spheroid-forming non-clonogenic feeder cells [64]. As spheroid environment can be controlled, effects on tumor cell viability can be carefully examined. This model is particularly adapted to high throughput screening in 96-well plate assays, and numerous solutions are commercially available.

Phenotypic and functional differences between lung tumor cells grown as 2D monolayer cultures, versus cells grown as 3D spheroids have been observed. Indeed, the 3D spheroid culture changed the cellular response to drugs and growth factors suggesting to be more accurately mimicking the natural tumor microenvironment than classical culture of lung cell line [65]. Multi-cell type tumor spheroids are a valuable model to reproduce cellular heterogeneity and provide more comprehensive assessment of tumor response to therapeutic strategies. 3D co-culture model using NSCLC cell lines in combination with lung fibroblasts can be prepared [66]. To date, co-cultures involving up to three different cell types in a single spheroid (tumor cells, fibroblasts and endothelial cells) have been established, but without any proof of micro-capillary functionality [67]. Recent studies report that NSCLC can acquire epithelial-mesenchymal transition and cancer stem-like phenotypes within chitosan-hyaluronan membrane-derived 3D tumor spheroids [68].

6. Microfluidic chip-based 3D co-cultures

In the continuity of the pioneering work of Donald Ingber (organ on chip), a series of 3D lung-on-a-chip microfluidic devices have been developed. Briefly, lung-on-a-chip is a biomimetic microsystem that reconstitutes the critical functional alveolar-capillary interface of the human lung, with periodic mechanical stretching and flow of the medium carrying immune cells. Using this micro-fluidic device, the authors were able to replicating the immune responses against bacterial infections *in vitro* [69]. Afterwards, devices were optimized as a drug screening platform to select individualized treatment for lung cancer. In these systems, lung cancer and stromal cell lines were co-cultured as 3D spheroids under continuous media supplementation, mimicking the circulation of nutrients and metabolic waste out of the cultures [70]. Another similar model has been developed for chemoresistive testing of pleural mesothelioma cancer spheroids. Interestingly, growth inhibitory concentration of cisplatin showed higher concentration in perfused tumor spheroids compared with spheroids cultured under static conditions [71]. These systems represent therefore valuable tools to get information about the efficacy of chemotherapeutic drugs in a dynamic microenvironment which recapitulate the actual *in vivo* situation, but they do not address side-toxicity on normal lung physiology. The challenge will be to improve the model so that it incorporates normal and functional tissues. That could be achieved by connecting such devices with other microphysiological organotypic chips, representative of healthy lung tissues.

7. *Ex vivo* 3D lung cancer model based on decellularized matrix

As it is not obvious to identify the ideal matrix components and conditions suitable for the development of various lung tumor types, an alternative strategy is to take advantage of existing natural matrices. This methodology relies on the initial work of Ott and colleagues that first succeed in regenerating a bioartificial organ from a rat cadaveric lung [72]. Briefly, in this model the organ of interest is perfused with a detergent in order to remove donor cells and leave the components of the extracellular matrix. The resulting decellularized matrix is then reloaded with human lung adenocarcinoma tumor cells. In addition to their well-adapted composition, decellularized matrices also display specific elasticity which has been pointed out as critical for tumor cell growth. To date, rat decellularized lung matrix [73] and porcine decellularized intestinal submucosa [17] have been used as scaffold. Interestingly, tumor cell lines (A549, H460 and H1299) engrafted in this microenvironment formed 3D lung tumor nodules and displayed histological features reminiscent of the original primary tumor [74]. They also recovered functionalities (e.g. MMP-9 production) that were lost in 2D culture [73]. These ex vivo 3D models can be kept in culture for up to 28 days and exhibit sensitivity to treatment comparable to what is observed in clinic [17]. Although relevant for fundamental research, current *ex vivo* 3D lung models clearly show limitations. First, they are difficult to produce, the cultivation of the cells must take place in a special incubator, and consequently they cannot be used for high-throughput screening. Second, they do not recapitulate the human – human interactions between tumor and stroma. Indeed, epithelial and mesenchymal cells have been removed from epithelial space by the decellularization process. Third, they necessitate large amount of tumor cells (~25 millions) in order to colonize the matrix, precluding personalized medicine. And finally, they required the sacrifice of animals for matrix supply. However, *ex vivo* 3D lung models must be seen as the gold standard to be reached by 3D bioprinting technologies combined to synthetic matrices.

8. Precision-cut lung tumor slices

As previously mentioned, the tumor microenvironment provides essential signaling necessary for establishing and maintaining tumor specific morphogenic programs. Precision-cut lung slices (PCLS) obtained from freshly isolated human lung cancer tissues maintain both the original cancer microenvironment and preserve the complexity of the tumor-stroma interaction [75, 76]. Usually thin tissue slices (~200 µM) are prepared with a vibratome and cultured submerged into medium for several days. PCLS constitute a valid tool for the *in vitro* evaluation of tumor morphology, proliferation, viability and resistance to therapy [75]. Moreover, a major advantage of this model is the preparation of multiple experimental replicates from a single tumor, allowing performing drug efficacy studies. Indeed, dose-response experiments with the PIK3 inhibitor LY294002 have shown that PCLS cultures from lung cancer may be used to predict tumor sensitivity to drugs in a patient-specific manner [75]. In a different study, tumor PCLS were used to investigate nanoparticles delivery of antisense as lung cancer treatment. The model was instrumental to demonstrate that nanoparticles could penetrate into tumor tissue and target telomerase activity, without disturbing adjacent tissue architecture or inducing significant side-toxicity [76]. PCLS established from human lung tumor tissue represent therefore a useful *in vitro* tumor model that has the potential to enhance preclinical drug evaluation studies. However, an obvious limitation of PCLS is their short lifespan, ~5 days, which prevents long-term exposure, and therefore chronic treatment evaluation.

9. Engineered 3D lung tumor tissues: The OncoCilAir™ model

Tissue engineering is an innovative technology designed at first to produce artificial functional tissues to repair or replace portion of injured tissues. While initially seen as unrealistic, this field has made tremendous progress over the past decade, and regenerative medicine will soon become a routine technique [77]. Today, it is possible by combining human cells with suitable bioscaffolds to produce *in vitro* tissue equivalents from many sources (e.g. corneal, cartilage, intestinal, muscle, respiratory, skin, etc...). More recently, this promising technology has been applied to the field of oncology with some attempts to develop engineered tumor tissues for pre-clinical research (e.g. human melanoma model) [78]. Here we took advantage of our tissue engineering know-how in the respiratory field [79] to develop a complex, but accessible, 3D lung cancer model: OncoCilAir™ [80, 81]. To this purpose, human primary bronchial cells, lung fibroblasts and lung adenocarcinoma cell lines were co-cultured at the air-liquid interface in a transwell insert (Fig.2). After appropriate differentiation, the system closely reproduces malignant pulmonary nodules invading a human functional airway epithelium (Fig.3).

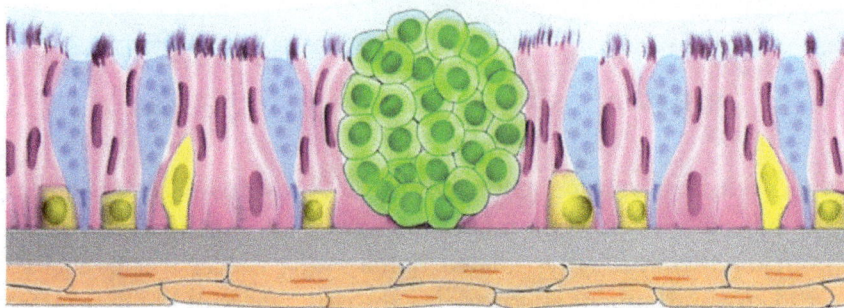

Figure 2. Schematic representation of the OncoCilAir™ lung cancer model. OncoCilAir™ is a complex cellular model based on the co-culture at the air-liquid-interface of three different human components: bronchial cells, lung fibroblasts and NSCLC cell lines. After 30 days, the cells differentiate into a functional respiratory epithelium which comprises ciliated cells (pink), goblet cells (blue) secreting mucus (light blue), basal cells (yellow), fibroblasts (brown) and tumor nodules (green).

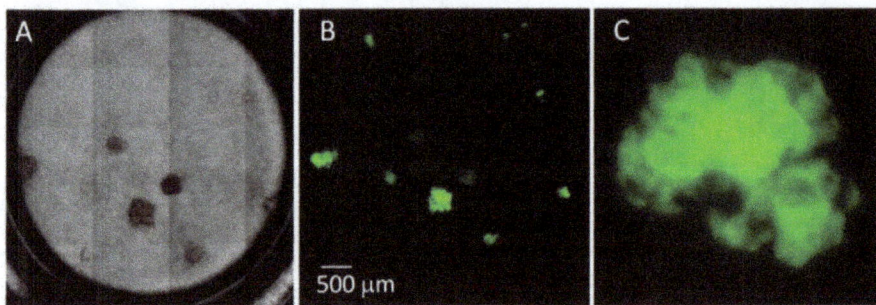

Figure 3. Cultured at the air-liquid interface in a convenient 24-wells format (A), the OncoCilAir™ model mimics the *in vivo* lung tissue of a patient with characteristic tumour lung nodules (B & magnification in C).

Several properties contribute to make OncoCilAir™ a relevant pre-clinical *in vitro* alternative: First, it is a 100% human three-dimensional model which summarizes human tumour-stroma interactions to assess therapies targeting host-tumor interactions (Fig.4). Second, it is a flexible system: depending on the cell line used to build its tumour component, OncoCilAir™ offers the possibility to recapitulate distinct molecular subsets of lung cancers (EGFR, KRAS, etc...) and thus to simulate patient stratification. Third, it is a bi-competency model: the fact that it includes both compromised and healthy tissues brings the possibility to experiment simultaneously drug efficacy and drug side-effect within a single culture. Lastly, its long lifespan (>3 months) allows to test chronic treatments and recurrence while reducing animal testing.

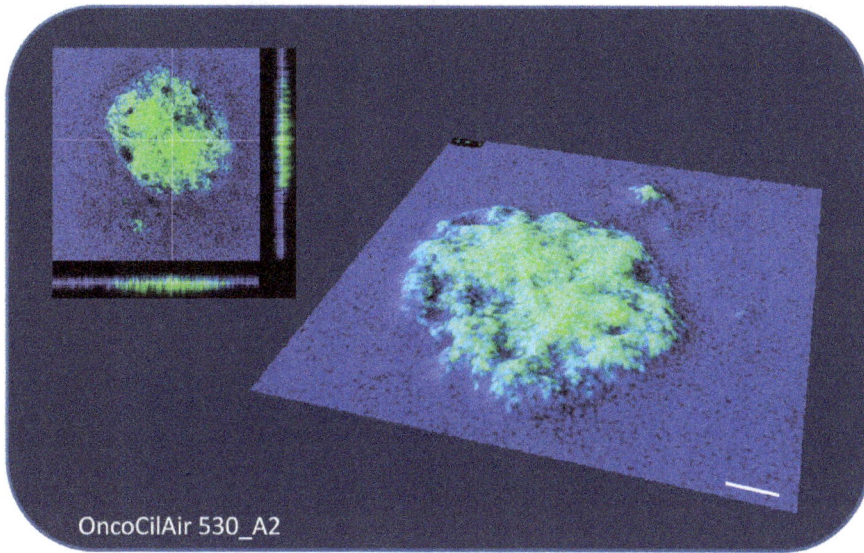

OncoCilAir 530_A2

Figure 4. A tumor nodule expanding within the OncoCilAir™ human airway epithelium. Adenocarcima cells GFP+ (green) and human bronchial epithelial cells nuclei DAPI+ (blue) were visualized by confocal laser scanning microscopy. Scale bar represents 100 μm.

Accordingly, a dose response efficacy study with the investigational MEK inhibitors selumetinib and trametinib demonstrated that OncoCilAir™ showed responsiveness to anticancer drugs in agreement with previously reported data, and therefore can be used as a predictive tool for anticancer drug evaluation [82].

10. Future perspective

Hanahans and Weinberg highlighted six cancer hallmarks which provide us with a framework to understand this complex disease. These hallmarks include (i) sustaining proliferative signaling, (ii) evading growth suppressors, (iii) resisting cell death (iv) enabling replicative immortality, (v) inducing angiogenesis, and (vi) activating invasion and metastasis [83, 84]. However, in essence, cancer is a genetic disease with germ or autosomal mutations affecting genes implicated in cell division and/or in tissue integrity. These genetic alterations lead to unrestricted cell division and formation of a clone of cells which undergo further genetic changes. Some of these mutations promote features that endow cells with a selective advantage over normal cells, thus creating a more aggressive subclone with an even higher mutation rate, eventually leading to tumor formation [85]. The clonal theory has been corroborated by several decades of cancer researches: we now know that mutation in some specific genes, so-called oncogenes and tumor supressors, are primary cause for cancers. For lung cancers, the components of EGF signaling, such as EGF receptor and its downstream effectors (KRAS, BRAF, ALK, etc...) are the main drivers [33]. With the advance in biotechnology, it is now possible to rapidly identify the underlying mutations of the lung cancers for diagnostics and for personalized treatment.

Cancer hallmarks	Barriers	Appropiate *in vitro* models
Sustaining proliferative signal	Inadequate growth promotion	Cell lines Spheroids 3D co-cultures *in vitro* PnP
Evading growth suppressors		
Resisting cell death	Apoptosis with loss of basement membrane	
Enabling replicative immortality	Senescence	
Inducing angiogenesis	Ischaemia	3D co-cultures *in vitro* PnP
Activating invasion and metastasis	ECM and epithelial barrier	
Deregulating cellular energetics	Acidosis	*in vitro* PnP

Table 2. Current and future *in vitro* lung cancer models sorted according to cancer hallmarks.

However, a genetic change is only one side of the same coin. It is generally recognized now that the microenvironment surrounding the cancer cells plays also a crucial role in cancer development [19, 83, 84]. Indeed, tumor cells have to overcome at least six barriers in order to become invasive [86]. The extracellular matrix, stroma cells, immune cells, etc... form an integral part of the tumor, therefore should be taken into account. In fact, not all the cancer cells can grow in standard cell culture conditions: out of 160 tumors, only 8 Chinese NSCLC cell lines have been established in culture [47].

Therefore, for tissue engineering, the most important, as well as the most challenging task is to recreate the *in vivo*-like tumor micro-environment.

Another important issue is to maintain the heterogeneity of the tumor populations. Despite of huge progresses made in cancer research, the toll cancer claims in both human lives and funds spent on health care has been only marginally reduced, and in some cases even increases [87, 88]. One of the reasons for this situation is the drug resistance. The underlying cause is the heterogeneity of the tumor cells: within a tumor several clones with different mutations may co-exist. Furthermore, another process termed the community effect may be involved. Studies have suggested that the ability of a cell to respond to a signal may be enhanced by, or even dependent on, other neighboring cells reacting in the same way at the same time [89]. This effect helps to explain the formation of blocks of tissue from sheets of cells, and could be of widespread occurrence and significance in various morphogenesis processes, including tumor development. The underlying mechanism of the community effect could be the autocrine or paracrine positive feedback loops, which have also been suggested and identified during tumor formation. Several studies have outlined the importance of autocrine IL-6 signaling in lung and breast cancers. For example, one group found a positive correlation between persistently activated tyrosine-phosphorylated STAT3, found in 50% of lung adenocarcinomas, and IL-6. Further investigation revealed that mutant EGFR could activate the oncogenic STAT3 pathway via upregulated IL-6 autocrine signaling [90].

The fact that most of the cancer cells, even the aggressive ones, cannot grow in culture once dissociated strongly supports this notion. In other words, all the cancer hallmarks are the hallmarks of the tumor as a whole, not that of individual cancer cells. This has to be taken into account during the development of *in vitro* cancer models.

	Cell lines	Spheroids	3D Co-culture Models	In vitro PnP
Pro	▶ Appropriate for identifying the mutations and for elucidating the signalling pathways. ▶ High throughput screening of drug candidates.	▶ Replicate only some features of cancer 3D environment (cell-cell interactions, community effect). ▶ Mechanistic studies. ▶ Drug screening and testing.	▶ Reflect closely *in vivo* situations, having relevant cell-cell and cell-stroma interactions. ▶ Possibility to study cancer metastasis and tumor invasion. ▶ Allow testing the efficacy and toxicity simultaneously. ▶ Allow chronic treatments and resistance studies. ▶ Provide insight about mechanistic at all levels. ▶ Identification and validation of drug candidate. ▶ Suitable for personalized medicine.	▶ An ideal model replicating most of the features of cancer development and cancer growth. ▶ Cell-cell and cell-stroma interactions, metastasis, immune responses, drugs circulation and metabolization, angiogenesis, etc...
Cons	▶ Do not reflect the original *in vivo* situations, lack of relevant cell-cell and cell-stroma interactions. ▶ loss of relevant biomarkers. ▶ Lack of mechanical constraints from the adjacent healthy tissue.	▶ Not cultured at ALI condition, these models are less relevant for *lung* cancers. ▶ Not possible to study metastasis. ▶ Lack of immune cells and no angiogenesis.	▶ Lack of immune cells and no angiogenesis.	▶ Could be difficult to standardize and to scale-up. ▶ Special expertise is needed. Often patent-protected.

Table 3. Strengths and weaknesses of the different human *in vitro* models for lung cancer.

Ideally, *in vitro* lung cancer models should recapture all the hallmarks of human lung cancer. Each model has its own strength and weaknesses (Table 3). But depending on the application, simple models may be more relevant and sufficient. Models can therefore be sorted by complexity:

1. Cell lines

2. As simplest 3D model, the tumor spheroids represent already a progress with regarding to monolayer culture of tumor cell lines or primary tumor cells: the cell-cell interaction is restored. Stroma cells and or matrix could also be added to better mimic the *in vivo* situation.

3. Since the lung tumor cells are located at air-liquid interface, co-culture with the normal airway epithelial cells and fibroblast cells at air-liquid interface, illustrated by OncoCilAir™, is another realistic scenario for modeling the lung tumors.

4. *In vitro* PnP (Plug and Play) models with primary tumor derived from the patient.

In addition, Table 2 summarizes how the current, as well as the future *in vitro* cancer models can replicate some or all the cancer hallmarks, their use and limitations for drug development.

Finally, we would like to propose an ideal *in vitro* lung cancer model based on the above considerations, so-called *in vitro* PnP (Plug and Play) model (Fig.5).

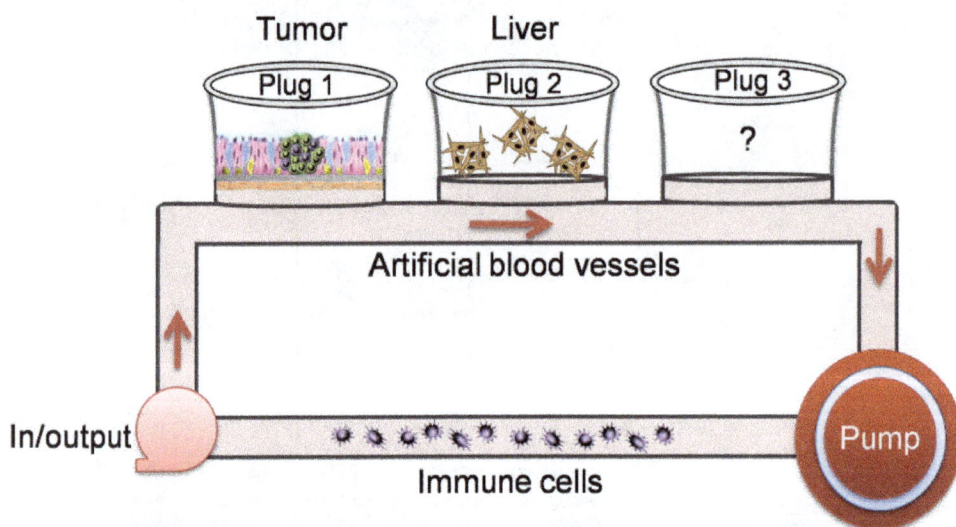

Figure 5. Schematic representation of an ideal *in vitro* PnP (Plug and Play) lung cancer model. A primary tumor derived from the patient is incorporated into a fully differentiated and healthy airway epithelium and cultured at air-liquid interface in a setting similar to OncoCilair™ (Mas et al., 2015); Then this co-culture model is plugged into a micro-fluidic device with artificial blood/or lymphatic vessels (pink color) containing circulating immune cells (blue color); liver cells (hepatocytes as spheroids, brown color) can also be integrated into the circuit through the plug number 2, providing metabolic capacity of drugs. If needed, other cells/organs can be further inter-connected in similar way. An input/output plug allows the addition of drug or the uptake of medium for analysis. The lung tissue culture remains accessible to apical exposure during all the experiment.

A primary tumor derived from the patient is incorporated into a fully differentiated and healthy airway epithelium and cultured at air-liquid interface, a setting similar to OncoCilair™ [82]. Then this co-culture model is plugged into a micro-fluidic device with artificial blood/or lymphatic vessels containing circulating immune cells; liver cells (hepatocytes as spheroids) can also be plugged into the circuit, providing metabolic capacity of drugs. If needed, other cells/organs can be further inter-connected in a similar way.

We are convinced that, with the development of new technologies such as microfluidic devices and 3D bio-printing, such models should quickly emerge and strengthen *in vitro* pre-clinical cancer research.

Author details

Samuel Constant, Song Huang, Ludovic Wisniewski and Christophe Mas*

*Address all correspondence to: christophe.mas@oncotheis.com

OncoTheis Sàrl, Geneva, Switzerland

References

[1] Malvezzi, M., et al., *European cancer mortality predictions for the year 2013.* Ann Oncol, 2013. 24(3): p. 792-800.

[2] Arrowsmith, J. and P. Miller, *Trial watch: phase II and phase III attrition rates 2011-2012.* Nat Rev Drug Discov, 2013. 12(8): p. 569.

[3] Scannell, J.W., et al., *Diagnosing the decline in pharmaceutical R&D efficiency.* Nat Rev Drug Discov, 2012. 11(3): p. 191-200.

[4] Rangarajan, A. and R.A. Weinberg, *Opinion: Comparative biology of mouse versus human cells: modelling human cancer in mice.* Nat Rev Cancer, 2003. 3(12): p. 952-9.

[5] Kung, A.L., *Practices and pitfalls of mouse cancer models in drug discovery.* Adv Cancer Res, 2007. 96: p. 191-212.

[6] Ruggeri, B.A., F. Camp, and S. Miknyoczki, *Animal models of disease: pre-clinical animal models of cancer and their applications and utility in drug discovery.* Biochem Pharmacol, 2014. 87(1): p. 150-61.

[7] Mak, I.W., N. Evaniew, and M. Ghert, *Lost in translation: animal models and clinical trials in cancer treatment.* Am J Transl Res, 2014. 6(2): p. 114-8.

[8] Odom, D.T., et al., *Tissue-specific transcriptional regulation has diverged significantly between human and mouse.* Nat Genet, 2007. 39(6): p. 730-2.

[9] Forsyth, N.R., W.E. Wright, and J.W. Shay, *Telomerase and differentiation in multicellular organisms: turn it off, turn it on, and turn it off again.* Differentiation, 2002. 69(4-5): p. 188-97.

[10] Rangarajan, A., et al., *Species- and cell type-specific requirements for cellular transformation.* Cancer Cell, 2004. 6(2): p. 171-83.

[11] Seok, J., et al., *Genomic responses in mouse models poorly mimic human inflammatory diseases.* Proc Natl Acad Sci U S A, 2013. 110(9): p. 3507-12.

[12] Dorman, G., et al., *Matrix metalloproteinase inhibitors: a critical appraisal of design principles and proposed therapeutic utility.* Drugs, 2010. 70(8): p. 949-64.

[13] Dong, X., et al., *Patient-derived first generation xenografts of non-small cell lung cancers: promising tools for predicting drug responses for personalized chemotherapy.* Clin Cancer Res, 2010. 16(5): p. 1442-51.

[14] Moro, M., et al., *Patient-derived xenografts of non small cell lung cancer: resurgence of an old model for investigation of modern concepts of tailored therapy and cancer stem cells.* J Biomed Biotechnol, 2012. 2012: p. 568567.

[15] Rong, S., et al., *Tumorigenicity of the met proto-oncogene and the gene for hepatocyte growth factor.* Mol Cell Biol, 1992. 12(11): p. 5152-8.

[16] Mestas, J. and C.C. Hughes, *Of mice and not men: differences between mouse and human immunology.* J Immunol, 2004. 172(5): p. 2731-8.

[17] Stratmann, A.T., et al., *Establishment of a human 3D lung cancer model based on a biological tissue matrix combined with a Boolean in silico model.* Mol Oncol, 2014. 8(2): p. 351-65.

[18] Lee, J.J., et al., *Stromal response to Hedgehog signaling restrains pancreatic cancer progression.* Proc Natl Acad Sci U S A, 2014. 111(30): p. E3091-100.

[19] Egeblad, M., E.S. Nakasone, and Z. Werb, *Tumors as organs: complex tissues that interface with the entire organism.* Dev Cell, 2010. 18(6): p. 884-901.

[20] Chen, W.J., et al., *Cancer-associated fibroblasts regulate the plasticity of lung cancer stemness via paracrine signalling.* Nat Commun, 2014. 5: p. 3472.

[21] Malvezzi, M., et al., *European cancer mortality predictions for the year 2014.* Ann Oncol, 2014. 25(8): p. 1650-6.

[22] Pesch, B., et al., *Cigarette smoking and lung cancer--relative risk estimates for the major histological types from a pooled analysis of case-control studies.* Int J Cancer, 2012. 131(5): p. 1210-9.

[23] Brambilla, E., et al., *The new World Health Organization classification of lung tumours.* Eur Respir J, 2001. 18(6): p. 1059-68.

[24] Ohe, Y., et al., *Randomized phase III study of cisplatin plus irinotecan versus carboplatin plus paclitaxel, cisplatin plus gemcitabine, and cisplatin plus vinorelbine for advanced non-small-cell lung cancer: Four-Arm Cooperative Study in Japan.* Ann Oncol, 2007. 18(2): p. 317-23.

[25] Reck, M., et al., *Tissue sampling in lung cancer: a review in light of the MERIT experience.* Lung Cancer, 2011. 74(1): p. 1-6.

[26] Nguyen, K.S., S. Kobayashi, and D.B. Costa, *Acquired resistance to epidermal growth factor receptor tyrosine kinase inhibitors in non-small-cell lung cancers dependent on the epidermal growth factor receptor pathway.* Clin Lung Cancer, 2009. 10(4): p. 281-9.

[27] Rosell, R., et al., *Screening for epidermal growth factor receptor mutations in lung cancer.* N Engl J Med, 2009. 361(10): p. 958-67.

[28] Sandler, A., et al., *Paclitaxel-carboplatin alone or with bevacizumab for non-small-cell lung cancer.* N Engl J Med, 2006. 355(24): p. 2542-50.

[29] Camidge, D.R., et al., *Activity and safety of crizotinib in patients with ALK-positive non-small-cell lung cancer: updated results from a phase 1 study.* Lancet Oncol, 2012. 13(10): p. 1011-9.

[30] Doebele, R.C., et al., *Mechanisms of resistance to crizotinib in patients with ALK gene rearranged non-small cell lung cancer.* Clin Cancer Res, 2012. 18(5): p. 1472-82.

[31] Shaw, A.T., et al., *Ceritinib in ALK-rearranged non-small-cell lung cancer.* N Engl J Med, 2014. 370(13): p. 1189-97.

[32] Chen, X., et al., *Clinical perspective of afatinib in non-small cell lung cancer.* Lung Cancer, 2013. 81(2): p. 155-61.

[33] Tsvetkova, E. and G.D. Goss, *Drug resistance and its significance for treatment decisions in non-small-cell lung cancer.* Curr Oncol, 2012. 19(Suppl 1): p. S45-51.

[34] Pao, W., et al., *Acquired resistance of lung adenocarcinomas to gefitinib or erlotinib is associated with a second mutation in the EGFR kinase domain.* PLoS Med, 2005. 2(3): p. e73.

[35] Engelman, J.A., et al., *MET amplification leads to gefitinib resistance in lung cancer by activating ERBB3 signaling.* Science, 2007. 316(5827): p. 1039-43.

[36] Katayama, R., et al., *Mechanisms of acquired crizotinib resistance in ALK-rearranged lung Cancers.* Sci Transl Med, 2012. 4(120): p. 120ra17.

[37] Ogawa, T., et al., *Methylation of death-associated protein kinase is associated with cetuximab and erlotinib resistance.* Cell Cycle, 2012. 11(8): p. 1656-63.

[38] Sequist, L.V., et al., *Genotypic and histological evolution of lung cancers acquiring resistance to EGFR inhibitors.* Sci Transl Med, 2011. 3(75): p. 75ra26.

[39] Yu, H.A., et al., *Analysis of tumor specimens at the time of acquired resistance to EGFR-TKI therapy in 155 patients with EGFR-mutant lung cancers.* Clin Cancer Res, 2013. 19(8): p. 2240-7.

[40] Mintz, B. and K. Illmensee, *Normal genetically mosaic mice produced from malignant teratocarcinoma cells.* Proc Natl Acad Sci U S A, 1975. 72(9): p. 3585-9.

[41] Mitra, A.K., et al., *MicroRNAs reprogram normal fibroblasts into cancer-associated fibro-blasts in ovarian cancer*. Cancer Discov, 2012. 2(12): p. 1100-8.

[42] Sherman, M.H., et al., *Vitamin d receptor-mediated stromal reprogramming suppresses pancreatitis and enhances pancreatic cancer therapy*. Cell, 2014. 159(1): p. 80-93.

[43] Rowley, D.R., *Reprogramming the tumor stroma: a new paradigm*. Cancer Cell, 2014. 26(4): p. 451-2.

[44] Gazdar, A.F., et al., *Lung cancer cell lines as tools for biomedical discovery and research*. J Natl Cancer Inst, 2010. 102(17): p. 1310-21.

[45] Oboshi, S., et al., *A new floating cell line derived from human pulmonary carcinoma of oat cell type*. Gan, 1971. 62(6): p. 505-14.

[46] Sugaya, M., et al., *Establishment of 15 cancer cell lines from patients with lung cancer and the potential tools for immunotherapy*. Chest, 2002. 122(1): p. 282-8.

[47] Zheng, C., et al., *Establishment and characterization of primary lung cancer cell lines from Chinese population*. Acta Pharmacol Sin, 2011. 32(3): p. 385-92.

[48] Gazdar, A.F. and H.K. Oie, *Cell culture methods for human lung cancer*. Cancer Genet Cytogenet, 1986. 19(1-2): p. 5-10.

[49] Lam, D.C., et al., *Establishment and expression profiling of new lung cancer cell lines from Chinese smokers and lifetime never-smokers*. J Thorac Oncol, 2006. 1(9): p. 932-42.

[50] Aurisicchio, L., et al., *The promise of anti-ErbB3 monoclonals as new cancer therapeutics*. Oncotarget, 2012. 3(8): p. 744-58.

[51] Sekine, I., et al., *Emerging ethnic differences in lung cancer therapy*. Br J Cancer, 2008. 99(11): p. 1757-62.

[52] Zhang, J., et al., *Intratumor heterogeneity in localized lung adenocarcinomas delineated by multiregion sequencing*. Science, 2014. 346(6206): p. 256-9.

[53] Lee, J., M.J. Cuddihy, and N.A. Kotov, *Three-dimensional cell culture matrices: state of the art*. Tissue Eng Part B Rev, 2008. 14(1): p. 61-86.

[54] Matsusaki, M., C.P. Case, and M. Akashi, *Three-dimensional cell culture technique and pathophysiology*. Adv Drug Deliv Rev, 2014. 74: p. 95-103.

[55] Sant, S., et al., *Biomimetic Gradient Hydrogels for Tissue Engineering*. Can J Chem Eng, 2010. 88(6): p. 899-911.

[56] Margulis, A., W. Zhang, and J.A. Garlick, *In vitro fabrication of engineered human skin*. Methods Mol Biol, 2005. 289: p. 61-70.

[57] Huang, S., et al., *Potential of in vitro reconstituted 3D human airway epithelia (MucilAir) to assess respiratory sensitizers*. Toxicol *In vitro*, 2013. 27(3): p. 1151-6.

[58] Schaller, M., et al., *Models of oral and vaginal candidiasis based on in vitro reconstituted human epithelia.* Nat Protoc, 2006. 1(6): p. 2767-73.

[59] Even-Ram, S. and K.M. Yamada, *Cell migration in 3D matrix.* Curr Opin Cell Biol, 2005. 17(5): p. 524-32.

[60] Vacanti, J.P. and R. Langer, *Tissue engineering: the design and fabrication of living replacement devices for surgical reconstruction and transplantation.* Lancet, 1999. 354 Suppl 1: p. SI32-4.

[61] Bohari, S.P., D.W. Hukins, and L.M. Grover, *Effect of calcium alginate concentration on viability and proliferation of encapsulated fibroblasts.* Biomed Mater Eng, 2011. 21(3): p. 159-70.

[62] Godugu, C., et al., *AlgiMatrix based 3D cell culture system as an in-vitro tumor model for anticancer studies.* PLoS One, 2013. 8(1): p. e53708.

[63] Zhao, Y., et al., *Three-dimensional printing of Hela cells for cervical tumor model in vitro.* Biofabrication, 2014. 6(3): p. 035001.

[64] Djordjevic, B. and C.S. Lange, *Clonogenicity of mammalian cells in hybrid spheroids: a new assay method.* Radiat Environ Biophys, 1990. 29(1): p. 31-46.

[65] Ekert, J.E., et al., *Three-dimensional lung tumor microenvironment modulates therapeutic compound responsiveness in vitro--implication for drug development.* PLoS One, 2014. 9(3): p. e92248.

[66] Amann, A., et al., *Development of an innovative 3D cell culture system to study tumour--stroma interactions in non-small cell lung cancer cells.* PLoS One, 2014. 9(3): p. e92511.

[67] Thoma, C.R., et al., *3D cell culture systems modeling tumor growth determinants in cancer target discovery.* Adv Drug Deliv Rev, 2014. 69-70: p. 29-41.

[68] Huang, Y.J. and S.H. Hsu, *Acquisition of epithelial-mesenchymal transition and cancer stem-like phenotypes within chitosan-hyaluronan membrane-derived 3D tumor spheroids.* Biomaterials, 2014. 35(38): p. 10070-9.

[69] Huh, D., et al., *Reconstituting organ-level lung functions on a chip.* Science, 2010. 328(5986): p. 1662-8.

[70] Xu, Z., et al., *Application of a microfluidic chip-based 3D co-culture to test drug sensitivity for individualized treatment of lung cancer.* Biomaterials, 2013. 34(16): p. 4109-17.

[71] Ruppen, J., et al., *A microfluidic platform for chemoresistive testing of multicellular pleural cancer spheroids.* Lab Chip, 2014. 14(6): p. 1198-205.

[72] Ott, H.C., et al., *Regeneration and orthotopic transplantation of a bioartificial lung.* Nat Med, 2010. 16(8): p. 927-33.

[73] Mishra, D.K., et al., *Human lung cancer cells grown on acellular rat lung matrix create perfusable tumor nodules.* Ann Thorac Surg, 2012. 93(4): p. 1075-81.

[74] Mishra, D.K., et al., *Human lung cancer cells grown in an ex vivo 3D lung model produce matrix metalloproteinases not produced in 2D culture.* PLoS One, 2012. 7(9): p. e45308.

[75] Vaira, V., et al., *Preclinical model of organotypic culture for pharmacodynamic profiling of human tumors.* Proc Natl Acad Sci U S A, 2010. 107(18): p. 8352-6.

[76] Dong, M., et al., *Tissue slice model of human lung cancer to investigate telomerase inhibition by nanoparticle delivery of antisense 2'-O-methyl-RNA.* Int J Pharm, 2011. 419(1-2): p. 33-42.

[77] Atala, A., F.K. Kasper, and A.G. Mikos, *Engineering complex tissues.* Sci Transl Med, 2012. 4(160): p. 160rv12.

[78] Walles, T., et al., *The potential of bioartificial tissues in oncology research and treatment.* Onkologie, 2007. 30(7): p. 388-94.

[79] Wiszniewski, L., et al., *Long-term cultures of polarized airway epithelial cells from patients with cystic fibrosis.* Am J Respir Cell Mol Biol, 2006. 34(1): p. 39-48.

[80] Mas C, Huang S, Wiszniewski L, Constant S., *A new 3D human airway tissue model for in vitro lung cancer research (OncoCilAir™).* ALTEX Proceedings, 2014. 3(1/14): p. I-4-204.

[81] Mas C, Huang S, Wiszniewski L, Constant S., *In vitro Human Airway Tissue Model For Lung Cancer Research.* Am J Respir Crit Care Med 2014. 189: p. A3455.

[82] Mas C, Boda B, CaulFuty M, Huang S, Wiszniewski L and Constant S., *Antitumour efficacy of the selumetinib and trametinib MEK inhibitors in a combined human airway-tumour-stroma lung cancer model.* J Biotechnol., 2015. in press.

[83] Hanahan, D. and R.A. Weinberg, *The hallmarks of cancer.* Cell, 2000. 100(1): p. 57-70.

[84] Hanahan, D. and R.A. Weinberg, *Hallmarks of cancer: the next generation.* Cell, 2011. 144(5): p. 646-74.

[85] Nowell, P.C., *The clonal evolution of tumor cell populations.* Science, 1976. 194(4260): p. 23-8.

[86] Gatenby, R.A. and R.J. Gillies, *A microenvironmental model of carcinogenesis.* Nat Rev Cancer, 2008. 8(1): p. 56-61.

[87] Siegel, R., et al., *Cancer statistics, 2011: the impact of eliminating socioeconomic and racial disparities on premature cancer deaths.* CA Cancer J Clin, 2011. 61(4): p. 212-36.

[88] Malakoff, D., *Can treatment costs be tamed?* Science, 2011. 331(6024): p. 1545-7.

[89] Gurdon, J.B., *A community effect in animal development.* Nature, 1988. 336(6201): p. 772-4.

[90] Gao, S.P., et al., *Mutations in the EGFR kinase domain mediate STAT3 activation via IL-6 production in human lung adenocarcinomas.* J Clin Invest, 2007. 117(12): p. 3846-56.

Permissions

All chapters in this book were first published in DDD&STDD, by InTech Open; hereby published with permission under the Creative Commons Attribution License or equivalent. Every chapter published in this book has been scrutinized by our experts. Their significance has been extensively debated. The topics covered herein carry significant findings which will fuel the growth of the discipline. They may even be implemented as practical applications or may be referred to as a beginning point for another development.

The contributors of this book come from diverse backgrounds, making this book a truly international effort. This book will bring forth new frontiers with its revolutionizing research information and detailed analysis of the nascent developments around the world.

We would like to thank all the contributing authors for lending their expertise to make the book truly unique. They have played a crucial role in the development of this book. Without their invaluable contributions this book wouldn't have been possible. They have made vital efforts to compile up to date information on the varied aspects of this subject to make this book a valuable addition to the collection of many professionals and students.

This book was conceptualized with the vision of imparting up-to-date information and advanced data in this field. To ensure the same, a matchless editorial board was set up. Every individual on the board went through rigorous rounds of assessment to prove their worth. After which they invested a large part of their time researching and compiling the most relevant data for our readers.

The editorial board has been involved in producing this book since its inception. They have spent rigorous hours researching and exploring the diverse topics which have resulted in the successful publishing of this book. They have passed on their knowledge of decades through this book. To expedite this challenging task, the publisher supported the team at every step. A small team of assistant editors was also appointed to further simplify the editing procedure and attain best results for the readers.

Apart from the editorial board, the designing team has also invested a significant amount of their time in understanding the subject and creating the most relevant covers. They scrutinized every image to scout for the most suitable representation of the subject and create an appropriate cover for the book.

The publishing team has been an ardent support to the editorial, designing and production team. Their endless efforts to recruit the best for this project, has resulted in the accomplishment of this book. They are a veteran in the field of academics and their pool of knowledge is as vast as their experience in printing. Their expertise and guidance has proved useful at every step. Their uncompromising quality standards have made this book an exceptional effort. Their encouragement from time to time has been an inspiration for everyone.

The publisher and the editorial board hope that this book will prove to be a valuable piece of knowledge for researchers, students, practitioners and scholars across the globe.

List of Contributors

Ken Yasukawa
School of Pharmacy, Nihon University, Funabashi, Chiba, Japan

Degenhard Marx and Matthias Birkhoff
Aptar Radolfzell GmbH, Radolfzell, Germany

Gerallt Williams
Aptar France SAS, Le Vaudreuil, France

Thales Kronenberger and Carsten Wrenger
Unit for Drug Discovery, Department of Parasitology, Institute of Biomedical Sciences, University of São Paulo, São Paulo, Brazil

Oliver Keminer and Björn Windshügel
Fraunhofer Institute for Molecular Biology and Applied Ecology IME, Hamburg, Germany

Simon A. Young and Terry K. Smith
Biomedical Sciences Research Complex, The North Haugh, The University, St. Andrews, Fife Scotland, U.K

Charles J. Malemud
Department of Medicine, Division of Rheumatic Diseases, Case Western Reserve University, School of Medicine, Cleveland, Ohio, USA

Adriana Ceci and Viviana Giannuzzi
Fondazione per la Ricerca Farmacologica Gianni Benzi onlus, Valenzano, Italy

Donato Bonifazi, Mariagrazia Felisi and Fedele Bonifazi
Consorzio per Valutazioni Biologiche e Farmacologiche, Pavia, Italy

Lucia Ruggieri
Gruppo Italiano per gli Studi di Farmacoeconomia, Pavia, Italy

Hrvoje Roguljic
Department of Mineral Research, Faculty of Medicine, J. J. Strossmayer University of Osijek, Croatia

Sonja Sarcevic and Nikola Raguz Lucic
Department of Pharmacology, Faculty of Medicine, J. J. Strossmayer University of Osijek, Croatia

Robert Smolic and Martina Smolic
Department of Mineral Research, Faculty of Medicine, J. J. Strossmayer University of Osijek, Croatia
Department of Pharmacology, Faculty of Medicine, J. J. Strossmayer University of Osijek, Croatia

Aleksandar Vcev
Department of Medicine, Faculty of Medicine, J. J. Strossmayer University of Osijek, Croatia
Department of Mineral Research, Faculty of Medicine, J. J. Strossmayer University of Osijek, Croatia

Elizabeth Hong-Geller and Sofiya N. Micheva-Viteva
Los Alamos National Laboratory, Bioscience Division, Los Alamos, NM, USA

Mark Voskoboynik
Sarah Cannon Research Institute UK, London, UK
Department of Medical Oncology, Guy's Hospital, London, UK

Hendrik-Tobias Arkenau
Sarah Cannon Research Institute UK, London, UK
University College London, London, UK

Samuel Constant, Song Huang, Ludovic Wisniewski and Christophe Mas
OncoTheis Sàrl, Geneva, Switzerland

Index

www.ingramcontent.com/pod-product-compliance
Lightning Source LLC
Chambersburg PA
CBHW061951190326
41458CB00009B/2849